W9-BEV-033

THE COMPLETE BOOK OF

Shoulders and Arms

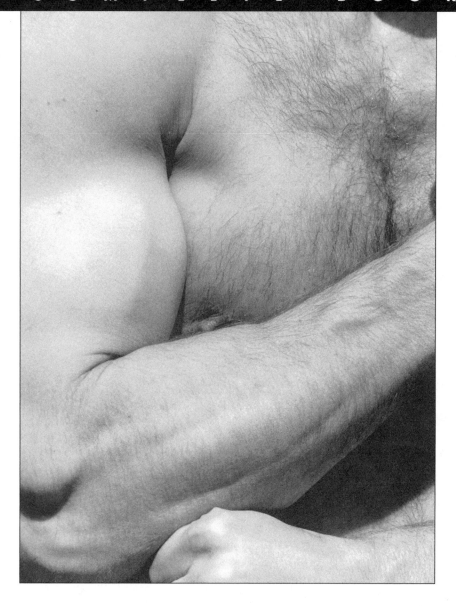

Shoulders and Arms

KURT, BRETT, AND MIKE BRUNGARDT

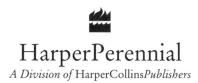

HarperPerennial

A Division of HarperCollins*Publishers*

THE COMPLETE BOOK OF SHOULDERS AND ARMS.
Copyright © 1997 by Kurt Brungardt. All rights reserved. Printed in the United
States of America. No part of this book may be used or reproduced in any manner
whatsoever without written permission except in the case of brief quotations
embodied in critical articles and reviews. For information address HarperCollins
Publishers, Inc., 10 East 53rd Street, New York, NY 10022.

HarperCollins books may be purchased for educational, business, or sales promo-
tional use. For information please write: Special Markets Department, HarperCollins
Publishers, Inc., 10 East 53rd Street, New York, NY 10022.

FIRST EDITION
Designed by BTD / Mary A. Wirth

Library of Congress Cataloging-in-Publication Data

Brungardt, Kurt
     The complete book of shoulders and arms/Kurt, Brett, and Mike
Brungardt.—1st ed.
          p. cm.
     Includes index
     ISBN 0-06-095166-4
     1. Exercise. 2. Arm. 3. Shoulder. I. Brungardt, Brett. II. Brungardt, Mike.
III. Title.
GV508.B789 1996
613.7'1—DC20   96-34138

97 98 99 00 01 ❖/CW 10 9 8 7 6 5 4 3 2 1

To our mother
who has carried us on her shoulders
all these years

CONTENTS

Part Three: The Exercises

Part Four: The Routines

ACKNOWLEDGMENTS

A book is always a collaborative effort, and most of the work and financial support is done by those behind the scenes—the ones who don't have their names and pictures in the book. At the top of this list is HarperCollins (their name, however, does go on the book), more specifically Diane Reverand and my editor Mauro DiPreta. Mauro has made working on this project pleasurable as opposed to a psychodrama. At the same time, they pushed the book to a polished final form. I would also like to thank Kristen Auclair and Molly Hennessy, who I know are going to be tired of shoulders and arms by the time this book goes through production. And I would like to thank my agent, Dan Strone, for his help in making this book a reality.

I would also like to thank Doug Levine and Sarah from Crunch Fitness in New York City for their support and the use of their state-of-the art facilities for shooting photos. Thanks also go out to Adolphus Fitness Inc. for use of their beautiful facility. I would like to thank Wheaton A.B. Mahoney for assisting and teaching me photography basics, doing the bulk of the printing, and contributing section photos. I would also like to thank Russ Oliver for assisting with the photography and printing for last-minute exercises that needed to be included, and for my author photo. Both are professional photographers—not assistants. I needed all the help I could get. And again I would like to thank Andrew Brucker for shooting the cover (as he did for the previous two books). He makes shooting bodies look so effortless that you think you could do it yourself. I tried it. It's a hard won art. I would also like to thank Kelly J. Batty for the photos she shot in Colorado, and Bulldogs Gym in Grand Junction for letting us use their facilities. And I would like to thank Karen Lander for her help throughout the project.

Above all, I would like to thank everyone who contributed routines and chapters to the book. Without your expertise and knowledge it would not have been possible. I would especially like to thank Bryon and Debbie Holmes, who unselfishly shared knowledge any time of the day or night (usually late at night), even after they had their first baby, Luke Owen Holmes.

Oh yes, and the two other authors, my brothers, Mike and Brett. It's easy to forget the obvious.

—Kurt Brungardt

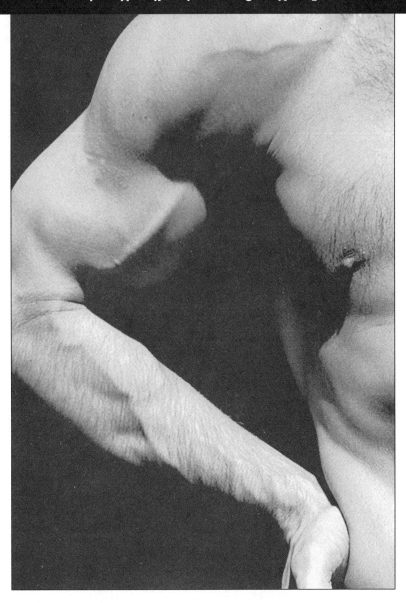

PART ONE

The Foundation

Working Out: The Truth

Aesthetics and Performance

The most commonly visible upper-body parts are the shoulders and arms. So it only makes sense that you want to keep these areas looking their best. Traditionally, for men, strong arms and broad shoulders are a sign of masculinity and power. And for women, one of the greatest areas of concern is flabby arms. In addition to their aesthetic value, these body parts work together in most sports and recreational activities: throwing, swinging, running, and swimming. Strengthening the shoulders and arms also improve performance by eliminating common injury. For both the serious and the recreational athlete, maladies such as tennis elbow, rotator cuff injuries, and shoulder separations can be greatly reduced by following an exercise plan based on muscle balance.

Purpose

The aim of this book is threefold: (1) It compiles all the major shoulder and arm exercises in a single volume, creating a complete resource for you; (2) it provides an organized and comprehensive battery of routines designed to fit the needs of almost every exerciser; and (3) it is a training manual in which you will learn the principles of working your shoulders and arms effectively and safely, allowing you to create your own individual program.

In addition, this book fortifies you with vital information about nutrition, the mind-body principles, and overall body wellness.

The Truth

From book to book, the basic truths still remain the same. There are no shortcuts in training. The only way to correctly work your shoulders and arms is through a combination of consistent, focused exercises, adherence to basic training principles (which also means taking time off), and proper nutrition. This book will give you all the tools you need. There is a light at the end of the tunnel. All you need is a map. No series of $19.95 gimmicks will eliminate the need to follow these basic and sound steps. We will take you step by step through the journey. Remember, a good plan is half the battle.

The other half is your commitment. Commitment is your fuel, the driving force behind your motivation. It's hard to nail down exactly why we procrastinate and stop pursuing goals; commitment is a very personal and intangible quality. The most important thing is to trust your first impulse to improve, and nurture that desire. Let it grow, allow it to overpower all the inner voices that try to hold you back. Allow it to overpower the outside voices of culture and society that try to pigeonhole you into their mass image, instead of our own individual image. You don't have to listen to the messages that say you're too old to work out, you don't have time, you'll feel too self-conscious in a gym, or you're just not the athletic or workout type. Instead, nurture that first impulse, that original spark of excitement you feel about your body and your potential, and let it grow, let it burn. Sometimes you have to start a fire to put out a fire. You have to start a new fire (a passion) to replace the old habits (unhealthy diet, inconsistent workouts, a defeatist attitude). These old habits are just that—habits. Not true wants. Let the real fire start to burn.

Myths and Facts

1. *If I lift heavy weights for my shoulders and arms, I will become muscle-bound.*

   Being muscle-bound is normally defined by a lack of flexibility—range of motion about a joint. The only ways you would become muscle-bound are if you become so huge that your range of motion is limited by the size of your muscles, or if you failed to lift through the prescribed range of motion. Adhering to the basic principles of resistance training and participating in a flexibility program will make your fears unwarranted.

2. *I can't do shoulder exercises because I have a bad lower back.*

   A bad back should in no way limit your ability to train your shoulders—or, for that matter, any body part. The first and most important factor is to eliminate your back problem (see Chapter 6). In conjunction with back rehab, shoulder exercises should be executed in a manner that places the back at minimal risk (seated or kneeling with proper back support).

3. *To get big arms, must I train them at the beginning of my workout?*

   If your only goal is to have big arms, then prioritizing them (doing them first) in a workout would make sense. But there are as many different theories as there are variables that affect arm size. None of them offers the absolute answer. Another theory would be prefatiguing your arms by working chest, back, and shoulders first. A systematic approach that includes training with high intensity and proper nutrition, coupled with periodizing (creating variety and steady adaptation in) your workouts (see Chapter 19: "Creating Your Own Routine") will bring you to your full potential.

4. *I don't want to exercise my traps because it will give me a big neck.*

So do you want to be a pencil-necked geek? Most important in training is the SAID principle—Specific Adaptations to Imposed Demands. For your neck to get bigger, you must train your neck. The purpose of exercising the traps is to help stabilize the shoulder girdle, to improve posture and to strengthen the trapezius muscles, not to increase the size of the neck. In an aesthetic sense, it would be true that big traps might make the neck look thick. If this is a concern, adjust your trap workout accordingly.

5. *I've tried every exercise to get rid of the sag in the back of my arms, and nothing works.*

Your exasperation is not uncommon, and the answer may not be pleasing. It requires discipline, dedication, and perseverance. A combination of a whole body workout combined with specific exercises for your triceps (as prescribed in this book), and stored body fat depletion (aerobic training and nutrition) will solve the problem.

6. *I do push-ups and pull-ups, so I don't need to weight-train my shoulders and arms.*

In a synergistic system (the body) all parts deserve their relative attention. The arms and shoulders are integral in the performance of a variety of movements and athletic endeavors. Their relative weakness would increase the potential of injury to a variety of connective and contractile tissue as well as to specific joints. Push-ups and pull-ups are both great exercises, but in these muscle movements, the shoulders and arms work as secondary, not primary muscles. Therefore, they do not get worked in isolation, allowing them to develop to their full potential.

7. *I don't use weights when I train shoulders and arms, because I don't want to get big like a man.*

The vast majority of women will not achieve the muscular size (hypertrophy) that a small number of men (elite bodybuilders) achieve, basically because of hormonal differences. By not using weights (either free weight or machines), you limit yourself and may make it more difficult to reach your full potential. The movements and intensity you can achieve with weights will introduce a variety into your training program that will keep you interested and improving for the rest of your life. If you feel that you are getting too big, adjust your workout (see Chapter 19). Don't use getting big as an excuse to avoid the weights.

8. *The bigger and more grueling the workout, the better the results.*

The answer to this lies in what you *shouldn't* do. Fifteen sets for any body part, let alone the biceps, is too much volume and not high enough intensity. If you can reach double figures in sets for any body part, your intensity level (weight used) is not high enough. For the biceps I would recommend 3 to 7 sets total with a variety of movements (see Biceps System).

9. *I have a shoulder injury, so I can't lift weights.*

Depending upon the severity of the injury, you may not be able to lift weights. But once rehabilitation starts, weight training can and should be an important component in its success and the future prevention of injury. After consulting with a doctor, start with light weights and proper technique.

10. *I'm too old to lift weights.*

Numerous studies show the benefits of weight training for "older" people. Improvements in body composition, injury prevention (including prevention of osteoporosis), and general well-being should far outweigh any fears or misconceptions you may have about age and weight training. The core of your problem lies in the preconceived notion of what it means to be old. Don't let these out-of-date notions keep you from making weight training one part of a healthy and active life.

11. *I train my biceps and triceps, so I don't need to train my forearms.*

   The body—and any movement—is only as strong as its weakest part or point, so if you neglect one area you cheat the rest of the body of its proper intensity. Consequently, you would probably be cheating your biceps or triceps because of forearm weakness. The forearms will give out before the biceps reach muscular failure.

12. *Training my arms won't improve my athletic performance because power is generated from the center of my body.*

   Movements are initiated from your center but they are finalized in your shoulders and arms. A balance of strength is one of the most important principles to keep in mind as you launch into your fitness journey.

Body Basics: Anatomy

This chapter gives you an overall view of the structural components that make up the shoulders and arms and will help you understand how the muscles of the shoulders and arms work, thus improving your ability to successfully train and visualize.

The shoulders and arms include numerous muscle groups that control movement, either working independently or working in some assisting capacity. The exercises in Part Three of this book will help you train and isolate each of these muscles. Other exercises will train two or more muscles at the same time, producing a synergistic relationship similar to what occurs in daily movements or athletic endeavors.

Movement/Anatomy Guidelines

This chapter looks at the components of movement: structure (skeletal), kinesiology (the science of movement), and muscle (how the muscular system works). Each section includes descriptions and anatomical drawings.

SKELETAL STRUCTURE

The science of osteology focuses on the structural, or skeletal, system. Each bone in the shoulders and arms plays an integral part in the functioning of its immediate area as well as in the total functioning of the overall skeletal system.

Functions: The skeletal system has five basic functions:

Support—It provides the structure that forms the framework to which the muscles and organs of the body are attached.

Protection—It protects the essential components of the body (heart, lungs, brain, central nervous system, etc.).

Movement—The bones of the skeletal system act as levers and the joints as axes when the muscles contract.

Hemopoiesis (blood cell production)—Bone marrow produces white blood cells, red blood corpuscles, and platelets.

Mineral storage—About 99 percent of the calcium and 90 percent of the phosphorus in the body is stored in the bones and the teeth.

The portion of the skeletal system we will focus on can be divided into three areas: (1) shoulder (shoulder girdle and shoulder joint), (2) upper arm (upper arm and elbow joint), and (3) lower arm (lower arm and wrist joint). See illustration on page 9.

KINESIOLOGY AND MUSCLE

Kinesiology is the science of human movement. Understanding how your body works—that is, which muscles contract and move the shoulders and arms—will help you visualize and enhance the mind-muscle link.

Muscle Action: We'll be using several different types of muscle action for shoulders and arms:

Prime mover—A muscle that is directly responsible for performing a movement (e.g., deltoid during a Lateral Raise)

Agonist—A concentric contraction resulting in joint action (e.g., biceps brachii during a Dumbbell Curl)

Antagonist—A muscle contracting in opposition to the agonist (e.g., triceps brachii during a Dumbbell Curl)

Synergist—A muscle that contributes to movement, but isn't the prime mover (e.g., brachioradialis during a Barbell Curl)

Fixator—A muscle that holds a part steady so that other muscles can function (e.g., deltoid during a Triceps Push-Down)

As mentioned, there are numerous muscles involved with the movement of shoulders and arms. To simplify this potentially complex endeavor we will identify muscles in relation to their location (shoulder, upper arm, and lower arm) and to anatomical movement. This will allow you to visualize how each muscle relates to the movement.

There are eight basic movements that encompass muscle anatomy: shoulder flexion and hyperflexion (shoulder complex), horizontal flexion and extension (shoulder complex), elevation and depression (shoulder complex), internal and external rotation (shoulder complex), arm abduction (shoulder complex), arm flexion and extension (upper arm), wrist flexion and extension (lower arm), supination and pronation (lower arm).

The muscle description and movement analysis for each designated segment will include a picture of the muscles and the movement. Also included are a performance and training section. This area will define more of the muscles' responsibilities as far as movement, and will be an index to specific exercises to train the muscles. Please remember that during a movement more than one muscle may be utilized in the movement in some assisting capacity. When we discuss muscles and movement we are talking about prime movers unless otherwise specified.

Note: In movements involving the shoulder complex, more than one muscle may be involved. We will try to focus on the muscles that are targeted for the movement.

Directional Movement Terms: Below are some directional terms that are used throughout this book.

Superior	the top, toward the top
Inferior	the bottom, toward the bottom
Anterior (ventral)	the front, toward the front
Posterior (dorsal)	the back, toward the back
Medial	toward the midline of the body
Lateral	away from the midline of the body, the side of the body
Proximal	nearer the principal mass of the body
Distal	away from the principal mass of the body

Skeletal Structure

SHOULDER

Complex in structure, the shoulder consists mainly of the shoulder girdle and the shoulder joint.

Shoulder Girdle: The main purpose of the shoulder girdle is to provide attachments for the numerous muscles that move the upper extremities, including the upper and lower arm. The shoulder girdle is composed of the clavicle, the scapulae, and the sternum.

Clavicle: The clavicle (collarbone) connects the shoulder to the axial skeleton and positions the shoulder joint for freedom of movement.

Scapula: The scapula (shoulder blade) is a flat, triangular bone on the posterior (backside) of the rib cage that provides numerous sites for muscle attachments.

Sternum: The sternum provides an attachment, or an articulation (where a joint forms or comes together), with the clavicle.

Joint Type: Within the shoulder girdle there are two joints, both of which are classified as gliding joints. The sternoclavicular joint articulates at the manubrium of the sternum. The acromioclavicular joint is lateral (away from the midline) and articulates with the acromion process of the scapula. Both joints are supported by numerous ligaments to prevent laxity and dislocation.

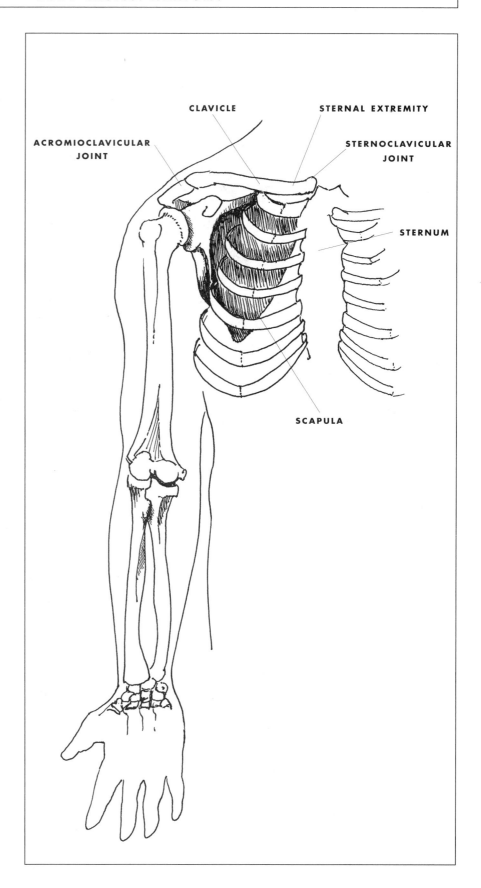

CLAVICLE

STERNAL EXTREMITY

ACROMIOCLAVICULAR JOINT

STERNOCLAVICULAR JOINT

STERNUM

SCAPULA

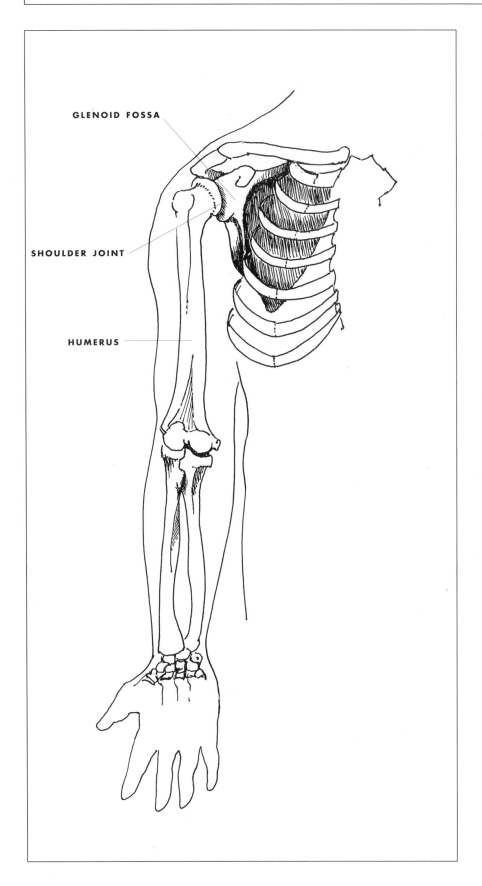

GLENOID FOSSA

SHOULDER JOINT

HUMERUS

Shoulder Joint: The shoulder (glenohumeral or humero-scapular) joint is a ball-and-socket joint and is the most freely movable joint in the body. The joint is formed by the articulation of the glenoid fossa of the scapula with the head of the humerus.

Three ligaments (coraco-humeral, glenohumeral, and transverse humeral) surround and support the joint, but the real strength and integrity of the joint comes from the rotator cuff muscles (subscapularis, supraspinatus, infraspinatus, and teres minor). See the muscular section of anatomy, page 13.

UPPER ARM AND ELBOW JOINT

Upper Arm: The humerus constitutes the longest bone of the upper extremity. The humerus articulates with the scapula (glenoid fossa) at the proximal (closest) head of the bone, while it articulates with the radial, olecranon, and coronoid fossa (lower arm) at the distal (farthest) end. The shape of the humerus is cylindrical at the proximal end and gradually changes to a triangular flat bone at the distal end.

Elbow Joint: The elbow joint is a hinge joint that allows flexion and extension. It is supported by the radial collateral (lateral) and the ulnar collateral (medial) ligaments.

Gender Difference: The forearms of both sexes are directed laterally (out). The carrying angle, the angle at which the arm hangs naturally, for males is usually 10 to 15 degrees, for females 20 to 25 degrees. Hence, females are generally more effective with arm flexion, and have a more difficult time with arm extension.

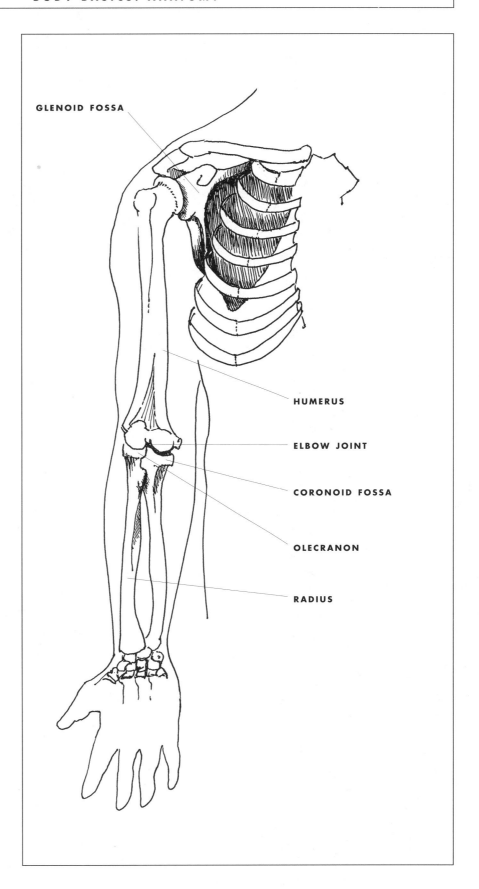

GLENOID FOSSA

HUMERUS

ELBOW JOINT

CORONOID FOSSA

OLECRANON

RADIUS

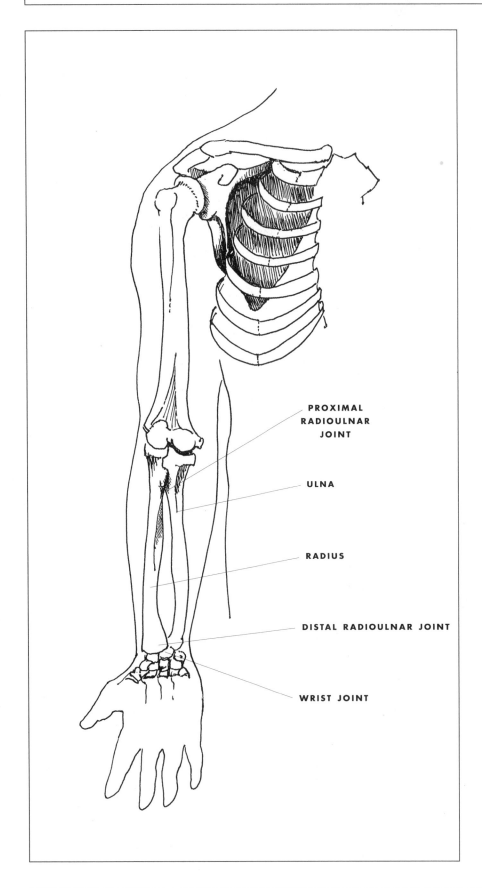

PROXIMAL
RADIOULNAR
JOINT

ULNA

RADIUS

DISTAL RADIOULNAR JOINT

WRIST JOINT

LOWER ARM AND WRIST JOINT

Lower Arm: The lower arm is made up of two bones, the ulna and the radius.

The ulna is the medial (inside) bone from the anatomical position (thumbs out) and articulates with the radius and the humerus at the proximal end. The ulna also articulates with the radius distally.

The radius is the lateral (outside) bone of the lower arm. Proximally, the radius articulates with the humerus and the ulna; distally, it articulates with the ulna.

Joint Type: Three joints are included in the lower arm:

Proximal radioulnar joint. This joint, located in the elbow region, is classified as a pivot joint (it rotates around a central axis). It is formed by the head of the radius articulating with the radial notch of the ulna.

Distal radioulnar joint. This joint, located above the wrist, is a slightly movable joint.

Both radioulnar joints are involved in supination (rotating the palms upward) and pronation (rotating the palms downward) of the forearm.

Radiocarpal joint or wrist joint. The wrist joint is a diarthritic condyloid joint (biaxial movement) formed by the distal end of the radius articulating with the carpal bones.

Kinesiology and Muscle

SHOULDER FLEXION AND HYPERFLEXION

Shoulder Flexion: Shoulder flexion involves the front/anterior portion of the shoulder complex. It is the movement of the arm upward and toward the front to shoulder level. Movement: front raise, lifting the arm while running (**A**).

Muscles Involved:
• anterior deltoid
• coracobrachialis

Shoulder Hyperflexion: This is a movement of the arm upward and toward the front to above the level of the head. Movement: front raise, lifting the arm to block a ball (**B**).

Muscles Involved:
• upper and lower trapezius, page 15
• serratus anterior

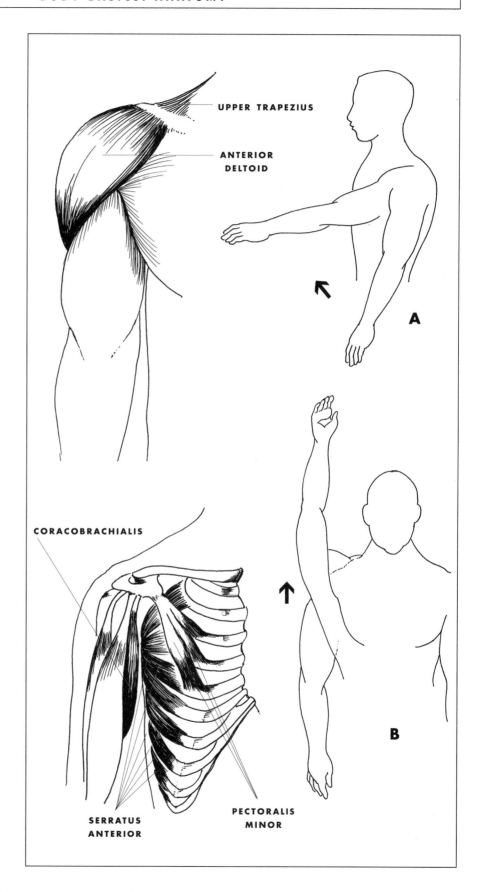

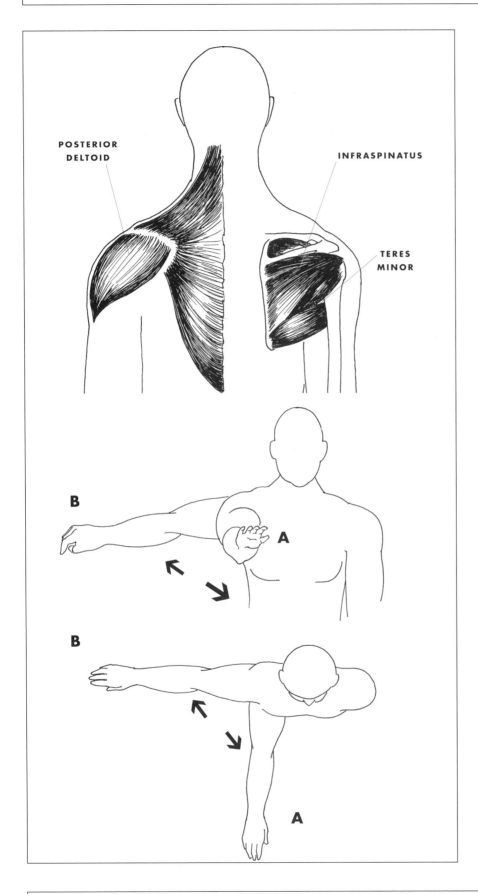

POSTERIOR DELTOID

INFRASPINATUS

TERES MINOR

B

A

B

A

A

HORIZONTAL FLEXION AND EXTENSION

Horizontal Flexion: Horizontal flexion involves the anterior/front portion of the shoulder complex. It's the movement of the arm from shoulder flexion or shoulder abduction toward the midline of the body along the transverse plane (parallel to the ground). Movement: discus throw (**A**).

Muscles Involved:
• anterior deltoid, page 13
• coracobrachialis, page 13

Horizontal Extension: This is a movement of the arm from shoulder flexion (in front and shoulder height) laterally (away from the midline) in the transverse plane to arm/shoulder abduction position. Movement: rear delt raise, backhand in tennis (**B**).

Muscles Involved:
• posterior deltoid
• medial/middle deltoid
• infraspinatus
• teres minor

SHOULDER ELEVATION AND DEPRESSION

Shoulder Elevation: Shoulder elevation involves the upper portion of the shoulder. It is the raising vertically of the shoulder girdle (clavicle and scapula) (**A**). Movement: shrugs, power cleans.

Muscles Involved:
• upper trapezius
• levator scapulae
• rhomboids

Shoulder Depression: Shoulder depression is the lowering vertically of the shoulder girdle (clavicle and scapula) (**B**). Movement: straight arm dips.

Muscles Involved:
• lower trapezius
• pectoralis minor, page 13

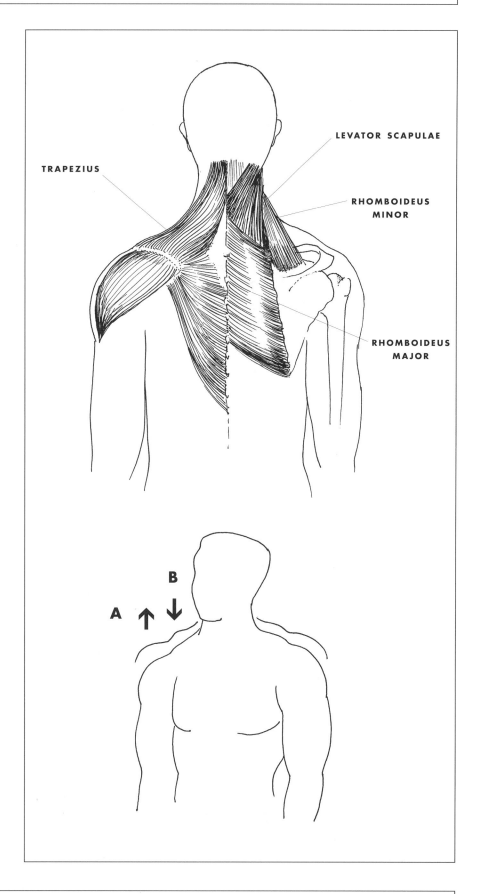

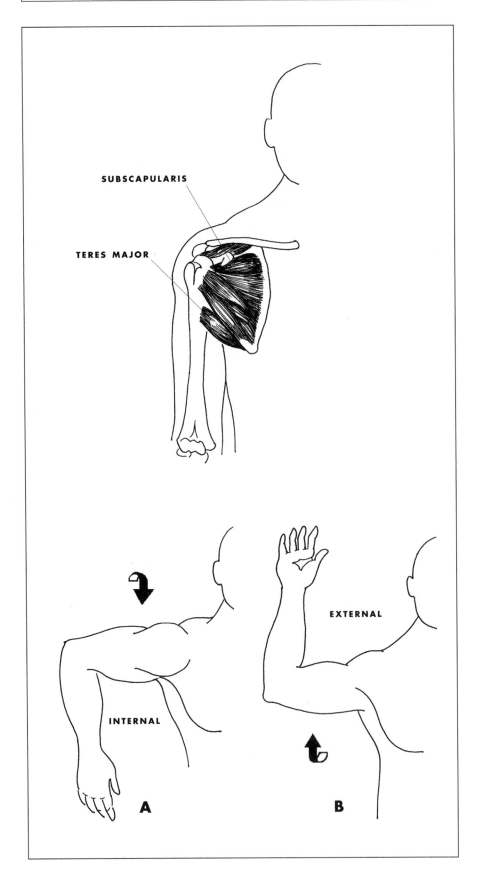

SUBSCAPULARIS

TERES MAJOR

INTERNAL A

EXTERNAL

B

INTERNAL AND EXTERNAL ROTATION

Rotator Cuff

Internal Rotation: Internal rotation occurs when the humerus (upper arm) is rotated inward, moving the arm downward. Movement: throwing (**A**).

Muscles Involved:
• subscapularis
• teres major

External Rotation: External rotation occurs when the humerus (upper arm) is rotated outward or if the arm is abducted, upward. Movement: preparation for throwing, stationary cleans (**B**).

Muscles Involved:
• infraspinatus, page 14
• teres minor, page 14
• supraspinatus, page 17

SHOULDER/ARM ABDUCTION

Shoulder/arm abduction involves the side/lateral part of the shoulder. It is the movement of the arm outward (away from the midline) and upward along the frontal plane.

Movement: lateral raises, movement of arm to shoulder level (**A**).

Muscles Involved:
• deltoid
• supraspinatus

Movement: upright rows, movement of arm above shoulder level (**B**).

Muscles Involved:
• upper and lower trapezius
• serratus anterior, page 13

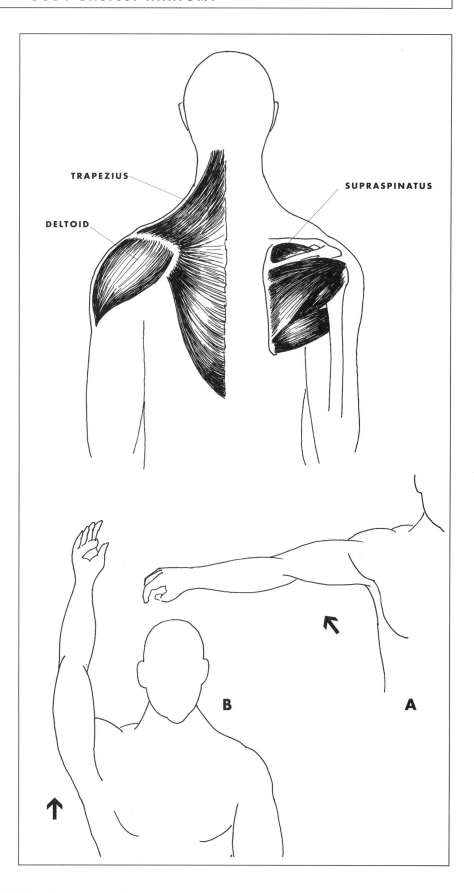

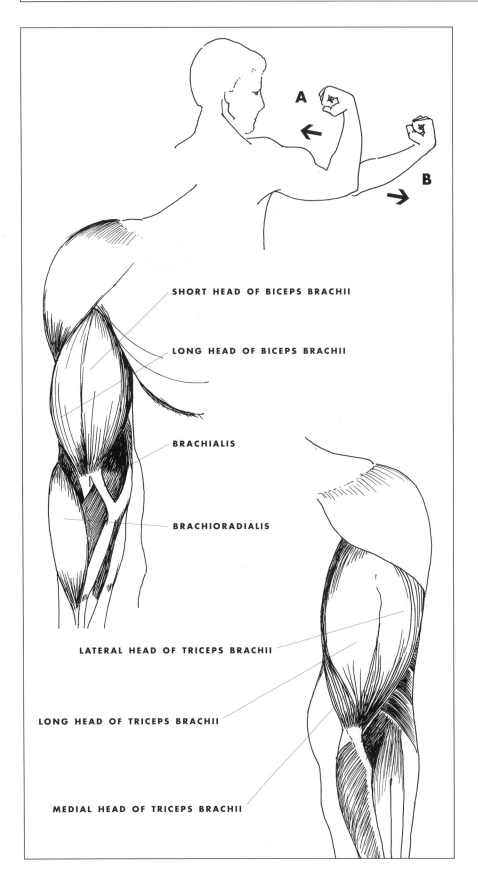

SHORT HEAD OF BICEPS BRACHII

LONG HEAD OF BICEPS BRACHII

BRACHIALIS

BRACHIORADIALIS

LATERAL HEAD OF TRICEPS BRACHII

LONG HEAD OF TRICEPS BRACHII

MEDIAL HEAD OF TRICEPS BRACHII

ARM FLEXION AND EXTENSION

Arm Flexion: Arm flexion involves movement of the lower part of the arm. It is the decreasing of the angle between the lower and upper arm (bringing the hand toward the shoulder or vice versa). Movement: biceps curl, pulling (**A**).

Muscles Involved:
• biceps brachii
• brachialis
• brachioradialis

Arm Extension: Arm extension involves movement of the lower part of the arm. It is the increasing of the angle between the lower and upper arm (movement of the hand away from the shoulder or vice versa). Movement: pushing and striking (**B**).

Muscle Involved:
• triceps brachii (three heads—long, lateral, and medial)

WRIST FLEXION AND EXTENSION

Wrist Flexion: Wrist flexion involves the palm side of the hand and forearm. It is the movement of the palm toward the biceps. Movement: pulling, wrist curls (**A**).

Muscles Involved:
• flexor carpi radialis
• flexor carpi ulnaris
• palmaris longus

Wrist Extension: Wrist extension involves the back side of the hand and forearm. It is the movement of the hand away from the biceps—opposite of flexion. Movement: reverse wrist curls (**B**).

Muscles Involved:
• extensor carpi radialis longus
• extensor carpi ulnaris
• extensor carpi radialis brevis

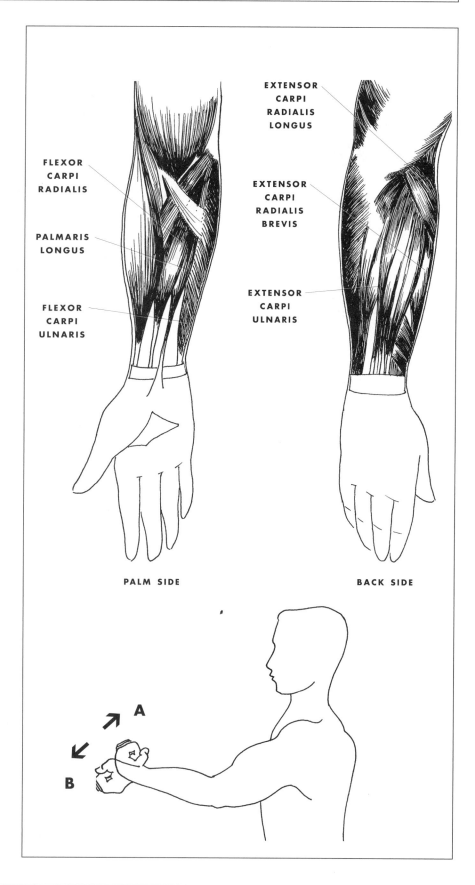

FLEXOR CARPI RADIALIS

PALMARIS LONGUS

FLEXOR CARPI ULNARIS

EXTENSOR CARPI RADIALIS LONGUS

EXTENSOR CARPI RADIALIS BREVIS

EXTENSOR CARPI ULNARIS

PALM SIDE

BACK SIDE

A

B

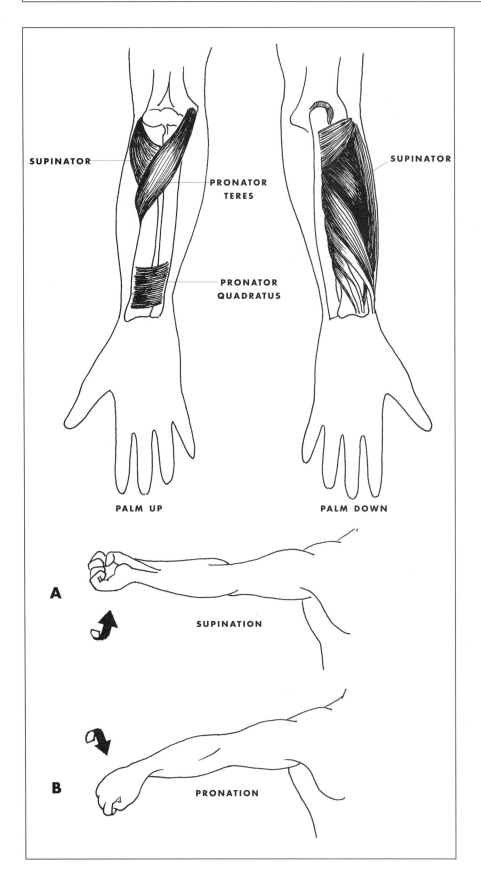

SUPINATOR

PRONATOR TERES

PRONATOR QUADRATUS

SUPINATOR

PALM UP

PALM DOWN

A

SUPINATION

B

PRONATION

LOWER ARM SUPINATION AND PRONATION

Supination: In lower arm supination, the lower arm is rotated so that the palm is up. Movement: tennis backhand stroke with overspin (**A**).

Muscle Involved:
• supinator
• biceps brachii, page 18

Pronation: In lower arm pronation, the lower arm is rotated so that the palm is down. Movement: tennis forehand stroke with overspin (**B**).

Muscles Involved:
• pronator teres
• pronator quadratus

References

O'Bryant, Harold, and Mike Stone. *Weight Training: A Scientific Approach.* 1st ed. Minneapolis: Burgess Publishing Co., 1984.

Rasch, Phillip. *Kinesiology and Applied Anatomy.* 7th ed. Philadelphia: Lea & Febiger, 1989.

Van De Graaff, Kent. *Human Anatomy.* Dubuque, Iowa: Wm. C. Brown Co., 1984.

Yessis, Michael. *Kinesiology of Exercise.* Indianapolis: Masters Press, 1992.

Proper Technique: The Body

Proper technique is essential for a successful training program. It is important for two reasons:

1. It helps you achieve the best results in the least amount of time.
2. It decreases the chance of injury during training. This chapter explains important training principles that are essential for complete shoulder, arm, and trap development.

Terms and Definitions

MUSCLE FUNCTION

The following are a few definitions of important concepts we will be using throughout this chapter:

Strength—The ability of a muscle to exert force; the maximum amount of effort that a muscle can apply in a contraction. Strength can be divided into two categories:

- *dynamic strength*—Involves the application of force through a full range of motion. Strength of this nature predominates in most skills and activities.
- *static strength*—The maximum amount of resistance that may be overcome involving little or no joint movement. An example would be isometric training.

Power—The rate at which work is performed (work/time), a combination of strength and velocity. Sometimes referred to as "explosive strength." An example would be the shot put.

Muscular Endurance—The ability to exert force, submaximally, repeatedly, over time. A very important component in that most activities involve repeated bouts of exercise.

Hypertrophy—Defined as an increase in size of muscle tissue.

Hyperplasia—A state in which muscle fibers actually split and multiply in number.

Atrophy—The exact opposite of hypertrophy. It results from submaximal training levels (below 30 percent intensity), extended layoffs, injury, or disease—three possible factors that would slowly cause you to lose the benefits from a healthy and consistent exercise program. An example of this would be the decrease in size of a limb that has been immobilized in a cast.

MUSCLE CONTRACTIONS

In muscular movement, there are basically three types of contractions:

1. *Isometric*—This involves no joint movement, but permits maximum muscular contraction. In this type of exercise, strength development is specific to the joint angle rather than through a full range of motion. Also referred to as "static" contractions.

2. *Isotonic*—Involves limb or body movement, with constant resistance throughout a full range of motion. The muscle either shortens or lengthens as the lifting movement is performed.

   • *concentric (positive) contractions* involve a shortening of the muscle as the resistance is overcome. An example of this would be the "raising" phase of a barbell curl exercise.
   • *eccentric (negative) contractions* occur when the muscle lengthens. An example would be the "lowering" phase of a barbell curl exercise.

3. *Isokinetic*—Refers to a contraction in which the speed of movement is controlled. This in theory eliminates biomechanical advantages and disadvantages that occur throughout a full range of motion, and may allow for maximum muscle contraction throughout a full range of motion.

Starting Out

The most frequently asked questions when beginning a training program are: "What should I do?", "How much should I do?", and "Where should I start?" There is no single, correct answer. Everyone is different. *You must experiment to find the answers.* Let's address these questions.

"What should I do?" First of all, you should include exercises that will train *all* the muscle groups in the body. The focus of this book is shoulders, arms, and traps, but by no means should we limit our training to just this area.

"How much should I do?" When starting out, you should do just enough to promote muscular failure for that exercise, no more. Your total exercise volume (sets and reps) should be minimal, probably no more than one set of 10 to 15 repetitions for each body part. This helps prevent three common problems: the negative physical and mental effects (burnout), excessive muscular soreness, and potentially serious injuries. Start slowly and build a foundation.

"Where should I start?" The following two principles will help you determine a proper starting weight and a place to begin:

• When learning a new exercise, use minimal weight (if possible) and perform the exercise while you are fresh.
• Once the exercise technique has been mastered, increase the intensity (weight) gradually each set, until you can no longer perform the movement for the prescribed number of repetitions or you have a breakdown in technique. Once this happens, drop back to the previous weight, and that will be your

starting point. When experimenting with finding a starting weight, perform no more than three sets per exercise, per session.

This is your starting place for the exercise. It may sound tedious, but remember: Technique is the key to success. Be patient. With proper execution you will be safer and the results will be greater in the long run. In the learning process there is no way to escape trial and error. Learn to love the process.

The Basic Principles

REPETITIONS (REPS)

A repetition is the completion of the entire movement of an exercise. If an athlete performs 10 triceps pushdowns, he has completed 10 repetitions.

SETS

A set is a series of consecutive repetitions. If you perform 10 repetitions of biceps curls, then rest, and then perform another 10 repetitions, you have performed two sets of 10 repetitions (2×10).

OVERLOAD

For a muscle to grow stronger it must be overloaded. Overloading means subjecting your muscles to more stress than they are accustomed to, causing them to adapt and get stronger. Adaptation is synonymous with development. Overloading muscles can be accomplished in two ways: by increasing volume and/or by increasing intensity.

Let's examine volume. This is done by either increasing the repetitions per set, adding sets, or by adding additional exercises for that muscle group.

The other way is by increasing the intensity of training. This can be accomplished by increasing the resistance (adding weight or doing a more difficult exercise) or by decreasing the rest time between sets and exercises.

These forms of progressive overloading should be done separately (increase either volume or intensity) or, on occasion, simultaneously. Beware: This form of simultaneous overloading can result in overtraining, injury, and burnout.

FULL RANGE OF MOTION

It is important to perform all exercises through the prescribed full range of motion, unless you are specifically performing special partial-range movements. Performing through the full range of motion is especially important for sports performance. Most performance skills are dynamic (i.e., in motion); therefore, your muscles need to be strengthened throughout their full range. You must maintain resistance on the muscles throughout the entire movement. A full range of motion means moving from full extension to complete contraction (or flexion) in any given exercise.

SPEED OF MOVEMENT

The speed at which you do an exercise is an important aspect of a successful training program. Generally, movement should be slow and controlled through the negative (eccentric) phase. The positive (concentric) phase of the movement should be as explosive as possible without creating momentum; it should keep constant tension on the muscles.

As you reach advanced levels of training, it is important to vary the speed of the exercise to achieve peak development.

CONSTANT TENSION

During a movement you must maintain constant tension on the muscle, feeling its contraction throughout the full range of motion. Do not let momentum take over; feel the muscle do the work.

WORKOUT LENGTH

The length of a training session is dependent on total volume, type of exercise, rest time taken, and goals of the individual. Another variable that determines workout length is intensity. High-intensity work will increase the need for recovery time, possibly increasing total workout length. Depending on your goals, you may spend anywhere between 10 minutes to one hour training your shoulders, arms, and traps. Part Four: "The Routines" offers a wide variety of routines from which to choose.

FREQUENCY OF TRAINING

Frequency of training is dependent upon many variables, including recovery time, level of experience, competition schedule, and goals of the trainee. Recovery time is key because strength gains and muscle growth occur during these periods. If recovery time between workouts is not adequate, strength gains will not be optimal, and overtraining will result.

EXERCISE ORDER

There are many factors to consider when choosing exercise order: individual weak areas, sports-specific routines, and your fitness level.

Generally, exercises are completed in order of highest energy expenditure to lowest, especially when starting out. In other words: You work from the largest muscles to the smallest muscles.

ROUTINES

The problems of exercise order, to a large extent, are already worked out for you in the routines. But as you progress, you will reach a stage when you must decide what variations you need to get peak results. You will have to determine your genetic strengths and weaknesses, and your overall goals including how you want to look, and then choose the exercises that will accomplish this fine tuning. As with everything else in life, at some point you will be left alone to face the truth about your shoulders and arms. But have no fear, you won't fall into the shoulders-and-arms abyss. Chapter 19: "Creating Your Own Routine" will guide you safely through this existential experience!

WARM-UP

It is always important to warm up your body before exercising. That prepares your body for action in three main ways:

1. It increases muscle blood flow and muscle metabolism.
2. The increase in muscle temperature allows the muscles to contract more forcefully and with greater speed. If the muscles are warm, contraction will be optimal.
3. It reduces injury potential.

A good general warm-up routine is five minutes of light aerobic work: biking, rowing, a brisk walk or slow jog.

BREATHING

As in all exercise, proper breathing is essential. The breathing technique to use for resistance training is as follows:

1. Inhale before the start of the negative contraction, when you are moving against the least resistance.
2. Exhale during the last two-thirds of the positive contraction.

For example, when performing a barbell curl you would inhale before you lower the resistance and exhale as you raise the resistance back up.

During long isometric and eccentric contractions, normal or pulsed breathing should take place. Pulsed breathing consists of short, pantlike breaths that create a quick exchange of oxygen.

INTENSITY

For our purposes, intensity means the amount of weight or degree of resistance used. Intensity can be decreased or increased by choosing easier or more difficult exercises or by subtracting or adding weight. You should aim for an intensity level that will produce momentary muscular exhaustion in the prescribed number of repetitions, and with each workout try to push the envelope by increasing intensity level.

VARIATION

Variation may be the most neglected training principle. People get comfortable in a routine and don't want to change; we are creatures of habit. But the body needs both structure and change. When you first begin a routine, the body hooks into this new structure and thrives on it. This will be a growth period. There will be gains in strength, endurance, and/or body appearance. But after a period of time, your body will adapt to this routine, and stagnate, or plateau. This means it's time for a change. The body wants something new. It needs a new routine that will challenge it, causing adaptation and growth.

Variation also prevents boredom and monotony in training. And hitting the muscles from a variety of angles gives better overall development. Chapter 17: "The System" has variety built into each level.

HOW MUCH DO I AIM FOR?

The number of repetitions and sets you do depends on your fitness level and your goals. There is no hard and fast rule. Professional bodybuilders and top athletes have gotten results using a wide variety of routines differing in numbers of sets, reps, and exercises. Chapter 19: "Creating Your Own Routine" will give you intelligent guidelines for achieving these goals, to meet your individual needs.

OVERTRAINING

Overtraining is doing too much and not giving yourself enough rest. It means you have worked the muscle too often and too intensely, not giving it enough time to repair itself. It is the same as being overworked at the office. You start to become less efficient at your work, and you start to burn out. It is easy to push yourself too hard, becoming too critical, always wanting more. Working out shouldn't become an unhealthy obsession. Sometimes less is more. Remember, the purpose of exercise is to improve the quality of your life both mentally and physically, not just your physical appearance. Be patient, train smart, and enjoy every repetition. Get into the process, not just the results.

QUALITY OF THE REP

The most important element in training is not quantity but quality. Don't sacrifice technique for heavier weight. Concentrate on quality and technique, keeping your technique strict and going through the prescribed range of motion on each repetition. Feel the contraction of each rep; keep constant tension on the muscles throughout the movement. Indulge in each and every repetition.

REST PERIODS

The purpose of a rest period between sets is to recover in order to perform the next set. In general, you should keep your rest time to a minimum, just long enough to allow recovery. But again, this depends on your goals and your fitness level. Beginners need more rest time. Any high-intensity training will generally require more rest time.

PAIN

An important part of working out is getting in touch with your body. Part of this journey is learning to distinguish between good pain and bad pain. So be smart and listen to your body.

Good pain is the feeling of being pumped, having the muscle fill with blood. And, yes, even that burning sensation that comes from lactic acid buildup is a good pain. It signals fatigue in the muscle or muscles you are working—which is the goal of exercise. These are feelings you will learn to thrive on and may even come to regard as pleasurable.

Bad pain is a warning sign. It means you've injured yourself. When you feel this type of pain, stop immediately. Warning signs include sharp pains, spasms, and periphery pain that moves into your legs, arms, feet, and hands. Do not push yourself through bad pain. It is a sign that you need to take time off and see a doctor, or change to exercises that don't cause problems. When in doubt, it's better to play it safe than risk injury. If you have lower back problems, be especially cautious. Be aware of your lower back at all times.

SORENESS

Muscle soreness is common after a workout. Don't worry if you're a little sore (good pain). Soreness may be caused by microscopic tears and stretching in muscle tissue. This is part of growth. Muscles need recuperation time and proper nutrition to repair (remodel).

If you are too sore to train during your next session, you have overdone it. Generally, it is good to train through mild soreness. Increased blood flow will help repair the area. Train hard and train smart—exercise is for a lifetime.

References

Brungardt, Brett. "Spring and Summer Four Week Mini Cycles," *National Strength & Conditioning Association Journal,* vol. 7, no. 5 (December/January 1986), 34–35.

O'Bryant, Harold, and Mike Stone. *Weight Training: A Scientific Approach.* 1st ed. Minneapolis: Burgess Publishing Co., 1984.

Proper Technique: The Mind

Imagine yourself as a movie on the screen. You are the story—your life as you experience it—but you are also the writer of the script, the director who brings the writer's vision into being, and the performer through whose actions and choices that vision becomes reality. Now think of your mind as the writer of your personal training script. It imagines—creates images of—and thus creates the body you wish to achieve. Your brain is the director, and your body is the performer or actor that brings the story to life. All three of these components must be fully developed and working in harmony to make a great script, body, and life. If these three components are not in harmony, or if one doesn't function up to its full capability, then the result will be a so-so script culminating in an average movie. But if your mind, brain, and body work in true harmony with each other, you can create the great body you are envisioning now. The body's job is covered in depth throughout this book. In this chapter, we'll look at how you can put the mind and brain into equal partnership with the body in the equation.

The Brain

The brain has two major functions in exercise: motivation and organization. These two play an important role in making your workout productive and successful. If you lack either of these functions, your ability to obtain optimal results will be hampered. It is therefore very important that you develop and incorporate the full potential of the mind/body connection in your exercise regimen.

MOTIVATION

Motivation is the desire to accomplish a goal. The question is, where do you find that desire? If you are reading this book, you obviously have a serious interest in training your shoulders and arms. Why do you have such an interest? In other words, what is the goal behind that desire? Is it to have enormously developed arms and shoulders in isolation from an otherwise unfit body? Probably not. The desire is the pathway to a more complex and organic goal. It is important to know why, to name it.

Take a moment to list the reasons that you want to make your shoulders and arms stronger or more pleasing to the eye. Do you feel you need extra strength, perhaps for some sport-specific goal? Or would you just like to be stronger overall? Would you like to look bigger? Or is your goal greater definition? Do you want to improve your posture to create or maintain shoulder and lower back health? Or do you want to improve your performance and avoid injury in a favorite sport? Often we follow desires without a clear understanding of where we actually wish to go with them.

Once you have evaluated why you want something, it is easier to accurately determine what it is you would like to accomplish or, in other words, set a goal. Goals need to be specific and they need to be written down. Now that you know *why* you are training your shoulders and arms, you need to look at two other important elements: the end result and the required investment of time.

When contemplating the end result of a given goal, be as specific as possible. Do you want bodybuilder biceps in a year? Or is your goal to be able to press a specific amount of weight over your head? Are you interested in balancing out the muscles in your shoulders to correct training problems and avoid injury? Be as detailed as possible in defining what it is you want to accomplish. Once you have the ultimate image in mind, it's time to break your goals down into specific time increments, making them both challenging and achievable. In other words you want to set your goals for the long term, the medium term, and for the short term.

Long-term goals can be viewed as those anywhere from two to three years and on. One of your most valu-able tools is a notebook in which you record your *goals* and log your progress toward them.

First, list your lifetime goals. Then list what you would like to accomplish ten years from now, five years from now, and two years from now. These are your long-term goals.

Medium-term goals can be viewed as those from six months to approximately twenty-four months from now. List where you would like to be within six months, by next year, and in six-month increments after that. Again, be as specific as possible.

Short-term goals consist of weekly and monthly goals to help you accomplish your medium- and long-term goals. List what you would like to have accomplished a month from now. Keep in mind what your medium- and long-term goals are when listing your short-term goals, so that everything is designed to help you achieve your master plan. Then list what you would like to accomplish each week. These goals must push you toward accomplishing your monthly goals.

Once you have set your weekly goal, you're ready to set up daily tasks for that week, which will help you achieve your goals. Be specific. List what you intend to eat each day. List what you will accomplish in a workout and set a specific time for that workout. An excellent tool to use for this is an appointment book. Do this every week. It may sound like a lot of work, but once you've established your initial long-, medium-, and short-term goals, it will take you only about 15 minutes a week. Following are examples of goal sheets you can utilize.

Now that you've established your goals, give yourself a pat on the back. You've performed a positive service for yourself! For many people, working out tends to bring up negative images. It takes too long. It's too hard. It hurts. It's no fun. However, if you look past these complaints for a moment to see the potential rewards that await you at the end of the journey, you will realize that the means justify the end. If you make the commitment to look at your end goal every day, if you maintain a positive workout attitude, and if you do this consistently for the proven period of about 21 days, your feelings about working out will begin to change profoundly. Although you may never be completely thrilled about working out, you will realize that the

LONG-TERM GOALS SHEET

I, _____(your name)_____ , in realizing the importance of setting long-term goals for myself, am committed to doing the very best I can to achieve the following goals (listed in order from the most important to the least important).

GOAL	DATE GOAL WILL BE ACCOMPLISHED
1._____	_____
2._____	_____
3._____	_____
4._____	_____
5._____	_____
6._____	_____
7._____	_____
8._____	_____
9._____	_____
10._____	_____

I, _____(your signature)_____ , resolve to have the discipline and perseverance to accomplish the goals I have written down here. _____(present date)_____

MEDIUM-TERM GOALS SHEET

I, _____(your name)_____ , in realizing the importance of setting medium-term goals for myself, am committed to doing the very best I can to achieve the following goals (listed in order from the most important to the least important).

GOAL	DATE GOAL WILL BE ACCOMPLISHED
1._____	_____
2._____	_____
3._____	_____
4._____	_____
5._____	_____
6._____	_____
7._____	_____
8._____	_____
9._____	_____
10._____	_____

I, _____(your signature)_____ , resolve to have the discipline and perseverance to accomplish the goals I have written down here. _____(present date)_____

rewards more than outweigh your resistance to training and you will begin to see measurable results. Just as desires point the way to specific goals, goals once achieved help fuel your desire to keep on going. It's a positive cycle.

Another good habit to adopt is to praise yourself after every workout. You've done something positive for yourself. You deserve a pat on the back, so give yourself one. Remember, every day that you work out is a personal victory. It takes you one step closer to your goals. Remind yourself of this before and after every workout. In this case the truth doesn't hurt; it helps.

Any day that you feel like blowing off a workout, take a time-out to stop and think of your goals. There are lots of tricks you can use; for instance, make a deal with yourself that whenever you consider skipping a workout you will at least dress out in gym clothes and shoes first. Nine times out of ten, the act of dressing for exercise will lead you straight to the gym. There are always a thousand excuses you can use not to work out. If you keep your goals at the forefront, it is easier to dismiss these excuses and overcome any lack of motivation you are experiencing at the moment. On the days you overcome these excuses, give yourself a double pat on the back. Realize what you've accomplished. You've pushed yourself past a previously perceived limit. You've broken one of your own boundaries, and pushed your own envelope.

ORGANIZATION

Organization means having a plan, a map. Once you've set goals, your destination is in sight. Now it's time to

SHORT-TERM GOALS SHEET

I, ____(your name)____ , in realizing the importance of setting short-term goals for myself, am committed to doing the very best I can to achieve the following goals (listed in order from the most important to the least important).

GOAL

DATE GOAL WILL
BE ACCOMPLISHED

1._____   _____

2._____   _____

3._____   _____

4._____   _____

5._____   _____

6._____   _____

7._____   _____

8._____   _____

9._____   _____

10._____   _____

I, ____(your signature)____ , resolve to have the discipline and perseverance to accomplish the goals I have written down here. ____(present date)____

plan the route you wish to take. By setting up your daily tasks you've already moved toward organizing that route, but you have to go further.

You need to know, specifically: (1) what exercises you will perform, (2) how many sets of each exercise you will perform, (3) how many reps in each set you will do, (4) what order you will perform the exercises, (5) how many times a week you need to perform these exercises, and (6) when you need to change to a new routine. In Chapter 17: "The System," all of this is planned for you. In Chapter 19: "Creating Your Own Routine," you learn how to do this yourself. Whether you use The System or tailor your own routine, the most important thing to remember is that you do need a plan.

Most people have to plan their workout around their day. Some people are fortunate enough to be able to plan their day around their workout. Whichever cate-

gory you fall into, it is important to find a time of day that works best for you and be as consistent as possible in sticking to that time. This will help to make your workout as much a habit as rising when the alarm clock goes off or brushing your teeth after a meal. For those who are just starting out, making your training an integral part of your regular routine is key.

The Mind

Trapping the power of the mind is an important step in taking your workouts to the next level. Two important skills to master are *visualization* and *focus*.

VISUALIZATION

You are what you perceive yourself to be. That is a truth that is hard to argue against. Throughout your life your experiences have shaped the way you view yourself. Every success and every failure you've experienced has had a tremendous impact on who you are, how confident you are, and what your chances for future success will be. Unfortunately, we all tend to have more failures than successes. It is the human condition. It starts at birth and continues through childhood and on into adolescence. The very nature of these phases—dependence on others, having to obey parents and teachers—reinforces the belief that people will always be bigger, stronger, wiser, and above all will possess more power than you. You quickly learn that you are powerless to do anything about this at the time. By the time you reach adulthood, you have experienced hundreds if not thousands of negative experiences that may program you to believe that you can't succeed. As an adult, these negative thoughts, feelings, and experiences continue to have a powerful impact on how you act, react, and feel about yourself. These early messages can also influence how high you set your sights and how willing you are to allow yourself to achieve them.

Visualization can be an effective method for reversing the negative beliefs that stem from your past experiences. Visualization allows you to overwhelm those past negative messages with a steady input of positive images. The brain is like a computer. It behaves exactly the way it has been programmed to act. The

WEEKLY GOALS AND DAILY TASKS SHEET

Week _____

Goals

1. _____

2. _____

DAILY TASKS

DAY/TIME	GOAL	WHEN IT WILL BE PERFORMED
MONDAY	1.	
	2.	
	3.	
	4.	
	5.	
TUESDAY	1.	
	2.	
	3.	
	4.	
	5.	
WEDNESDAY	1.	
	2.	
	3.	
	4.	
	5.	
THURSDAY	1.	
	2.	
	3.	
	4.	
	5.	
FRIDAY	1.	
	2.	
	3.	
	4.	
	5.	
SATURDAY	1.	
	2.	
	3.	
	4.	
	5.	
SUNDAY	1.	
	2.	
	3.	
	4.	
	5.	

only way to erase a bad program is to reprogram a better one. You can overcome your past failures by programming for future success.

For years, many of the world's greatest athletes have been using visualization successfully. In fact, athletes were visualizing long before anyone gave the process a name. Jack Nicklaus always previews his golf shot mentally before ever beginning the swing. Divers, dancers, and gymnasts all know the value of practicing mentally before performing. Most successful athletes use some form of visualization to help them perform better, as do most successful businesspeople. In fact, successful people in all walks of life usually include some form of visualization among their techniques for achieving their goals. We all do it when we dream of the future: a new car, a big house in the country, kids.

The reason it works is simple. The brain can't tell the difference between a real and imagined event. You can fool the brain, and create new patterns of behavior. As you train yourself to imagine success you cease to concentrate on failure. This reverses the usual scenario in which negative thoughts overwhelm you, especially at critical times. Instead, as you consistently feed your brain with positive images you begin to neutralize the negatives.

Visualization is a tool that will both motivate and program you for success. As with any other tool, first you have to become skilled at using it before you can expect results. This takes practice—consistent practice. Visualization should become a daily part of your mental training routine. When you write down your daily tasks at the beginning of each week, be sure to note when and how long you plan to visualize. Plan on visualizing—and nothing else—for at least 15 minutes each day. A good time is in the morning after you awaken or in the evening before you go to bed. Avoid visualizing right after you eat, as your visualization may turn into a nap! Give yourself two to three hours after a meal before you visualize.

To visualize effectively, first find a quiet spot where you won't be distracted or disturbed. Sit or lie down and close your eyes. The most important skill for you to master is relaxation. A good method to use for this is Deep Abdominal Breathing.

Deep Abdominal Breathing: In this method you will take five deep breaths. The goal is to become deeply relaxed in about 15 seconds. If you consistently practice it several times a day, you will become fairly adept at it in a couple of weeks.*

1. Breathe through your nostrils. Breathing through the mouth isn't very relaxing. The only exception is if your nose is clogged.
2. Inhale slowly, letting your abdomen expand out naturally. Breathe deeply but not forcefully (forceful breathing defeats the purpose of relaxation and can cause hyperventilation). Take slower and shallower breaths if you feel dizzy.
3. Once you feel your abdomen completely expanded, draw your shoulders back and raise or extend your head. Continue to breathe in to expand the upper portion of your lungs.
4. Hold the breath for five seconds.
5. Exhale slowly through your nose allowing your abdomen to deflate. Wait two seconds before inhaling again.
6. Repeat for five breaths (or more if needed), counting 5-4-3-2-1 after each breath. Feel yourself relaxing more and more deeply after each breath.
7. When coming out of this relaxed state (after the last breath), count slowly 1-2-3-4-5. After 5 say to yourself, "I am relaxed, alert, and full of energy."
8. When you have become skillful at this technique, try relaxing yourself in just three breaths.

Use steps 1 through 6 of this technique before every visualization. Use step 7 to come out of every visualization. Here are two sample visualizations you may use before workouts:

Preworkout Visualization: Imagine yourself in your club or gym. See all the equipment, smell the smells, notice the temperature in the room. What are you wear-

* Chungliang Al Huang and Jerry Lynch, *Thinking Body, Dancing Mind* (New York: Bantam Books, 1992), pp. 18–19.

ing? What is your mind-set? Feel yourself walking to the first area where you're going to lift. Hear the activity around you. Imagine yourself preparing for your first exercise. Visualize yourself picking the dumbbells up off the rack or setting up the bar or machine. Imagine yourself getting in the proper position to perform the lift. Perform one repetition in your mind of your first exercise, using perfect form. Feel your muscles working as you imagine the exercise. See the muscles work. See them contract and move. Repeat this procedure for every exercise you plan to perform this day. Be as detailed and specific as you can be, using as many senses as you can. When you are finished visualizing your last exercise, remember to count up to 5 and then say to yourself, "I am relaxed, alert, and full of energy."

Goal Visualization: Picture yourself having accomplished your goals. Imagine how you will look. See yourself in detail. Observe the definition and shape of your body. Feel strength and health radiate through your body. Imagine yourself performing tasks that you would like to perform with relative ease: playing your favorite sport, working out, walking on the beach or hiking in the mountains with a loved one. Notice how much energy and confidence you have. Imagine how different your perception of yourself is due to the way you now look, feel, and perform. Praise yourself for having worked and accomplished your goals. When you are finished visualizing, remember to count up to 5 and then say to yourself, "I am relaxed, alert, and full of energy."

Perform the Preworkout Visualization on every workout day, as close to your workout as possible. Perform the Goal Visualization every day, either in the morning before starting your day or just before you go to sleep.

FOCUS

Focus involves being aware of your body, understanding how it works, and concentrating on the task at hand. For most of us, body awareness doesn't come naturally. We have been raised in a culture that doesn't encourage us to develop intimacy with our own bodies, especially when it involves feeling our muscles work. A good way to focus during exercise is to consciously

put the mind in the muscle. Try to feel the muscle working. If, for example, you are trying to focus on your biceps, concentrate on two things. First, concentrate on the muscle shortening as you bend your arm. Notice how your biceps appears to get harder as you bend. Keeping the arm bent, try to make the muscle even harder. The longer you try, the more of a burning sensation you will feel in your biceps. Keep this in mind, because this is the feeling (the famous "burn") that you want when working any muscle. Second, concentrate on the muscle lengthening as you straighten your arm. Feel the biceps stretch. Notice how the muscle doesn't feel as hard as when it was bent. It seems to relax, and the straighter you try to make the arm, the more of a stretch you feel in the biceps. Keep this in mind also because it will give you a way to compare two different aspects of muscle movement, the sensation of a contraction (hardness and burning) and the sensation of flexion (stretching and often relaxation). This allows you to become aware of your body as it exercises. And the more aware and focused you are during your workouts, the better the results will be.

Body Scan: Try the following exercise to check your own body awareness. It will allow you to compare your perceptions with the reality of what is going on physically with your body. For example, many of us have bad posture without being aware of it. The first step to change, in the body as in life, is to develop awareness.

Lie on your back with your arms at your sides, palms down. Close your eyes. Try to discover through your other senses how your body is placed. Is your body aligned or twisted? If you're twisted, how much are you twisted? Is your head aligned with your body or is it tilted to the side? Are your feet locked back with the toes pointed up or are they tilted to the side forming a V? Are your knees locked or slightly bent? Are your arms straight or slightly bent? Open your eyes. Are you looking straight up or slightly to the side? This tells you your head position. Now lift your head and check your arms. How are they positioned? Next check your torso. Finally, check your legs and feet. Lower your head and close your eyes. Now notice what happened to your breathing during the scan. If you stopped paying attention to your breath, notice it now. Is it relaxed? Is it steady? Are you breathing through your nose? Many people tend to hold their breath unconsciously while concentrating. You need to be aware of your breathing.

How did you do? Was your awareness of your body's placement accurate? Partly accurate? Completely inaccurate? Perform this check every day for two to three weeks. You'll be amazed at your increased awareness of simple things regarding your body, and as your awareness increases, so will your focus.

THE BODY

The body receives instructions from the brain and carries out those instructions to the best of its ability. If the body is not developed to its capacity, then it may be limited in carrying out the instructions it receives. Like an automobile, you can turn the ignition key and send the message to start, but if the engine isn't finely tuned, it cannot run at peak performance. It is therefore imperative that the body be developed to its fullest potential to allow it to perform whatever is asked.

We have discussed the mind, body, and brain as separate entities, but you may be better served in thinking of them as a chain whose links are constantly interacting with each other. But remember that a chain is only as strong as its weakest link. It would therefore greatly benefit you to develop each link to the fullest. If you do, the sky is the limit.

References

Brungardt, Brett, and Mike Brungardt. *The Strength Kit.* 2nd ed. Grand Junction, Colo.: Strength Advantage, Inc., 1987.

Feldenkrais, Moshe. *Awareness Through Movement.* New York: HarperCollins, 1990.

Huang, Chungliang Al and Jerry Lynch. *Thinking Body, Dancing Mind.* New York: Bantam Books, 1992.

Masters, Robert, and Jean Houston. *Listening to the Body.* New York: Dell Publishing, 1978.

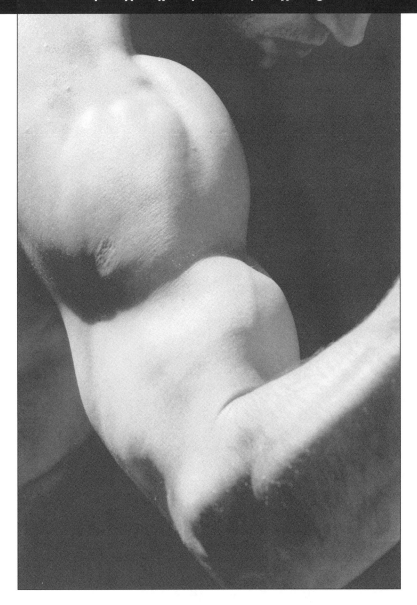

PART TWO

Wellness

Power Nutrition: Eating to Fuel Fitness

BY BECKY CHASE, M.S., R.D.

Everywhere you turn today, you run into advice about how to eat—what is good, what is bad, what will make you thin or fat, and what will make you fit. What you read in one magazine is contradicted by what you see on television. One fitness "expert" recommends high carbohydrates while another recommends high protein. How are you supposed to figure out what is right for you?

The field of nutrition is nothing if not controversial. Nutrition research has exploded over the last quarter century. This new interest in how food affects health is a double-edged sword—we are learning more every day about nutrition, but the field is growing so fast it is hard to keep up with current information. Recommendations change as new information becomes available. When a new study is completed, it becomes headline news the next day, interfering with the scientific process of review and replication by other members of the scientific community. If a new finding does not pan out, a new headline is born—leading to the confusion of what is *really* known about nutrition.

What do we know for sure about food and exercise? Actually, quite a lot. We know that nutrition can make the difference between having enough energy to get by and feeling really good. That's a fact that won't change! We know there are no magical foods or nutritional supplements that will single-handedly give you a strong, lean body. There is no "triceps diet" to skinny down your arms or bulk them out. But eating well *will* maximize your efforts in the gym. To achieve the shape you want, you have to *work off what you eat* and *eat what you work off*. This simply means working off excess calories and body fat and replacing the essential nutrients used during those workouts with the right foods.

The information in this chapter applies to all healthy, adult exercisers. It is not, however, intended to replace medical advice. Nor will it necessarily apply to children or people with chronic health problems. If you have any medical problems, consult your physician before making significant changes in your exercise or diet. Whatever your sport or fitness goal, the nutrition basics have to be followed to achieve lasting results. Remember, *food is fuel.* Choosing the right fuels, in the right proportions, will enhance your exercise effectiveness and help you achieve a healthy, fit body. That's the power of Power Nutrition. Next, you will find a step-wise system for implementing Power Nutrition and guidelines for both body building and endurance training.

Training Your Tastebuds for Fitness

A STEP-WISE SYSTEM FOR POWER NUTRITION

Okay, so you're determined to eat healthier, get fit, and change your life, right? If this isn't the first time you have vowed to clean up your act, perhaps it would help to take a moment to evaluate your plan of attack. Just how are you going to *really change* this time?

There are two schools of thought about change. One school advocates the "cold turkey" approach. You make all your changes in one big, giant step. You switch from whole milk to nonfat, bypassing the low-fat options. You give up all animal fat and never look back. And you begin an aggressive exercise routine. Zero to 100 in nothing flat. This approach works well for some people. It is simple and clear-cut; no ifs, ands, or buts. The downside to this approach is that sudden, drastic change often results in burnout and giving up because it is too hard, too demanding.

The second school of thought advocates slow, gradual change that allows you to adapt to each step before going on to the next. You don't have to change all your unhealthy habits at once, you just have to be consistent. Make small, relatively easy changes, such as reducing your fat intake in small ways and working out for a few minutes every day. Gradually lengthen your

workouts and increase their intensity as you become more fit. Every small change is considered success, progress. Permanent changes sort of sneak up on you, but if you look back over a year you recognize how much healthier you are. This is the "slow but steady" approach.

The right approach for you depends on your personality, on what actually works for you in the long run. Physical and nutritional fitness are a way of life requiring an ongoing commitment to health. The bottom line is to develop healthy habits that you can sustain for your life, not just for a few weeks. You can start by trying the following:

10 EASY THINGS YOU CAN DO TODAY TO IMPROVE YOUR FITNESS!

1. Eat a real breakfast—with fruit, whole grains, and a protein or milk/yogurt.

2. Drink a tall glass of water before you have your first cup of coffee.

3. Use evaporated skimmed milk in your coffee instead of creamer or half and half.

4. Pack a healthy snack to have when you get hungry this afternoon—fresh or dried fruit and baby carrots.

5. Park an extra two blocks from your office.

6. Use the stairs in your building.

7. On your coffee break, go outside and walk around the block.

8. Get away from your desk at lunch and enjoy a satisfying meal.

9. Eat that healthy snack you brought to work when you get hungry this afternoon.

10. Do some stretching exercises while watching TV tonight.

The Power Nutrition System

The following Power Nutrition System is divided into three segments or steps. Each step assumes you are spending more time and energy working out. This progressive system is designed to be used in conjunction with the workout system, giving you a complete program. The meal plans reflect that by containing different amounts of carbohydrate (CHO), protein, and fat to meet your exercise needs. If you are just beginning to exercise (or getting back to it after a long absence), start with Step One and progress to the next level as your body becomes more fit. Step Two can be either a maintenance plan or a stepping stone to more competitive pursuits. If you are already reasonably fit, start at Step Two or Three, depending on your exercise level and goals.

TOOLS FOR SUCCESS

For change to occur, you must stay committed and focused on your goals *and* enjoy the process. These tools will help you do that. The time it takes to use them is minimal, especially if you compare it to the time you lose when you don't stay focused.

A Food Composition Book or Software: Use it to look up the nutrient content of the foods you are eating. You will be surprised at what you learn when you have the facts instead of guessing or assuming you already know. These books come in a variety of sizes, content, and ease of use. They can be found in any bookstore. You want at least the following nutrient breakdown for foods: calories, carbohydrate, protein, fat, cholesterol, and dietary fiber. Brand names and fast foods should be included, too. Nutrition software, though more expensive than a book, is easy to use and gives a more complete nutritional breakdown of your diet. It often includes a component for tracking exercise, too. Some suggested titles are: *The Complete Book of Food Counts* by Corinne T. Netzer (New York: Dell Publishing, 1991), *Food Values of Portions Commonly Used*, 15th ed., by Jean A. T. Pennington (New York: Harper-Perennial, 1993), *Dine Healthy* for Windows or Macintosh by Dine System, 1-800-688-1848.

A Notebook or Diary: Recording food intake and exercise are essential tools for success. It's important to record as you go, instead of trying to remember tomorrow what you ate today. You're too busy for that and it is impossible to be accurate in retrospect. The note-book can be as simple or elaborate as you choose—a pocket notebook, a printed diary, or a three-ring binder. I use my Day Runner because it is always with me. I make my own log sheets to meet my needs. If I'm tracking only a couple of things, like fruit/vegetable intake and stretching, I use plain sheets and track each day with tally marks. If I want to do a more thorough nutrient evaluation, I write down everything I eat and drink. You will find a sample food/exercise log in the back of this chapter. Copy it and shrink it to fit your needs. Or make up your own.

Small Insulated Cooler or Lunch Bag with a Freezer Pack: Eating healthy is easiest when you plan ahead and take food with you for lunch and snacks. You can pack more variety if you have a way to keep perishable foods safe. You should be able to find what you need in a large grocery store or a discount department store.

Master Menus: Write out 5 to 10 simple meals each for breakfast, lunch, and dinner that you can make without thinking. Use these when you are too busy or too stressed to plan meals. Include easy, frozen or packaged foods you can keep on hand and some healthy take-out meals from a nearby restaurant. See the section on Planning Tips later in this chapter for ideas.

Master Shopping List: This consists of the items you need for your master menus. Always keep these items stocked in your freezer and pantry.

Goals/Affirmation Sheet: The number one reason people give for not eating healthy or exercising is, "I don't have time." Well, you have all the time there is, just like the rest of us! So, to help you keep your focus on fitness, keep a goal and affirmation sheet by your bed, such as the one at the end of this chapter. Read it right before you go to sleep and again when you wake up. It is very reinforcing. The affirmation will help you believe in yourself.

Rewards for Short-Term Goals: It takes time to fully realize a fit body. To stick with the process of making permanent changes, make it fun! Set short-term goals and establish a reward for yourself for meeting them. Rewards can be all kinds of things, except food! New exercise clothes or equipment, a long-distance phone call to a close friend, a day of play, whatever feels really good to you. Rewards are *not* self-indulgence, but a critical component of success. They reinforce the positive behavior changes you have worked so hard on. If you earn it, get it. Don't blow off rewarding yourself.

GETTING STARTED: SELF-EVALUATION OF EATING HABITS

In order to figure out how to get where you're going, you must know where you are. Don't assume you already know your habits; you may be surprised. Start by writing down *everything* you had to eat or drink over the last 24 hours. Do it now, even if you think yesterday's

intake was unusual. And be honest with yourself. Evaluating a day when you didn't know anyone would be looking can be very telling!

POWER NUTRITION FOOD GROUPS

At the top of each food group, the average amount of carbohydrate and protein for each serving within the group is given. Recommended intakes in *servings per day* and serving sizes are listed, too. Foods are divided within each group by the *average* amount of fat present. Brands vary in fat content, so read food labels.

You won't find every food that exists in these food groups. That doesn't mean you have to limit your food choices to those on the lists. Just categorize your foods based on their ingredients.

24-HOUR FOOD RECALL EVALUATION

How many servings of the following did you eat? Compare your intake to the servings recommended in the Servings Goal column.

FOOD GROUP	SERVINGS EATEN	SERVINGS GOAL
CEREAL, BREAD, GRAINS (1 slice bread, ½ bagel, ½ cup cooked rice)	_____	6 to 11
VEGETABLES (½ cup cooked, 1 cup raw)	_____	3 to 5
FRUITS (½ cup canned, 1 small piece, 6 oz. juice)	_____	2 or more
PROTEIN (1 oz. meat, chicken, fish; ½ cup beans; 1 egg; 1 oz. cheese)	_____	3 to 6
MILK AND YOGURT (1 cup of either)	_____	2 to 3
FATS (1 tsp. margarine, butter, oil; 1 Tbsp. mayo, sour cream, half & half)	_____	0 to 3
SUGARS (1 Tbsp. sugar, honey, syrup; 2 cookies; small piece cake or pie; 12 oz. soda)	_____	0 to 2
ALCOHOL (12 oz. beer, 5 oz. wine, 1½ oz. liquor)	_____	0 to 2

NUTRITIONAL FITNESS QUIZ

Now, think about your *typical* or *average* food day. Consider weekends, late nights at work, restaurant meals, and snacks. With those in mind, take the Nutritional Fitness Quiz.

DO YOU EAT, ON AVERAGE:	YES	NO
Meals or snacks in the morning, midday, *and* evening?	_____	_____
Some sort of grain or bread at every meal?	_____	_____
100 percent whole grain bread more often than wheat or white bread?	_____	_____
Whole grain or bran cereal more often than other cereals?	_____	_____
Brown rice more often than white rice?	_____	_____
Mostly low-fat crackers (saltines, Wasa, etc.) instead of regular snack crackers?	_____	_____
Chips (potato, tortilla, etc.) less than twice a week?	_____	_____
Muffins, donuts, croissants, and pastries less than twice a week?	_____	_____
At least 2 to 3 cups of vegetables every day?	_____	_____
Deep yellow or green leafy vegetables every day?	_____	_____
At least 2 pieces of fruit or glasses of fruit juice every day?	_____	_____
Berries, melons, citrus fruit, or other high vitamin C foods every day?	_____	_____
Mostly 100 percent fruit juices instead of fruit drinks?	_____	_____
Mostly skim or 1% dairy products (milk, yogurt)?	_____	_____
Milk or yogurt daily (either cow, goat, or fortified soy)?	_____	_____
Fat-free or low-fat cheese more often than regular cheese?	_____	_____
Packaged luncheon meats less than twice a week?	_____	_____
Less than 8 ounces total of meat, chicken, and fish per day?	_____	_____
Bacon, sausage, and hot dogs less than once a week?	_____	_____
Beans, peas, or lentils at least twice a week?	_____	_____
Skinless poultry most of the time?	_____	_____
4 or fewer whole eggs a week?	_____	_____
Only water-packed canned tuna?	_____	_____
Deep-fried foods or gravy less than once a month?	_____	_____
Mostly low-fat tub margarine instead of butter or stick margarine?	_____	_____

(table continues)

NUTRITIONAL FITNESS QUIZ, continued

	YES	NO
Mostly low-fat or fat-free mayonnaise, sour cream, and salad dressings?	_____	_____
Low-fat frozen desserts more often than regular ice cream?	_____	_____
Fewer than two high-sugar foods, including regular sodas, candy, desserts, daily?	_____	_____

DO YOU DRINK, ON AVERAGE:

3 or fewer cups of coffee per day?	_____	_____
At least 8 glasses of water, including milk and juice, every day?	_____	_____
2 or fewer servings of alcohol per day?	_____	_____
TOTALS	_____	_____

Total the number of answers in each column. The ideal answer to all of the questions is Yes. Although the quiz is not a scientific test, it is designed to help you see where you can make positive changes in your usual diet. The Power Nutrition plan is aimed at helping you convert the No answers to Yes answers.

SCORING:

> Very fit: 28 to 31
> Fit, but can do better: 24 to 27
> Good intentions, now get serious!: 18 to 23
> A nutritional disaster waiting to happen: less than18

Combination Foods: How do you categorize foods like pizza, enchiladas, macaroni and cheese, etc.? Simply break them down by ingredient. For example, pizza contains **grain** (the crust), small serving of **vegetables** (tomato sauce and veggie toppings), and **high-fat animal protein** (cheese and meat toppings). Use a fat gram counter (available in bookstores) to get a more accurate fat gram count of foods.

Alcohol = Fat: Because of the way alcohol is metabolized in the body, it can increase storage of body fat. So, include alcohol in your fat gram budget, as follows: Count every drink as 9 grams of fat!

A "drink" is a 12 oz. beer, 4 oz. wine, or 1 cocktail made with 1.25 oz. of 80 proof liquor.

GUIDELINES TO HEALTHY, LOW-FAT EATING
BREADS, CEREALS, GRAINS

Each serving of grains provides, on average, 15 grams carbohydrate and 3 grams protein. Foods are divided by fat content. Exact nutrient content may vary with brands. Check food labels. Note: The serving size specified on a food label may be different from the serving size listed here. Eat at least 6 to 11 servings of grains every day.

0 TO 2 GRAMS OF FAT	SERVING SIZE
Breads:	
Whole grain or enriched breads w/o egg or cheese	1 slice
Bagels or pita bread, small	½ each
Corn tortillas**	1 each
English muffins, hard rolls, hamburger buns	½ each
Saltines	6 crackers
Fat-free crackers	¾ ounce
Baked tortilla chips	15 chips (¾ ounce)
Pretzels	¾ ounce
Cereals:	
Dry cereals w/o nuts or oils, Shredded Wheat, Cheerios, etc.	1 ounce (⅓ to 1 cup usually)
Low fat granola, Grape-Nuts	¼ cup
Fat-free granola bars	1 bar
Wheat germ	3 tablespoons
Cooked cereals:	
Oatmeal, grits, Zoom, etc.	½ cup cooked
Grains:	
Whole grain or enriched noodles, quinoa, buckwheat, kasha, bulgur	½ cup cooked
Whole-grain crackers w/o added fat: RyKrisp, Wasa, Kavli, etc.	2 to 5 crackers (¾ ounce)
Flour	3 tablespoons
Rice, millet, couscous	⅓ cup cooked
Rice milk (Enriched Rice Dream**)	½ cup
Rice cakes, large	2
Popcorn, air popped and no added fat	3 cups popped

2 TO 5 GRAMS OF FAT	SERVING SIZE
Breads:	
Biscuit	1 biscuit
Corn bread	2-inch square
Croutons	1 cup
Dinner roll, flour tortilla	1 each, small

(table continues)

GUIDELINES TO HEALTHY, LOW-FAT EATING, continued
BREADS, CEREALS, GRAINS

2 TO 5 GRAMS OF FAT	SERVING SIZE
Muffin, small	1 small
Pancakes	4-inch pancake
Popcorn, low fat	3 cups, popped
Snack crackers, butter-type	6 crackers
Snack crackers, cheese or peanut butter	3 crackers
Taco shell	2 6-inch shells
Waffle, frozen	4-inch waffle
Cereals:	
Granola bar	1 bar
Muesli or granola cereal	¼ cup
Soups: Low-fat cream or vegetable soups	1 cup

10 GRAMS OF FAT	SERVING SIZE
Croissant	1
Snack chips (corn, potato)	15 chips (1 ounce)
Tabbouleh (tabouli)	½ cup
Waffle, homemade	7-inch waffle

**Nondairy source of calcium

VEGETABLES: LOW CARBOHYDRATE

Each serving provides, on average, 5 grams carbohydrate and 2 grams protein. Foods are divided by fat content. Eat at least 3 to 5 servings of vegetables every day.

0 TO 1 GRAM OF FAT	SERVING SIZE
Broccoli**, kale**, leaf lettuce**, seaweed**	½ cup cooked, 1 cup raw
Artichoke, artichoke hearts, asparagus, green beans, bean sprouts, beets, brussels sprouts, cabbage, carrots, cauliflower, celery, cucumber, eggplant, greens, leeks, mushrooms, okra, onions, pea pods, peppers, radishes, radicchio, sauerkraut, spinach, summer squash, tomato, tomato sauce, turnips, water chestnuts, zucchini	½ cup cooked, 1 cup raw
Vegetable juices (V-8, tomato)	½ cup

5 GRAMS OF FAT	SERVING SIZE
Cole slaw	½ cup
Marinara sauce	½ cup

10 TO 15 GRAMS OF FAT	
Artichoke hearts, marinated in oil	¼ cup
Avocado	½ medium

**Nondairy source of calcium

GUIDELINES TO HEALTHY, LOW-FAT EATING
VEGETABLES: HIGH CARBOHYDRATE

Each serving provides, on average, 15 grams carbohydrate and 4 grams protein. Foods are divided by fat content. Eat at least 3 to 5 servings of vegetables every day.

0 TO 1 GRAM OF FAT	SERVING SIZE
Winter squash (acorn, butternut)**	1 cup cooked
Sweet potato and pumpkin**	½ cup cooked
Baked potato	1 small
Corn, plaintain	½ cup cooked
Corn on cob	1 medium ear
Baked beans	⅓ cup
Beans (pinto, black, lima, etc.)**	½ cup cooked
Peas and lentils	½ cup
Miso	3 tablespoons

5 GRAMS OF FAT	SERVING SIZE
Baked french fries	10 fries
Candied sweet potatoes	½ cup
Mashed potatoes	½ cup

10 TO 15 GRAMS OF FAT	SERVING SIZE
Fried french fries	10 fries
Hash brown potatoes	½ cup

**Nondairy source of calcium

NOTE: Beans and peas are also on the plant protein list. Count as either a high carbohydrate vegetable *or* a protein.

FRUITS AND FRUIT JUICES

Each serving provides, on average, 15 grams of carbohydrate, no protein, and a trace of fat. Eat at least 2 servings every day.

	SERVING SIZE
Bananas, oranges, peaches, pears	1 small piece
Berries, fresh or frozen without sugar	¾ cup
Canned fruit (in juice)	½ cup
Grapefruit	½
Melons	1 cup
Dried fruits	2 tablespoons
Fruit juices (no sugar added)	⅓ to ½ cup
Fruit juice cocktails (with sugar)	⅓ cup
Grapes	1 cup

(table continues)

GUIDELINES TO HEALTHY, LOW-FAT EATING, continued
PLANT PROTEIN

Each serving provides, on average, 7 grams of protein (equal to 1 ounce of meat). Legumes also provide about 22 grams of carbs/cup. Foods are divided by fat content. Use plant protein several times a week in place of animal protein.

0 TO 3 GRAMS OF FAT	SERVING SIZE
Legumes: beans, peas and lentils, dried or canned, and cooked without added fat**	½ cup cooked
Low-fat hummus	½ cup
Low-fat veggie burgers (such as Boca Burgers)	½ burger
Seitan (White Wave or Meat of Wheat)	1 ounce

6 TO 9 GRAMS OF FAT	SERVING SIZE
Miso	¼ cup
Tempeh	1½ ounces
Tofu (firm, raw, or baked without fat)	1½ ounces

**Nondairy source of calcium
NOTE: Legumes are also listed on high CHO vegetable list. Count them as either a protein *or* a vegetable.

ANIMAL PROTEIN

Each food listed here provides, on average 7 grams protein *per ounce* and no carbohydrate. Food is divided by fat content. Use within protein budget, usually 3 to 9 ounces per day. (3 ounces of cooked meat is about the size of a deck of cards.)

0 TO 2 GRAMS OF FAT	SERVING SIZE
1% or 2% cottage cheese*	½ cup (2 ounces)
Egg whites	2 whites (1 ounce)
Fat-free cheese*	2 ounces
Flounder or sole, baked	3 ounces cooked
Oysters, raw	3 ounces
Shrimp, boiled	3 ounces
Tuna, packed in water	¼ cup (2 ounces)

3 TO 5 GRAMS OF FAT	SERVING SIZE
Regular cottage cheese*	½ cup (2 ounces)
Chicken or turkey, no skin, baked or roasted	3 ounces
Most fish and shellfish, grilled or cooked without fat	3 ounces
Egg, whole	1 egg (1 ounces)
Low-fat luncheon meats	3 ounces
Salmon, pink, canned w/bones**	3 ounces

GUIDELINES TO HEALTHY, LOW-FAT EATING
ANIMAL PROTEIN

8 TO 12 GRAMS OF FAT	SERVING SIZE
Cheese, low-fat*	2 ounces
Chicken with skin, roasted	3 ounces
Ham, lean, baked or canned	3 ounces
Kippered herring	3 ounces
Mackerel, canned	3 ounces
Meatballs	2 to 3 ounces
Oysters and scallops, fried	3 ounces
Sardines	3 ounces
Salmon, sock-eye, grilled	3 ounces
Shrimp and squid, fried	3 ounces
Steak, broiled or grilled, fat trimmed	3 ounces

15 TO 25 GRAMS OF FAT	SERVING SIZE
Beef, ground or roasts	3 ounces
Cheese*	2 ounces
Chicken, fried	3 ounces
Hot dogs	2 to 3 ounces
Lamb	3 ounces
Luncheon meats	2 to 3 ounces
Pork	3 ounces
Sausages	2 to 3 ounces

*Source of calcium
**Nondairy source of calcium

MILK/YOGURT PROTEIN

Each serving provides, on average, 12 grams carbohydrate and 8 grams protein. These are all excellent sources of calcium. Food is divided by fat content. Eat 2 to 3 servings a day to meet calcium needs.

0 TO 1 GRAM OF FAT	SERVING SIZE
Nonfat milk powder	⅓ cup
Nonfat or skim milk	1 cup
Nonfat yogurt, plain or artificially sweetened	¾ cup (6 ounces)
Evaporated skim milk	½ cup
Skim Lactaid milk	1 cup
Fat-free soy milk, calcium fortified	1 cup

3 GRAMS OF FAT	SERVING SIZE
1% milk	1 cup
Low-fat soy milk, calcium fortified	1 cup
Low-fat fruited yogurt (contains 35 grams carbs)	¾ cup

(table continues)

GUIDELINES TO HEALTHY, LOW-FAT EATING, continued
MILK/YOGURT PROTEIN

5 GRAMS OF FAT	SERVING SIZE
2% milk	1 cup
Soy milk, calcium fortified	1 cup
Low-fat yogurt, plain	¾ cup

10 GRAMS OF FAT	SERVING SIZE
Whole milk	1 cup
Yogurt, plain, from whole milk	¾ cup
Milk shake, whole milk	1¼ cup
Goat's milk	1 cup

NOTE: Fruited or sweetened yogurts count as 1 milk plus 1 sweet.

SUGARS/SWEETS

Each serving provides about 15 to 40 grams carbohydrate and 0 to 4 grams protein. Foods divided by fat content.
SERVING SIZES: Eat no more than 2 servings daily.

0 TO 1 GRAM OF FAT	SERVING SIZE
Angel food cake	1 medium slice
Blackstrap molasses*	1 tablespoon
Fat-free cakes	1 medium slice
Fat-free cookies	2 cookies
Fat-free frozen yogurt or ice cream, sorbet	½ cup
Hard candy	2 pieces
High-sugar dry cereal	1 cup
Nonfat fruited yogurt*	¾ cup
Jelly, jams, preserves	1 tablespoon
Soft drinks	12-ounce can
Sugar, honey, syrup	2 tablespoons

2 TO 5 GRAMS OF FAT	SERVING SIZE
Graham crackers, vanilla wafers, fig cookies, sugar cookies	2 to 3 cookies
Low-fat fruited yogurt	¾ cup
Low-fat ice cream and frozen yogurt	½ cup
Low-fat cakes	1 medium slice
Pudding, from mix*	½ cup
Sherbet*	½ cup

*Source of calcium
NOTE: Fruited or sweetened yogurts count as 1 milk plus 1 sweet.

GUIDELINES TO HEALTHY, LOW-FAT EATING
SUGARS/SWEETS, continued

6 TO 15 GRAMS OF FAT	SERVING SIZE
Brownies	1 medium
Candy, chocolate	1 ounce
Chocolate chip cookies	1 to 2 cookies
Donuts and eclairs	1
Most cakes	1 small piece
Fruit pies	1 small piece
Whole yogurt, fruited	¾ cup

> 15 GRAMS OF FAT	SERVING SIZE
Bread pudding*	½ cup
Cheesecake	1 small slice
Fried pies	1
Pecan pie	1 small slice

*Source of calcium

NOTE: Fruited or sweetened yogurts count as 1 milk plus 1 sweet.

FATS/OILS

Each serving provides little or no carbohydrate and protein and 5 grams of fat. Use within daily fat gram budget.

	SERVING SIZES
Avocado	⅛ medium
Bacon	1 slice, cooked
Butter	1 teaspoon
Cream, half and half	2 tablespoons
Cream cheese, regular	1 tablespoon
Cream cheese, low-fat	2 tablespoons
Sour cream	2 tablespoons
Margarine, low-fat	2 teaspoons
Margarine, regular	1 teaspoon
Mayonnaise	1 teaspoon
Mayonnaise, low-fat	1 tablespoon
Nayonaise (soy mayo)	2 tablespoons
Nuts and seeds	6 to 10 nuts
Olives	5 large
Peanut butter	2 teaspoons
Salad dressing, regular	1 tablespoon
Salad dressing, low-fat	2 tablespoons
Vegetable oils: olive, canola, sunflower, corn, etc.	1 teaspoon

(table continues)

GUIDELINES TO HEALTHY, LOW-FAT EATING, continued
LOW-CALORIE EXTRAS

Use in moderation. Each serving provides no fat and few carbs. Serving sizes are small, so provide few calories.

0 GRAMS OF FAT	SERVING SIZES
Diet soft drinks	12-ounce can
Fat-free cream cheese	1 to 2 tablespoons
Fat-free margarine	1 to 2 teaspoons
Fat-free salad dressings, mayo, and sour cream	1 to 2 tablespoons
Sugar substitutes (e.g., Equal)	1 packet
Coffee or tea	1 cup
Spray-on oils (e.g., Pam)	to coat pan
Butter substitutes (Molly McButter, Butter Buds)	½ to 1 teaspoon

Power Nutrition Step One

Step One is designed for the beginning exerciser. It assumes you are including a combination of strength training (two to three times a week) and aerobic or cardiovascular exercises in your workout schedule. It also assumes your aerobic workouts are in the mild-to-moderate intensity range for 20 to 40 minutes each.

Goals of Step One Meal Plan: To provide adequate carbohydrate to fuel cardiovascular activity. To provide adequate protein intake for strength training. To keep fat intake within a healthy range, without being too rigid.

Step One Meal Plan: Calorie mix equals 55 to 60 percent carbohydrate, 20 to 25 percent fat, and 20 percent protein (or about 0.7 grams protein per pound body weight). Food is divided into three mixed meals and one to two snacks, with a substantial breakfast. Presented below are meal plans and sample menus for three calorie levels: 1700, 2000, and 2500. If none of these seems right for you, create your own using the Diet Worksheet at the end of this chapter.

STEP ONE: 1700 CALORIES
234 TO 255 GRAMS CHO
85 GRAMS PROTEIN
38 TO 47 GRAMS FAT

Calories are divided into the following servings from each Power Nutrition food group per day. You can mix the food up any way you like, but eat at least three meals and one snack.

TOTAL SERVINGS PER DAY:

- 6 grains
- 4 low CHO vegetables
- 2 high CHO vegetables
- 4 fruits
- 2 milk/yogurt
- 4½ protein
- 1 sweet/sugar
- 3 fats

SAMPLE MEAL PLAN	SAMPLE MENU
Morning	**Morning**
2 grains	Large glass of water
3 fruits	1 small bagel, toasted, with 2 Tbsp. low-fat cream cheese
1 milk/yogurt	¾ cup plain fat-free yogurt with 1 cup mixed fruit, canned in juice
1 fat	½ cup orange juice
Midday	**Midday**
2 grains	2 slices whole-grain bread with 1½ ounces sliced turkey, tomato slices, leaf lettuce, and 1 Tbsp. low-fat mayonnaise
2 low CHO vegetables	
1 milk/yogurt	4 to 6 baby carrots
1½ protein	1 cup 1% milk
1 fat	
Snack	**Snack**
2 grains	1½ ounces pretzels
1 fruit	small can pineapple juice
Evening Meal	**Evening Meal**
2 low CHO vegetables	large baked potato topped with 2 Tbsp. sour cream and chives
2 high CHO vegetables	1 cup steamed broccoli
3 protein	½ skinless chicken breast (3 ounces)
1 sweet/sugar	2 fig cookies (such as Fig Newton)
1 fat	

STEP ONE: 2000 CALORIES
275 TO 300 GRAMS CHO
100 GRAMS PROTEIN
44 TO 56 GRAMS FAT

Calories are divided into the following servings from each Power Nutrition food group per day. You can mix the food up any way you like, but eat at least three meals and one snack.

TOTAL SERVINGS PER DAY:

- 8 grains
- 4 low CHO vegetables
- 3 high CHO vegetables
- 4 fruits
- 2 milk/yogurt
- 5 protein
- 1 sweet/sugar
- 4 fats

SAMPLE MEAL PLAN	SAMPLE MENU
Morning	**Morning**
3 grains	large glass of water
3 fruits	1 cup Apple-Raisin Oatmeal*
1 milk/yogurt	1 slice whole-grain toast with 1 tsp. margarine
1 fat	1 cup 1% milk
Midday	**Midday**
2 grains	Veggie Burritos: 2 flour tortillas, *each one* filled with ¼ cup fat-free refried beans; ½ cup mixture of tomato, leaf lettuce, and salsa; ⅛ avocado, sliced; and 4 Tbsp. fat-free grated cheese
2 low CHO vegetables	
1 high CHO vegetable	
1 fruit	
2 protein	
2 fat	1 orange
Snack	**Snack**
2 grains	6-oz. container fat-free vanilla yogurt topped with ½ cup low-fat granola
1 milk/yogurt	
1 sweet/sugar	
Evening	**Evening**
1 grain	3-oz. portion of Grilled Tuna*
2 low CHO vegetables	1 cup green beans
2 high CHO vegetables	1 large ear corn on the cob
3 protein	1 small dinner roll with 1 tsp. margarine
1 fat	

* Power Nutrition Recipe at end of chapter.

STEP ONE: 2500 CALORIES
344 TO 375 GRAMS CHO
125 GRAMS PROTEIN
56 TO 69 GRAMS FAT

Calories are divided into the following servings from each Power Nutrition food group per day. You can mix the food up any way you like, but eat at least three meals and one snack.

TOTAL SERVINGS PER DAY:

- 11 grains
- 4 low CHO vegetables
- 4 high CHO vegetables
- 4 fruits
- 3 milk/yogurt
- 6 protein
- 1 sweet/sugar
- 5 fats

SAMPLE MEAL PLAN	SAMPLE MENU
Morning	**Morning**
4 grains	large glass of water
3 fruits	1 cup Apple-Raisin Oatmeal*
1 milk/yogurt	1 whole English muffin, toasted,
1 fat	with 1 tsp. margarine
	1 cup 1% milk
Snack	**Snack**
1 grain	2 large caramel corn rice cakes,
1 fat	*each one* topped with 1 tsp.
	peanut butter
Midday	**Midday**
2 grains	2 slices whole grain bread
2 high CHO vegetables	spread with ½ cup Low-Fat
2 low CHO vegetables	Hummus*, 2 slices low-fat
1 fruit	mozzarella cheese, and
3 protein	several tomato slices
1 fat	12 Sweet Potato Fries*
	small can V-8 juice
	1 small apple
Snack	**Snack**
1 high CHO vegetable	1¼ cup Pumpkin Yogurt*
1 milk/yogurt	
1 sweet/sugar	
Evening	**Evening**
4 grains	2 cups Stir Fry Chicken and
2 low CHO vegetables	Veggies* over 1½ cups
1 high CHO vegetables	fettuccini noodles
1 milk/yogurt	1 slice french bread dipped in
3 protein	1 tsp. olive oil
2 fats	1 cup 1% milk

* Power Nutrition Recipe at end of chapter.

Power Nutrition Step Two

Step Two is for those with better than average fitness, who exercise consistently, four or more times a week. It assumes a fitness routine that includes a maintenance-level weight training workout one to three times a week plus moderate- to high-intensity aerobic activities three or more times a week, 45 to 60 minutes per session. It may also include occasional endurance workouts lasting at least 90 minutes, such as long bike rides or cross-country skiing trips.

Goals of Step Two Meal Plan: To provide slightly more carbohydrate than in Step One to fuel the aerobic activity. To provide adequate protein for maintenance of muscle mass and maintain a healthy fat intake. To provide guidelines for carbohydrate/protein recovery following endurance activities.

Step Two Meal Plan: Calorie mix of 60 to 65 percent carbohydrate, 15 percent protein (at least 0.5 grams protein per pound body weight), and 20 to 25 percent fat. Food is divided into three mixed meals and one to two high-carbohydrate snacks. You will need an additional post-exercise recovery meal on the days you work out for more than 90 minutes. See "Maximizing Workouts: What to Eat Before, During, and After Exercise" (page 77).

Presented below are meal plans and sample menus for three calorie levels: 1700, 2000, and 2500. If none of these seems right for you, create your own using the worksheet at the end of this chapter. Notice the changes between Step One and Step Two. You now need more carbohydrate to fuel more frequent, higher-intensity exercise. You are used to the demands of weight training, requiring less protein. So, the meal plans include more vegetables and fruit and fewer protein foods.

STEP TWO: 1700 CALORIES
255 TO 276 GRAMS CHO
64 GRAMS PROTEIN
38 TO 47 GRAMS FAT

Calories are divided into the following servings from each Power Nutrition food group per day. You can mix the food up any way you like, but eat at least three meals and one snack.

TOTAL SERVINGS PER DAY:

- 6 grains
- 5 low CHO vegetables
- 3 high CHO vegetables
- 4 fruits
- 2 milk/yogurt
- 1 protein
- 1 sweet/sugar
- 5 fats

SAMPLE MEAL PLAN	SAMPLE MENU
Morning	**Morning**
3 grains	large glass of water
2 fruits	6 oz. fat-free vanilla yogurt with
1 milk/yogurt	½ cup low-fat granola
1 fat	1 slice whole-wheat toast with
1 sweet/sugar	1 tsp. margarine
	1 cup orange juice
Midday	**Midday**
2 grains	small toasted bagel topped with
3 low CHO vegetables	½ cup Low-Fat Hummus,*
1 fruit	tomato slices, and leaf lettuce
1 protein	12-oz. can Light'n Tangy V-8 juice
1 fat	½ cup unsweetened applesauce
Snack	**Snack**
1 milk/yogurt	1 cup 1% milk
1 fruit	1 banana
Evening	**Evening**
1 grain	1 2-inch square corn bread or
2 low CHO vegetables	small cornbread muffin
3 high CHO vegetables	1½ cups Easy and Yummy Beans*
3 fats	Large dinner salad made of leaf
	lettuce and 1 cup mixture of
	any low CHO veggies, 5
	sliced olives, and 2 Tbsp. low-
	fat salad dressing

STEP TWO: 2000 CALORIES
300 TO 325 GRAMS CHO
75 GRAMS PROTEIN
44 TO 56 GRAMS FAT

Calories are divided into the following servings from each Power Nutrition food group per day. You can mix the food up any way you like, but eat at least three meals and one snack.

TOTAL SERVINGS PER DAY:

- 8 grains
- 5 low CHO vegetables
- 3 high CHO vegetables
- 5 fruits
- 2 milk/yogurt
- 2 protein
- 1 sweet/sugar
- 5 fats

SAMPLE MEAL PLAN	SAMPLE MENU
Morning	**Morning**
3 grains	large glass of water
2 fruits	3 toaster low-fat waffles topped
1 milk/yogurt	with 6 oz. fat free vanilla
1 fat	yogurt and ¾ cup berries
1 sweet/sugar	½ cup grapefruit juice
Midday	**Midday**
1 grain	1 can Healthy Choice Clam
2 low CHO vegetables	Chowder
3 high CHO vegetables	6 saltine crackers
1 fruit	medium garden salad, about
1 protein	2 cups topped with 2 Tbsp.
2 fats	low-fat salad dressing
	1 small banana
Snack	**Snack**
2 grains	4 multigrain Wasa Crispbreads
1 low CHO vegetable	spread with 2 Tbsp. low-fat
1 fruit	flavored cream cheese
1 fat	4 to 6 baby carrots
	small can apple juice
Evening	**Evening**
2 grains	2⅔ cups Shrimp Cowpot*
2 low CHO vegetables	1 cup 1% milk
1 fruit	½ cup canned peaches, in juice
1 milk/yogurt	
1 protein	
1 fat	

* Power Nutrition Recipe at end of chapter.

STEP TWO: 2500 CALORIES
375 TO 406 GRAMS CHO
94 GRAMS PROTEIN
56 TO 69 GRAMS FAT

Calories are divided into the following servings from each Power Nutrition food group per day. You can mix the food up any way you like, but eat at least three meals and one snack.

TOTAL SERVINGS PER DAY:

- 11 grains
- 5 low CHO vegetables
- 4 high CHO vegetables
- 7 fruits
- 2 milk/yogurt
- 2½ protein
- 1 sweet/sugar
- 6 fats

SAMPLE MEAL PLAN	SAMPLE MENU
Morning	**Morning**
4 grains	large glass of water
2 fruits	1 container Fantastic Foods
1 milk/yogurt	Hot Cereal**
1 fat	1 slice toast with 1 tsp. margarine
	1 large banana
	1 cup 1% milk
Snack	**Snack**
1 grain	2 large flavored rice cakes
1 fruit	1 orange, sliced
Midday	**Midday**
2 grains	large baked potato topped with
3 low CHO vegetables	2 tsp. low-fat margarine
2 high CHO vegetables	large green salad, 3 cups, with
3 fruits	any mixture of low CHO
1 protein	veggies, 1½ oz. baked tofu,
2 fats	and 2 Tbsp. low-fat salad
	dressing
	12 saltine crackers
	12-oz. can cranberry juice
	cocktail
Snack	**Snack**
1 grain	6 oz. plain fat-free yogurt topped
1 fruit	with ¼ cup fat-free granola
1 milk/yogurt	and 2 Tbsp. raisins

Evening
3 grains
2 low CHO vegetables
2 high CHO vegetables
1½ protein
3 fats
1 sweet/sugar

Evening
2 cups Black Beans and Rice*
   topped with 1½ links
   turkey Italian sausage
1 cup steamed carrots
2 fat-free Snackwell cookies

* Power Nutrition Recipe at end of chapter.
** Found in natural foods section of grocery store.

Power Nutrition Step Three

Step Three is for the serious exercise enthusiast interested in either bodybuilding or endurance sports. It assumes a training schedule of six days a week, with higher intensities than in Step Two. Because these sports require somewhat different calorie distributions, this step is divided into two parts. Also, the calorie levels provided in the sample meal plans are higher: 2500, 3000, and 3500 calories.

Goals of Step Three Meal Plan for Bodybuilding: To provide adequate protein intake for increasing muscle mass. To provide adequate carbohydrates to fuel workouts and spare protein. To provide an overall low-fat diet. If you plan to participate in bodybuilding competitions, you will need to change your diet several weeks beforehand to maximize muscle definition.

Some general guidelines for precompetition diet follow, but I recommend you work with a sports nutritionist experienced in this area for a personalized plan, beginning three months before a competition.

Step Three Meal Plan for Bodybuilding: Calorie mix is 20 to 25 percent protein (or about .7 to 1.0 gram protein per pound body weight), 60 to 65 percent carbohydrate, and 10 to 20 percent fat. Food is divided into three mixed meals and two to three snacks, including a recovery snack to eat after training sessions. The primary change from Step Two is an increased need for protein for bodybuilding, resulting in less room for fat calories.

Precompetition Diet Guidelines for Bodybuilders:

- Begin working toward peak condition 10 to 12 weeks before a contest. You should be within 10 pounds of competition weight by then. Your goal is to be at competition weight by two to three weeks precompetition.
- Do not drop calorie intake below 1200 to 1500 as you work your body fat down. Going lower than 1200 calories per day will compromise muscle store.
- Follow a low-fat, balanced diet of high-quality food.
- In the last week, cut sodium intake to a minimum by cutting out all added salt and salty foods. Eat primarily complex carbohydrates from vegetables with a small amount of high-carbohydrate starches, such as rice and potatoes. Drink plenty of low-sodium fluids.
- The last two to three days, begin eating primarily high-carbohydrate starches with small amounts of lean protein. Eliminate vegetables to reduce gas and bulkiness in the stomach. Eat small, frequent meals to avoid bloating.
- The night before the competition, begin limiting water intake to just enough to prevent dehydration.

For more information about competition diets, I recommend the book *Built on Balance*, by Carol Emich, R.D., available through Emich Ensembles in Golden, Colorado.

STEP THREE FOR BODYBUILDERS:
2500 CALORIES
375 TO 406 GRAMS CHO
125 TO 156 GRAMS PROTEIN
28 TO 56 GRAMS FAT

Calories are divided into the following servings from each Power Nutrition food group per day. You can mix the food up any way you like, but eat at least three meals and one snack.

TOTAL SERVINGS PER DAY:

- 11 grains
- 5 low CHO vegetables
- 4 high CHO vegetables
- 7 fruits
- 2 milk/yogurt
- 10 protein
- 1 sweet/sugar
- 1 fat

SAMPLE MEAL PLAN	SAMPLE MENU
Morning	**Morning**
3 grains	large glass of water
2 low CHO vegetables	Spinach Omelette*
3 fruits	large toasted bagel, topped with fat-free cream cheese
3 protein	½ cup orange juice
	1 cup fruit, canned in juice
Snack (Recovery Meal)	**Snack**
½ grain	Blueberry/Strawberry Crunchy "Milkshake"*
4 fruits	
1 milk/yogurt	
1 sweet/sugar	
Midday	**Midday**
4 grains	2 tuna fish sandwiches, made with a total of 4 slices multi-grain bread, ½ cup water-packed tuna mixed with 1 Tbsp. low-fat mayonnaise, and sliced tomato and leaf lettuce
3 low CHO vegetables	
4 protein	
1 fat	
	12-oz. can Light'n Tangy V-8 juice
Snack	**Snack**
3½ grains	Clif Bar
Evening	**Evening**
4 high CHO vegetables	3 oz. baked chicken (1 small breast)
1 milk/yogurt	1 large baked potato with Molly McButter
3 protein	1 cup green peas
	1 cup 1% milk

* Power Nutrition Recipe at end of chapter.

STEP THREE FOR BODYBUILDERS:
3000 CALORIES
450 TO 488 GRAMS CHO
150 TO 188 GRAMS PROTEIN
33 TO 67 GRAMS FAT

Calories are divided into the following servings from each Power Nutrition food group per day. You can mix the food up any way you like, but eat at least three meals and one snack.

TOTAL SERVINGS PER DAY:

- 12 grains
- 6 low CHO vegetables
- 4 high CHO vegetables
- 9 fruits
- 2 milk/yogurt
- 12 protein
- 2 sweet/sugar
- 1 fat

SAMPLE MEAL PLAN	SAMPLE MENU
Morning	**Morning**
2 grains	large glass of water
1 low CHO vegetable	Breakfast Beans* with Pico
2 high CHO vegetables	de Gallo*
4 fruits	2 flour tortillas
1 milk/yogurt	1 cup 1% milk
2 protein	1 cup orange juice
	1 cup unsweetened canned
	peaches
Snack (Recovery Meal)	**Snack**
3½ grains	1 Clif Bar
3 fruits	12 oz. fruit juice blended with
1 protein	¼ cup cottage cheese
Midday	**Midday**
2 grains	chicken sandwich made with
3 low CHO vegetables	1 small can (5 oz.) Swan-
2 high CHO vegetables	son White Premium Chicken
1 fruit	mixed with 1 Tbsp. low-fat
4 protein	mayonnaise on 2 slices multi-
1 fat	grain bread, with tomato and
	leaf lettuce
	1 cup corn kernels
	1 small apple
Snack	**Snack**
1 grain	6 oz. fat-free plain yogurt mixed
1 fruit	with ¼ cup fat-free granola
1 milk/yogurt	and 1 small banana

Evening
3½ grains
2 low CHO vegetables
5 protein
2 sweet/sugar

Evening
5-oz. portion of Grilled Tuna*
1 cup brown rice with Molly McButter
1 cup green beans
1 cup low-fat pudding topped with 2 Tbsp. fat-free granola

STEP THREE FOR BODYBUILDERS:
3500 CALORIES
525 TO 569 GRAMS CHO
175 TO 219 GRAMS PROTEIN
39 TO 78 GRAMS FAT

Calories are divided into the following servings from each Power Nutrition food group per day. You can mix the food up any way you like, but eat at least three meals and one snack.

TOTAL SERVINGS PER DAY:

- 14 grains
- 6 low CHO vegetables
- 6 high CHO vegetables
- 10 fruits
- 2 milk/yogurt
- 15 protein
- 2 sweet/sugar
- 1 fat

SAMPLE MEAL PLAN	SAMPLE MENU
Morning	**Morning**
2 grains	large glass of water
2 low CHO vegetables	2 Breakfast Burritos*
2 high CHO vegetables	6-oz. can tomato juice
2 fruits	1 cup unsweetened applesauce
4 protein	
1 fat	
Snack	**Snack**
3 grains	1 container Fantastic Foods Hot
1 milk/yogurt	Cereal**
	1 cup 1% milk
Midday	**Midday**
2 grains	large chicken breast (5 oz.) sliced
2 low CHO vegetables	on top of green salad with leaf
2 high CHO vegetables	lettuce and 1 cup mixture of
3 fruits	low CHO vegetables, fat-free
5 protein	salad dressing
1 sweet/sugar	12 saltine crackers

* Power Nutrition Recipe at end of chapter.
** Found in natural foods section of grocery store.

Midday, continued

1 medium-large baked sweet
potato, topped with Molly
McButter and 2 Tbsp. maple
syrup
12-oz. can orange juice

Snack (Recovery Meal)
5 fruits
1 milk/yogurt

Snack
6 oz. fat-free plain yogurt
blended with 2 cups apple
juice and 1 small banana

Evening
6 grains
2 low CHO vegetables
2 high CHO vegetables
6 protein

Evening
2 Boca Burgers** with low-fat
cheese, leaf lettuce, tomato,
mustard, and ketchup on
whole-grain buns
⅔ cup baked beans
1½ oz. (30) baked tortilla chips

Snack
1 grain
1 sweet/sugar

Snack
1 Zucchini Health Muffin*

* Power Nutrition Recipe at end of chapter.
** Found in natural foods section of grocery store

Goals of Step Three Meal Plan for Endurance Sports: To provide adequate carbohydrate and protein to fuel endurance activities, to replenish glycogen stores, and to maintain muscle mass. To provide a low-fat diet. To provide adequate carbohydrate during training and recovery meals following endurance training sessions. To provide carbohydrate-loading guidelines for preparation for endurance events.

Step Three Meal Plan for Endurance Sports: Calorie mix of 65 to 70 percent carbohydrate, 15 to 20 percent protein (or about 0.5 to 0.7 grams protein per pound body weight) and 10 to 20 percent fat. Food is divided into three meals and two to three snacks, including a postexercise recovery snack. Information about carbohydrate loading follows the menus. You will notice higher CHO levels and less protein in the following meal plans, to fuel endurance training.

**STEP THREE FOR ENDURANCE:
2500 CALORIES
406 TO 438 GRAMS CHO
94 TO 125 GRAMS PROTEIN
28 TO 56 GRAMS FAT**

Calories are divided into the following servings from each Power Nutrition food group per day. You can mix the food up any way you like, but eat at least three meals and one snack.

TOTAL SERVINGS PER DAY:

- 12½ grains
- 4 low CHO vegetables
- 3½ high CHO vegetables
- 8 fruits
- 2 milk/yogurt
- 2 protein
- 2 sweet/sugar
- 3 fats

SAMPLE MEAL PLAN	SAMPLE MENU
Morning	**Morning**
6 grains	large glass of water
1 fruit	1 large bagel w/ 2 Tbsp. low-fat cream cheese
1 milk/yogurt	1 container Fantastic Foods Hot Cereal**
1 fat	½ cup orange juice
Snack (Recovery Meal)	**Snack**
1 grain	16 oz. apple juice
4 fruits	1 Zucchini Health Muffin*
1 sweet/sugar	
Midday	**Midday**
2 grains	1 can Healthy Choice Split Pea and Ham Soup
3½ high CHO vegetables	4 multigrain Wasa Crispbreads
2 fruits	1 large banana
2 protein	
Snack	**Snack**
1 fruit	Blueberry Frozen Yogurt* topped with 2 Tbsp. low-fat granola
1 milk/yogurt	
½ grain	
1 sweet/sugar	
Evening	**Evening**
3 grains	1½ cups cooked pasta shells topped with 1 cup marinara sauce and 5 sliced olives
4 low CHO vegetables	
2 fats	15 to 20 steamed asparagus spears

* Power Nutrition Recipe at end of chapter.
** Found in natural foods section of grocery store.

STEP THREE FOR ENDURANCE:
3000 CALORIES
488 TO 525 GRAMS CHO
113 TO 150 GRAMS PROTEIN
33 TO 67 GRAMS FAT

Calories are divided into the following servings from each Power Nutrition food group per day. You can mix the food up any way you like, but eat at least three meals and one snack.

TOTAL SERVINGS PER DAY:

- 14 grains
- 5 low CHO vegetables
- 5 high CHO vegetables
- 10 fruits
- 2 milk/yogurt
- 3 protein
- 2 sweet/sugar
- 3 fats

SAMPLE MEAL PLAN	SAMPLE MENU
Morning	**Morning**
4 grains	2 cups MultiGrain Cheerios with
3 fruits	1 large banana and 1 cup
1 milk/yogurt	nonfat milk
1 sweet/sugar	2 slices whole-wheat toast with
	1 Tbsp. jam
	½ cup orange juice
Snack (Recovery Meal)	**Snack**
3½ grains	1 Clif Bar
3 fruits	12-oz. can cranberry juice
	cocktail
Midday	**Midday**
4 grains	turkey sandwich made with
3 low CHO vegetables	2 slices bread, 3 oz.turkey,
1 high CHO vegetable	1 Tbsp. low-fat mayonnaise,
1 milk/yogurt	tomato slices, and leaf lettuce
3 protein	2 cups garden salad with ½ cup
1 fat	green peas and fat-free salad
	dressing
	1½ oz. pretzels
	1 cup 1% milk
Snack	**Snack**
1 grain	2 large rice cakes topped with
2 fruits	2 tsp. peanut butter
1 fat	small box (1½ oz.) raisins
Evening	**Evening**
1½ grains	3-oz. portion of Easy
2 low CHO vegetables	Microwave Fish*
4 high CHO vegetables	1 cup green beans

2 fruits	1 cup corn
3 protein	1 large baked potato with
1 sweet/sugar	1 tsp. margarine
1 fat	1 slice french bread
	1 Baked Apple*

STEP THREE FOR ENDURANCE:
3500 CALORIES
569 TO 613 GRAMS CHO
131 TO 175 GRAMS PROTEIN
28 TO 56 GRAMS FAT

Calories are divided into the following servings from each Power Nutrition food group per day. You can mix the food up any way you like, but eat at least three meals and one snack.

TOTAL SERVINGS PER DAY:

- 16 grains
- 6 low CHO vegetables
- 6 high CHO vegetables
- 10 fruits
- 2 milk/yogurt
- 5 protein
- 2 to 3 sweet/sugar
- 3 fats

SAMPLE MEAL PLAN	SAMPLE MENU
Morning	**Morning**
4 grains	large glass of water
1 low CHO vegetable	½ grapefruit
2 fruits	1 Better Than Egg-A-Muffin*
1 milk/yogurt	½ cup orange juice
1 protein	1 cup 1% milk
1 fat	
Snack (Recovery Meal)	**Snack**
2 grains	2 fat-free granola bars (Barbara
4 fruits	or Health Valley)
1 milk/yogurt	16 oz. apple juice blended with
1 sweet/sugar	6 oz. fat-free vanilla yogurt
Midday	**Midday**
3 grains	1 can Healthy Choice Clam
2 low CHO vegetables	Chowder with ½ cup corn
4 high CHO vegetables	kernels added
1 fruit	18 saltine crackers
1 protein	4 to 6 baby carrots and
	Jicama Sticks*
	1 cup grapes
Snack	**Snack**
1 grain	3 cups low-fat popcorn
3 fruits	12-oz. can orange juice
1 sweet/sugar	3 ginger snap cookies

* Power Nutrition Recipe at end of chapter.

Evening

4 grains
3 low CHO vegetables
2 high CHO vegetables
3 protein
2 fats

Snack

2 grains
1 sweet/sugar

Evening

½ Poached Salmon Fillet* (3 oz.)
2 cups Quinoa Salad*
1 cup green peas
3 cups salad with mixture of low
    CHO vegetables and fat-free
    salad dressing

Snack

½ cup low-fat granola on top of ½
    cup fat-free frozen yogurt

* Power Nutrition Recipe at end of chapter.

Carbohydrate Loading: If you plan to participate in an endurance event, such as a marathon, half-marathon, or triathlon, use the carbohydrate-loading techniques to maximize your glycogen stores for the event. Carbohydrate loading takes one week. It works only if you are well trained and otherwise prepared for the event. It is not a substitute for training.

The goal of CHO-loading is to force your muscles to fill up with more glycogen than you normally carry around. The extra glycogen allows you to maintain a racing pace longer; it doesn't increase speed or strength, but endurance. Old methods of CHO-loading involved severe depletion of muscles before loading. This caused many side effects for athletes, such as muscle fatigue, ketosis, dehydration, and hypoglycemia. The current method has prevented those problems by not including the drastic depletion phase.

CHO-loading is accomplished by changes in both diet and training. During the week prior to the event, training sessions begin with an exhaustive workout and are then gradually shortened until you are doing very little light exercise on day six, the day before the event (some trainers recommend *no* exercise the day before). The first three days of CHO-loading eat only 350 grams of CHO, or about 2.3 grams CHO per pound body weight. The last three days, eat 550 grams of CHO/day or 4.5 grams per pound body weight, divided into six meals. The last three days are more like a regular high CHO diet with 70 percent CHO calories.

It is a good idea to practice the CHO-loading method before an important competition, so you don't make mistakes when they can cost you. Packing away extra glycogen requires extra water. So, be sure to be on top of your hydration at all times.

Each gram of glycogen carries almost 3 grams of water! So, CHO-loading allows you to start the competition with excesses of both water and CHO. This is a plus in an endurance event lasting longer than two hours. However, in shorter events, such as a 10K race, the extra weight will just slow you down and make you feel sluggish. CHO-loading is appropriate only for true endurance events.

The Nutrients

There are more than 50 nutrients and food compounds required for optimum health in humans. At least 44 of those nutrients must be supplied by the diet, because the body cannot make them. Nutrients fall into one of six categories: water, carbohydrate, fat, protein, vitamins, minerals. All of these are important players in the game of nutritional fitness.

THE ENERGY NUTRIENTS AND WATER: PRIMARY PLAYERS IN FUELING FITNESS

Energy from food is measured in the form of calories. Fat, carbohydrate (CHO), and protein all contain calories in varying amounts, as shown in Table 1. Food energy is used to do the work of the body, both involuntary functions and physical activities. In addition to providing energy, protein and fat have other functions in the body as well.

While all calories count, research indicates that all calories are not created equal when it comes to their effect on body weight. The body is more efficient in storing excess fat calories than excess carbohydrate calories, at least in most people. If you eat 100 calories of *extra* fat—say, a tablespoon of margarine—the body stores about 97 of those calories in your fat cells. The other 3 are lost as heat. (This process is called the TEF, or thermal effect of food.) However, if you eat 100 calories of *extra* CHO, about 2 tablespoons of jam, the body stores only 77 calories as fat and loses 23 as heat. And those extra carbs are first stored in the muscle and liver as glycogen, the storage form of CHO, especially if you exercise regularly. Only when the glycogen stores are full will the carbs be stored as fat. But even if you are not eating any *extra* calories, a low-fat diet (10 to 30 percent of calories) may allow for a leaner body. There will be more about the CHO vs. fat debate later in this chapter, in Balancing Energy.

CARBOHYDRATES (CHO)

Carbohydrates have to be eaten daily to meet energy demands and keep active muscles primed. They are the preferred fuel for most body functions, especially those of the brain and central nervous system. Carbohydrates spare protein from being used as a fuel source and are necessary to burn fat efficiently. For optimum health and energy, eat at least 55 to 60 percent of your total calories from CHO, about 275 to 375 grams of CHO for most mild to moderately active adults. If you perform a lot of endurance exercise, you will need even more. A training diet for an endurance athlete should consist of 3½ to 4 grams of carbohydrate for every pound of body weight, daily, or 65 to 70 percent of total calories. Table 2 lists the carbohydrate content of various common foods.

There are two types of carbohydrates in food: simple and complex. Simple carbs are found predominantly in

TABLE 1. ENERGY NUTRIENTS AND WATER

NUTRIENT	MAIN FUNCTIONS	RECOMMENDED INTAKES	FOOD SOURCES
CARBOHYDRATE provides 4 calories per gram.	Energy; preferred fuel for most body functions, especially of brain and central nervous system. Primary fuel during high-intensity exercise.	55 to 70 percent of total calories, depending on exercise demands. Minimum of 250 grams per day for active people.	Whole and refined grains, breads, and cereals, milk, yogurt, fruit, vegetables, sugar, syrup, candy, soft drinks, desserts.
PROTEIN provides 4 calories per gram.	Growth and maintenance of body tissue; building of enzymes, hormones and antibodies; maintaining fluid and electrolyte balance and acid-base balance. Energy.	0.4 gram/pound body weight if sedentary. 0.5 grams to 0.7 grams per pound for endurance and strength athletes. 0.9 grams per pound for bodybuilding, especially if new to the sport.	Meat, poultry, fish, milk, yogurt, cheese, legumes, tofu, nuts and nut butters, whole grains and vegetables.
FAT provides 9 calories per gram.	Energy; maintenance of body temperature; protection of organs; to make hormones, cell membranes, prostaglandins, and other essential compounds; provide essential fatty acids; carry fat-soluble vitamins.	10 to 30 percent of total calories.	Oils, butter, margarine, shortening, mayonnaise, salad dressing, olives, nuts, nut butters, avocado.
WATER	Participates in many reactions in the body. Carries nutrients and waste products; lubrication and shock absorption; solvent for many compounds; maintaining body temperature.	1 to 1.5 ml of water per calorie expended. Usually 8 to 10 cups per day, more when exercising.	Drinking water, fruit and vegetable juices, milk, soup, herbal tea, noncaffeinated and nonalcoholic beverages, watery fruits and vegetables.

TABLE 2. CARBOHYDRATE CONTENT OF FOODS

FOOD ITEM	TOTAL	CARBOHYDRATE CONTENT IN GRAMS		
		COMPLEX	SIMPLE	FIBER
Bagel, small	31.0	27.8	2.0	1.2
Spaghetti, 1 cup cooked	39.0	35.2	1.7	2.1
Baked potato, medium, with skin	26.7	22.9	0.8	3.0
Carrot, medium, raw	7.3	0.2	4.8	2.3
Apple, medium, with skin	21.1	0.3	17.8	3.0
Banana, medium	26.7	7.1	17.8	1.8
Grape-Nuts, ½ cup	46.8	40.1	4.0	2.7
Raisin bran, ½ cup	21.4	9.8	8.6	3.0
Oatmeal, 1 cup cooked	25.3	22.3	0.9	2.1
Raisins, 2 Tbsp.	14.4	1.6	11.8	1.0
Orange juice, ½ cup	13.4	0.2	13.0	0.2
Acorn squash, ½ cup, cooked	15.0	8.9	3.9	2.2
Pumpkin, canned, ½ cup	9.0	0	4.0	5.0
Whole wheat bread, 1 slice	11.3	7.5	1.0	2.8
White bread, 1 slice	12.2	10.5	1.0	0.7
Broccoli, ½ cup, cooked	3.9	0.8	1.1	2.0
Black beans, canned, ½ cup	19.0	12.0	0	7.0
Brown rice, ½ cup, cooked	22.9	21.2	0	1.7
English muffin, 1 whole	29.8	26.3	2.0	1.5

Data taken from N-Squared Computing, programs NIII, 7.0, and NIV, 2.0 and from product labels.

sugars, milk, and fruit. They are simple in their chemical structure, just two molecules hooked together. Simple carbs are digested and absorbed into the bloodstream quickly, which is why people talk about getting an *energy high* from sugary foods. One downside to simple carbs is that some people also get a corresponding *energy low* (from a drop in blood sugar) if they eat too many simple carbs or eat them without other foods.

Sugars are basically devoid of any nutritional value other than the carbohydrate, making them *empty calories*. Because calories require vitamins and minerals to be burned for fuel, too many empty calories will zap your energy. A little sugar is okay if you are active enough to afford the empty calories, say one or two servings of sugary junk food a day. More than that will compromise nutritional fitness.

Complex carbs consist of long strings of molecules, often referred to as *starch*, and are the best source of energy for active people. Breads, noodles, cereals, potatoes, corn, beans, and peas are excellent sources. Plenty of grains, vegetables, and legumes should fill your plate. Fruits are important too because, even though they are mostly simple carbs, they provide necessary fiber, vitamins, and minerals.

Oh, yes, did I mention fiber? This brings me to a word about *refined* versus *whole* foods. Whole foods, such as whole grains, have been prepared with the fiber portion intact. Refined foods, such as enriched white bread, have been stripped of their fiber and nutrient-rich germ layer. Dietary fiber, undigestible carbohydrate, is essential for a healthy gut. Some types of fiber, like oat bran and legumes, aid in lowering blood cholesterol levels. Other types, such as wheat bran, makes it easier to pass stools and are associated with lowering the risk of developing colon cancer. Whole grains, vegetables, and fruits (but not juice) all contain dietary fiber. You need roughly 20 to 35 grams per day of dietary fiber. To accomplish that, eat five to nine servings of fruits and vegetables a day. Also, at least two-thirds of your grain products should be whole grain. See Table 2 for the fiber content of various foods.

FATS—A LITTLE DAB WILL DO YA!

If you are working hard to have a lean body, the last thing you want to do is re-feed your fat cells. Any extra calories can become stored fat, but remember that fat calories are stored most readily. Thanks to a media-driven obsession with fat-free foods, many people have the mistaken idea that they should not eat *any* fat. This is simply not true! Fat is a necessary part of a well-balanced diet, but a little goes a long way.

How Much Fat and What Kind of Fat Should You Eat? You need some food fat to supply essential fat-soluble vitamins and fatty acids required to make hormones and other compounds necessary for life and optimum health. The essential fatty acids are known as linolenic acid and linoleic acid. Without them, your immune system would suffer, you would not make critical hormones, and the membranes of your cells would not be properly constructed. Technically, we can meet our need for essential fats with a healthy diet of only 5 percent fat calories. Practically speaking, a diet that low in fat would have problems. It would eliminate many nutritious foods from the diet. Plus, food fat helps you feel satisfied after eating. It slows down digestion and keeps you from being hungry all the time. Fat contributes a lot of flavor to food, too.

Fat is in nearly all foods, except pure sugars—honey, table sugar, molasses, etc. So every piece of whole-grain bread and every ounce of lean tuna will provide some fat. For good health and disease prevention, limit fat intake to no more than 30 percent of calories. If you need to lose body fat, shoot for about 20 percent fat calories. For optimum health don't go lower than 10 percent fat calories, or 25 grams of fat.

Figuring Your Recommended Fat Intake: Knowing what percentage of fat calories to eat is not as helpful as knowing how many fat *grams* to eat. Food labels and calorie charts list grams of fat in foods, so you can count your fat intake easily. Table 3 provides a quick method for estimating how many grams of fat you can eat and still be within the percentage of fat calories you want.

Types of Food Fat: Three types of fatty acids give us calories: saturated (SAT), polyunsaturated (POLY), and monounsaturated (MONO). The difference between the three, chemically, has to do with the number of hydrogen ions attached. If a fat has all the hydrogens it can hold, it is considered saturated. If one hydrogen is missing, it is a monounsaturated fat, and if several hydrogens are missing, it is polyunsaturated.

The significance, healthwise, is that SATs tend to increase blood cholesterol, especially LDL cholesterol—the harmful kind. SATs are found predominantly in fatty animal products, such as cheese, butter, whole milk, and fatty meats. The recent good news about fat is that the predominant saturated fatty acid in beef and chocolate, stearic acid, does not seem to affect LDL cholesterol. So lean beef and the occasional chocolate bar can be part of a healthy diet.

POLYs are the type of fat in most plants, except coconut and palm oil, which are saturated. When POLYs replace saturated fats in the diet, LDL-cholesterol goes down. The same is true if MONOs replace SATs. Olive oil and canola oil are two predominant sources of MONOs.

You have probably seen the term *hydrogenated* on labels of shortening, margarine, and other foods. *Hydrogenated* is the term used when man *saturates* a plant oil by adding hydrogens. Controversy exists about the health effects of hydrogenated fats. The hydrogenation process creates *trans* fatty acids, which have a chemical structure different from the original fat and suspected of being just as harmful as other saturated fats. It is probably a good idea to use oil instead of shortening when possible, but the most important point is to not use very much of either.

This fatty acid stuff can get pretty technical. The

TABLE 3. HOW MUCH FAT CAN I EAT?

First, estimate your total calorie needs and the number of fat calories. Then figure grams of fat to eat daily. It is best to calculate a range of intakes instead of a single number.

EXAMPLE

1. Multiply your present weight by the appropriate factor to estimate baseline calorie needs.

135-pound female who is normal weight and moderately active

Men: 11   _____ pounds × 11 = _____

Women: 10   _____ pounds × 10 = _____   135 pounds × 10 = 1350 baseline calories

2. Multiply your weight by the appropriate *activity factor** to estimate calories needed for activity.

	Sedentary	Light	Moderate	Heavy
Men:	3.2	6	7.2	10.5
Women:	3.0	5	6	9

_____ pounds × _____ (factor) = _____   135 pounds × 6 = 810 activity calories

3. Add together the calories from 1 and 2 to estimate *total calorie needs* per day.

_____ + _____ = _____   1350 + 810 = 2160 total calories

(Add 500 calories to total if currently underweight. Subtract 300 calories from total if currently overweight.)

4. Multiply the total calories by .20 or .30 for 20% or 30% fat calories.

_____ × .20 = _____   2160 × .20 = 432 fat calories

_____ × .30 = _____   2160 × .30 = 648 fat calories

5. Divide the calories from fat by 9 to get your *daily fat gram allotment.*

20% = _____ ÷ 9 = _____   432 ÷ 9 = 48 fat grams

30% = _____ ÷ 9 = _____   648 ÷ 9 = 72 fat grams

*Sedentary = little exercise and sit-down job; Light = some exercise or standing job; Moderate = exercises 3 to 5 times a week and/or moderately active job; Heavy = exercises 5 or more times a week or very active job (e.g., construction work).

important thing for you to know is that too much of *any* fat is too much. The fats you do eat should be about half MONOs and one-quarter each from POLYs and SATs. This means, use small amounts of olive or canola oil in cooking and salad dressings, eat only lean animal products, and the POLYs will take care of themselves through the fat naturally present in grains and vegetables.

Cholesterol: Dietary cholesterol is another type of fat that affects heart health but does not provide calories. Many experts consider total fat in the diet more important than total cholesterol, but limiting cholesterol intake to 300 milligrams per day is still recommended. This is especially important if you already have a high blood cholesterol level or if it runs in your immediate family. Cholesterol is made in the liver of animals, including humans. Since plants do not have livers, they have no cholesterol. It is possible for a food to be high in fat and low in cholesterol—oil for example. It is also possible to have a high-cholesterol, low-fat food—boiled shrimp. Shrimp, calamari (squid), organ meats, and egg yolks are some of the biggest contributors of cholesterol in our diet, so go easy on them.

PROTEIN BUILDS MUSCLE, RIGHT?

You've seen the advertisements. An extremely well-developed man with perfect *cut* is touting protein powder as the reason for his incredible physique. Everyone knows muscle is made of protein, so it is logical to assume you need to eat more protein if you want to build muscle. The logic has some merit, but *the amount of extra protein needed is smaller than most athletes imagine.*

Protein requirements are still debated among sports nutritionists; however, exercisers probably do require more protein than nonexercisers, with endurance athletes and bodybuilders requiring the most. Sedentary adults need 0.4 gram of protein per pound of body weight. Exercisers require 0.6 to 0.9 gram/pound. That means, if you are a 150-pound bodybuilder, your maximum protein requirement is 135 grams. I often see men who eat that much protein without even trying! Virtually all foods, except pure sugars and pure fats, contain some protein. Table 4 gives the protein content of some common foods.

Although we burn a little protein to supply energy, the body has to spare most of its protein for more important functions, such as the building and repair of tissue and the formation of enzymes, hormones, and other important compounds. Weight training and body-building require a little extra protein to build lean body mass. At rest, the body uses protein for only 2 to 5 percent of its calories. Endurance activities will increase protein's usage to 5 to 10 percent of energy because protein can be converted into glucose. If an exerciser fails to eat adequate carbohydrate, his usage of protein for energy will increase. This takes protein away from its other duties and can lead to dehydration and calcium losses. Generally, protein intake is safe and adequate at 10 to 20 percent of total calories.

TABLE 4. PROTEIN CONTENT OF SELECTED FOODS

FOOD	PROTEIN (GRAMS)
Canned tuna, 6½-ounce can	45.5
Chicken breast, 4 ounces	36.0
Refried beans, 1 cup	15.8
Broccoli, cooked, 1 cup	5.8
Brown rice, 1 cup	4.9
Whole wheat bread, 2 slices	4.8
Green beans, 1 cup	2.4
Baked potato, 1 medium	2.0
Banana, 1	1.0

Protein/Meat Eaters Versus Vegetarians: The debate is lively and often heated. Should humans eat meat or not? Research indicates many of the life-threatening diseases in the United States could be diminished if we ate fewer animal products, both animal fats and animal proteins. The key word here is *fewer*, not *none*. Since the Stone Age, humans have been omnivorous, able to digest and absorb nutrients from animals as well as plants. (Of course, there were no processed foods then, so diets were lower in fat, sugar, and salt.) A healthy diet can be achieved *with or without* animal flesh or animal milk. The key is knowing how to choose a nutrient-rich diet.

Body protein is made by putting together various amino acids according to specific directions from DNA. Your body is programmed to do this, assuming all the necessary amino acids are available. Most amino acids can be produced by the body, but there are several that have to be supplied from food, the so-called *essential amino acids* (EAA). The advantage of animal protein is that it contains all of the EAA, in optimum proportions, and is therefore known as *complete protein.* Some plant foods, such as corn, are missing one or more essential amino acids and are known as *incomplete proteins.* Other plants, such as rice, contain all the essentials, but in very small quantities and less optimum proportions.

After eating any protein food, whether it be steak or beans, the process of digestion breaks apart the protein and you absorb individual amino acids and pairs of amino acids. These enter the body's amino acid pool. When you need a protein built, the body will draw the necessary amino acids from this pool. As long as you obtain all the essential amino acids in enough quantity over the course of a few hours, it doesn't matter if they originally came from an animal or a plant.

Combining Proteins: Is it important to eat a complete protein, whether from animals or a combination of plants, at each meal? The answer depends in part on how much total protein you eat. Of course, it isn't an issue for meat eaters. If you eat no animal protein and limited amounts of vegetable sources, protein combining with plants becomes more important. You need to insure that all the essential amino acids are not only present, but present in the right amounts to support optimum protein metabolism.

Protein combining has developed spontaneously in places where animal protein is limited. It is very easy to *combine,* so if you are a vegetarian, you might as well make it a habit. Any combination of grains and legumes, legumes and seeds, or dairy protein and plant protein make a complete protein. See Table 5 for examples of complete protein dishes common to the vegetarian diet.

Pros and Cons of Plant and Animal Proteins: Plant proteins, except for nuts and seeds, are usually very low in fat. However, today many red meats are also quite lean, as are certain fish, skinless poultry, and nonfat dairy products. Vegetarians are not guaranteed a low-fat diet; they have to select foods as carefully as meat eaters do.

An advantage to plant proteins is that most of them, such as beans and whole grains, are also high in complex carbohydrates. Of course you have to eat 2 cups of beans to get the same amount of protein found in 4 ounces of chicken. So you have to consume more vol-

TABLE 5. COMPLETE VEGETARIAN PROTEINS
Black Beans and Rice
Peanut Butter Sandwich
Bean Taco
Hummus on Pita Bread
Macaroni and Cheese
Rice Pudding
Noodles with Tofu Sauce
Lentil Curry on Rice
Cereal and Milk
Veggie Burger on Bun

ume of plant protein than animal protein to meet your protein needs. This is not a handicap. We need lots of grains and vegetables to meet other nutritional needs anyway. Also, vegetarians are less likely to overdo it on protein unless large amounts of eggs, milk, and cheese are consumed.

Let's not forget the nutritional advantages of *lean* animal protein. Red meat and dark poultry are excellent sources of iron. Also, animal flesh improves the absorption of iron from plant foods. Animal protein, especially meat, poultry, and fish, is also high in many B vitamins, zinc, and phosphorus. Ounce for ounce, lean beef contains four times as much zinc as tofu and eight times as much as pinto beans. Vitamin B_{12} is extremely limited in the plant world, but plentiful in animal foods.

Arguments can be made in favor of both vegetarian and meat-based diets. Both can be highly nutritious or disastrous, depending on food choices. The important thing is to eat adequate, not excessive, protein that provides all your essential amino acids.

WHAT ABOUT ALCOHOL?

Alcohol is a concentrated source of calories, providing 7 calories per gram. When alcohol enters the body, it forces the liver to process it while other work comes to a standstill. As a result, fat metabolism slows down, leading to a buildup of fat in the liver. Also, alcohol metabolism ties up niacin and thiamine, B vitamins necessary for energy production. Carbohydrate metabolism is also affected by alcohol, leading to lower levels of muscle glycogen. This can make it difficult to exercise after a night of drinking. Also, muscle cells do not use alcohol for energy, so you cannot burn off a martini in the same way you can burn off a donut. And remember, alcohol has a *diuretic* effect on the body, forcing you to lose precious water. If you are going to drink, don't do it right before or after exercise. When participating in a beer-sponsored sports event, be sure to rehydrate your body with plenty of water before hitting the free beer!

A drink or two may help you feel calm and better able to handle the world. It might even decrease your risk of having a heart attack, if you drink red wine. But it can also increase your risk of other diseases, such as breast cancer. Alcohol stimulates appetite and makes it harder to exercise, interfering with efforts to lose weight. So, go easy on the stuff!

Balancing Your Fuel Sources

How you balance your intake of energy nutrients will affect your energy level—in and out of the gym. What works best? The optimum combination of carbohydrate, fat, and protein is dependent on several factors: the type and intensity of exercise you do, how sensitive you are to changes in blood sugar levels, how well you metabolize carbohydrate, how your body responds to various food combinations, and personal preference. Before we look at these factors, you need to understand how the different energy nutrients are utilized for fuel.

As you sit and read this book, 50 to 80 percent of the calories you are using come from fat and the rest are mostly carbohydrate. Of course, you aren't burning enough of either one to produce weight loss, which is why the *read-books-and-lose-weight* diet was never a success. Now, if you jump up and sprint to the corner, your body shifts into burning mostly carbs. Should you then decide to walk briskly to the store four miles away, you will start to burn significant amounts of fat, too,

after about the first mile and a half. If you sprint hard the last quarter mile, you switch back to using mostly carbs for energy.

Carbohydrate inside the body is in the form of glycogen, stored in the muscles and liver, and glucose, or blood sugar. We can store pounds and pounds of fat, but glycogen stores are limited to 1 pound for the average adult and up to 2 to 3 pounds for highly trained athletes. Brain cells and nerve tissue rely almost exclusively on glucose for energy. And since carbs are stored in the muscle, they are the most readily available source of energy. So they get used in large amounts during the early stages of exercise, such as during the sprint to the corner. After the body gets *revved up* (the four-mile walk to the store), fat stores begin to break down for energy also. If you continue to increase the intensity of the exercise, you switch back to using your reserve of carbs (glycogen). As shown in Figure 1, as the intensity of an exercise increases, you tend to burn proportionately more carbohydrate and less fat. Of course, as intensity increases, you tend to burn more total calories, too, so you are still using significant amounts of fat. (Since protein provides relatively few calories during exercise, it isn't included in Figure 1.)

The body uses up more grams of carbohydrate than any other fuel. Since our storage volume of glycogen is

FIGURE 1. FUELS BURNED DURING EXERCISE

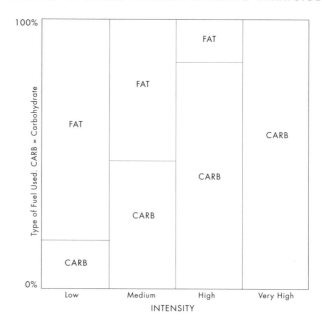

limited, we need to replace the glycogen used during exercise as well as provide plenty of glucose to maintain optimum blood sugar levels. The only effective way to replace carbs is to eat carbs. We don't need to worry about replacing the fat we burn; we will always have plenty of fat on board. Of course, as mentioned earlier, we need some fat in the diet for essential functions and satiety.

For better energy levels, the goal is to keep your blood sugar level within its optimum range. Your body works hard to do that by making you hungry when it needs glucose. After eating, hormones are stimulated to put the glucose where it is needed for immediate energy or into storage for later use. You can assist this process by not skipping meals.

I have found that most people feel more energetic and in better control of their appetite when they eat *mixed* meals, a combination of carbohydrate, protein, and a little fat. Mixed meals offer a longer-lasting supply of blood sugar. Some people are more sensitive to the normal fluctuations in blood sugar than others. If you tend to *crash* when you haven't eaten in four hours, you may feel better when you make the effort to eat mixed meals. A mixed CHO/protein meal would be a turkey and vegetable sandwich with fruit and skim milk, as opposed to a bagel and fruit, which is mostly CHO.

A currently popular approach to nutrition, called *food combining*, is to *not* combine starches and protein, and to eat only fruit in the mornings. A few of my clients swear by this approach, but the majority do not, especially if they are exercising hard. Energy levels are not well maintained by eating just fruit, and the menu limitations with this approach are unnecessary for most people.

GLYCEMIC INDEX—
ADDITIONAL CONSIDERATIONS FOR
EXERCISE AND WEIGHT MANAGEMENT

A phenomenon known as the *glycemic effect of foods* is gaining attention from sports nutritionists. *Glycemic effect* refers to the way a food affects one's blood sugar level: how quickly, how high, and how long it raises blood glucose. Scientists have managed to measure this effect and assign a *glycemic index* to various foods,

mostly carbohydrates. A food with a high glycemic index (G-I) causes a rapid rise in blood glucose levels, providing an energy boost for exercising muscles. Foods with a low G-I tend to offer a more gradual and sustained rise in blood sugar, which might be helpful if you plan to do a long workout or activity. Table 6 divides foods into high, moderate, or low G-I.

Many factors affect the G-I of a food, such as cooking, density, and digestion. Also, if you eat a carbohydrate food along with fat or protein foods, its G-I will be lowered. Since very active people often eat meals or snacks made up of mostly carbohydrate, choosing

TABLE 6. GLYCEMIC INDEX OF SELECTED FOODS

HIGH G-I	MODERATE G-I	LOW G-I
Bagel	Grapes	Apples
Banana	Noodles	Applesauce
Chocolate bar	Oatmeal	Cherries
Corn	Orange	Chickpeas
Corn flakes	Potato, sweet	Coarse rye or
Corn syrup	Sponge cake	wheat
Cracker, plain	Yam	bread, European style
Honey		
Molasses		Dates
Muesli		Figs
Potato, white		Fructose
Raisin		Grapefruit
Rice, white		Ice cream
Rice, brown		Milk
Rye bread		Navy beans
Shredded wheat		Peaches
Sucrose		Plums
White bread		Red lentils
Whole-wheat bread		Yogurt

foods according to the G-I may be useful. Theoretically, one should eat low to moderate G-I foods in the meal prior to a long workout. Eat moderate to high G-I foods during and after that workout to maintain blood glucose and replace glycogen stores.

There is some evidence that eating foods with a low G-I can help suppress hunger and therefore decrease overall calorie intake. This will be useful if you need to lose excess body fat or if you suffer from food cravings that undermine your weight-loss efforts. I know of no clinical trials using the G-I approach to weight management. But you can give it a try by eating low G-I foods versus high G-I foods at breakfast and at snacks. For example, eat chickpea spread (hummus) on coarse rye bread, low G-I foods, instead of corn flakes, a high G-I food. Experiment with this method and see if it is helpful.

The Zone (Or the Carbohydrate Backlash)

If you read fitness magazines, you are probably familiar with diets promoting higher protein and lower carbohydrates to keep your body in its *fat burning zone.* The theory behind this approach is based on the concern that a diet high in carbohydrate keeps insulin levels high in your blood and triggers unstable blood sugar levels. Insulin is a hormone involved in getting glucose from your blood into your cells and also aids in storing fat in fat cells. The theory continues to claim that eating fewer carbohydrate (40 percent of total calories) and more protein and fat (30 percent each) will force your body to burn its stored body fat as fuel.

This theory catches the attention of anyone trying to lose body fat. However, it doesn't make physiological sense for most exercisers. True, a diet high in carbohydrate will cause the body to secrete more insulin, but unless you have a faulty metabolism, the body accommodates carbohydrate very well. It is also true that the body will burn what it is fed. If you eat a high-carb diet the body burns more carb. If you eat a high-fat diet, the body adapts to burn more fat as fuel. The primary determinant of fuel burned during exercise is the exercise you do: type, duration, and intensity. When more oxygen is available, such as during low to moderate exercise, the body will burn fat readily. In greater intensity of exercise, oxygen is less available. The body can't burn fat without oxygen, so it relies on glycogen. And, as your glycogen stores get low, such as in endurance exercise, you get fatigued unless you eat more carbohydrate. You need carbs to be able to train at greater intensity for longer duration, allowing you to become fit. The more fit you are, the better your body is at conserving glycogen and burning fat. A diet too low in carbs will not keep glycogen stores replaced; it will result in dehydration and general fatigue. Forty percent carbs is too low for most of us.

CARBOHYDRATE SENSITIVITY/INSULIN RESISTANCE

Some people, primarily the obese, have a condition known as *carbohydrate sensitivity* (or insulin resistance), where the body doesn't metabolize carbohydrate normally. If unresolved, this condition can lead to problems such as high cholesterol, diabetes, and obesity. The treatment includes a diet with less carbohydrate, usually 45 to 50 percent of total calories instead of the 60 percent minimum recommended for exercisers. Most of the carbohydrate should come from vegetables, fruits, and whole grains instead of sugars and refined grains.

Symptoms of carbohydrate sensitivity can include sugar cravings, excess hunger after meals, inability to stop eating, difficulty losing weight even with exercise, sudden onset of weight gain, dizziness, weight loss only with very-low-calorie diets, and elevated triglyceride levels. The dietary recommendations for this condition are 45 to 50 percent CHO, 20 to 25 percent protein, and 30 percent fat at every meal. Regular aerobic exercise is necessary, too.

WHAT MIX IS RIGHT FOR YOU?

Table 7 compares the different fuel mixes presented so far. You will need to do some experimenting to find out which combination of energy nutrients makes you feel the most energized *and* the most satisfied. You should be able to go four to six hours between meals, assuming you have eaten a reasonable-sized meal instead of a snack. You should be able to experience hunger creeping up on you instead of suddenly crashing due to low

TABLE 7. COMPARISON OF FUEL MIXES		
FOR MOST ACTIVE ADULTS	THE ZONE	CHO SENSITIVITY
CHO: 55 to 65%	CHO: 40%	CHO: 45 to 50%
Protein: 10 to 20%	Protein: 30%	Protein: 20 to 25%
Fat: 10 to 30%	Fat: 30%	Fat: 25 to 30%

blood sugar. At the end of each meal, you should feel a sense of satiety, not just a full belly. Satiety is what you experience when your meal has that sense of having "hit the spot" or your stomach feels "just right." If you think you may suffer from carbohydrate sensitivity, try eating protein at every meal and increase your fat intake to 25 to 30 percent of total calories. Talk to your physician or sports nutritionist about your symptoms.

WATER—The Single Most Important Nutrient

Sixty percent of an adult's body weight is water. Every metabolic reaction in the body involves water, including the burning of body fat and other fuels for energy. The body's dependence on water is reflected in the fact that a person can live only three days without it, whereas he could survive many days without food. When a person is low on water—dehydrated—all body functions suffer, including the ability to exercise. Losing as little as 1 to 2 percent of your body weight (1.5 to 3 pounds in a 150-pound person) through sweat can cause a 10 percent decrease in aerobic capacity—your ability to use oxygen for energy production. Fatigue sets in, and you lose coordination skills. As a result, your stamina and performance go down. You can easily lose that much water in one hour of hard exercise. Severe dehydration, of course, has fatal consequences. But even mild levels will cause you to feel sluggish and "not your best."

HOW MUCH IS ENOUGH?
The average adult uses 6 to 12 cups of water daily to take care of essential tasks such as removing waste products, transporting nutrients and oxygen throughout the body, and maintaining normal body temperature. This water is lost through urine, breath, sweat, and stools. Exercisers lose even more water, especially if working out in high altitudes or in hot, humid weather. Remember the advertisements for *sweat suits* in the back of magazines and on late-night TV? "Lose an inch a day while walking your way to slimness in our new exercise-enhancement suits." Well, the term *sweat suit* is appropriate. The heavy suits trapped water, preventing the body from cooling itself through sweat evaporation. The body produced more sweat in an effort to compensate. The inches lost were inches of water! A dehydrated body *appears* slimmer, right up to the moment it collapses from lack of water.

So be good to yourself and drink plenty of water daily to replace normal fluid losses and to replace the water used during exercise. Most people need 8 to 10 cups of water daily. This may sound like you will be drowning yourself. Once you get used to drinking plenty of water, you won't mind, because the reward is feeling more energetic.

FLUID OPTIONS
While it is important to drink several glasses of plain water each day, you can use other beverages too—juices, soups, skim milk, herbal tea, decaffeinated coffee, seltzer water, and sports drinks. Even juicy foods help, such as oranges, tomatoes, and cucumbers. Caffeine and alcohol have a *diuretic* effect on the body, meaning they cause you to make more urine and lose more water. If you drink caffeinated or alcoholic beverages, do so in moderation and do not count them as part of your water intake.

How can you be sure you are getting the fluids you need? Your sense of thirst is not always reliable, so monitor your urine output. You should make frequent trips to the bathroom and have clear urine, except for the first void in the morning. (Note: Vitamin supplements may cause your urine to be yellowish-green in color, whatever your hydration status.) To optimize hydration, drink small amounts of liquid throughout the day rather than slugging down large amounts over a short period of time. Follow the guidelines below for water intake during exercise.

FLUID REPLACEMENT GUIDELINES

MODERATE TO HEAVY WORKOUTS
(1 TO 1½ HOURS LONG)

Before: Drink 1 to 2 cups of plain cool water 30 minutes
before exercise.

During: Drink ½ cup of water every 15 minutes.

After: Drink 1½ to 3 cups after exercising, over a 1- to 2-
hour period of time.

ENDURANCE EVENTS

Before: Weigh yourself before the event!

Drink 2 to 4 cups of plain cool water during the
2 hours before the event.

During: Drink ½ cup of water every 15 minutes.

Also drink ½ cup of carbohydrate sports drink after
1 hour of exercise and every 20 to 30 minutes.

After: Drink 1 cup of water, fruit juice, or sports drink every
20 minutes until your pre-event weight is reached,
about 2 cups per pound lost.

Vitamins, Minerals, and Quasi-Nutrients

Tables 8 to 10 summarize 39 nutrients and quasi-nutrients, 30 of which are known to be essential to humans. Vitamins and minerals are intricately involved in all reactions that occur in the body, including energy metabolism. Many of the vitamins act as coenzymes, facilitating metabolism in numerous ways. The minerals are often a part of our physical structure. Amazingly, your vitamin and mineral requirements total less than 4 grams' worth of these vital nutrients, compared to 400 to 700 grams' worth of the energy nutrients. Yet you can consume all the fuel you need (energy nutrients) but without the necessary support from vitamins and minerals, you're going nowhere.

The amount of vitamins and minerals present in your diet depends on your food choices and preparation. Many nutrients are lost in the processing of foods.

Making a whole potato into potato chips, for example, wipes out most of the naturally present vitamin C, potassium, and dietary fiber. Turning whole wheat into bleached, white flour reduces the wheat to practically nothing but carbohydrates. A diet high in processed foods results in unhealthy ratios of sodium to potassium and phosphorus to calcium. The goal of Power Nutrition is to have a diet high in nutrient density—meaning you get a lot of vitamins, minerals, and fiber per calorie.

You may have heard that the American food supply is devoid of nutrients because farming practices have stripped the soil. Though this is probably true to some extent, certainly we still get many nutrients from our food, if we make healthy choices of minimally processed foods. Processed foods typically provide fewer nutrients per calorie than whole foods. Eating foods that are close to their original form is the best way to increase nutrient density.

Some people complain that eating well is too complicated and others say healthy foods don't taste good. As for the *how-to* part, follow this rule: *Choose more of the best and less of the rest*, meaning choose mostly wholesome, *real* foods and eat the processed junk food less often. Instead of instant macaroni and cheese, eat noodles topped with chicken and veggies. Have pudding made with skim or low-fat milk for dessert instead of creme-filled sandwich cookies. As for good taste, you may have to reacquaint your taste buds with the flavor of real food. But what could taste better than a juicy peach, fresh steamed asparagus, a salad of mixed greens, or a bowl of pasta with spaghetti sauce? The spaghetti sauce can even contain meatballs and still be lean, healthy, and delicious.

If you cannot or will not eat a nutrient-dense diet, be sure to take a vitamin/mineral supplement daily. Even if you eat well most of the time, you may choose to use some supplements. Nutritional supplements are discussed later in this chapter.

SODIUM—HOW BIG AN ISSUE IS IT?

Clearly, most Americans eat far more sodium than our bodies require. Due to the prevalence and dangers of high blood pressure (HBP), many health experts recommend eating no more than 2400 milligrams of

TABLE 8. VITAMINS

NUTRIENT	WHAT IT DOES (MAIN FUNCTIONS)	RDIs AND PROBABLE SAFE SUPPLEMENTAL DOSES*	SOME MAJOR FOOD SOURCES**	TOXICITY LEVELS/CONCERNS
VITAMIN A (retinol; beta-carotene)	Antioxidant; involved in maintenance of skin, mucous membranes, bones, teeth; vision and hormone regulation.	5000 IU (1000 RE). Probable safe supplemental intake: up to 25,000 IU (with half from beta-carotene).	Liver, fortified milk, cheese, egg yolk, carrot, sweet potato, spinach, dried apricots, broccoli, pumpkin, kale.	25,000 to 50,000 IU. Excesses are stored in the liver and can be quite dangerous.
VITAMIN B$_1$ (thiamine)	Necessary component of energy metabolism; supports normal functioning of muscles, heart, and nervous system.	1.5 mg. Probable safe supplemental dose: up to 300 mg. Up to 500 mg for some treatments.	Organ meats, pork, whole grains, brewer's yeast, dried beans, salmon, wheat germ, sunflower seeds, egg yolks.	No known toxicity for oral doses. Headache, insomnia, and irritability can occur from large doses. Accentuates action of muscle relaxants.
VITAMIN B$_2$ (riboflavin)	Necessary component of energy metabolism; supports normal vision, skin, and nervous system; interacts with other B vitamins.	1.7 mg. Probable safe supplemental dose: up to 300 to 500 mg.	Milk, milk products, liver, oysters, avocado, chicken, salmon, collard greens, spinach, whole or enriched grains, brewer's yeast, almonds.	Conflicting information. Possibly 1000 mg. Symptoms can include nausea and vomiting. May interfere with some anticancer medications.
VITAMIN B$_3$ (niacin, niacinamide, nicotinamide)	Necessary component of energy metabolism; supports skin, nervous system and digestive system; involved in synthesis of DNA.	20 mg. Probable safe supplemental dose: up to 300 mg. Up to 1000 mg in some treatments.	Beef, pork, fish, milk, cheese, whole wheat, potato, eggs, broccoli, tomato, carrot, peanut butter, peas, Brewer's yeast, orange juice.	Conflicting information. Possibly 1000 mg. Can cause body flush, weakness, headache, disturbances in heart rhythms. Large doses can interfere with many medications.
VITAMIN B$_5$ (pantothenic acid)	Necessary in energy metabolism; involved in nerve transmission and formation of steroids and hemoglobin.	10 mg. Probable safe supplemental dose: up to 500 mg.	Present in many foods, especially potato, eggs, milk, red meat, saltwater fish, legumes, fresh vegetables.	Toxicity is vary rare, but has been seen with doses of 10,000 mg. Symptoms include diarrhea and water retention.
VITAMIN B$_6$ (pyridoxine)	Involved in metabolism of protein and fat; formation of niacin and serotonin from tryptophan; production of red blood cells.	2 mg. Probable safe supplemental dose: up to 300 mg; 500 mg for some treatments. (Dependency can develop with doses of 200 mg.)	Navy beans, potato, fish, poultry, meat, banana, green and leafy vegetables, whole or enriched grains.	2,000 mg, less in some individuals. Symptoms usually involve the nervous system. Can cause depression when taken with oral contraceptives.
FOLATE (folic acid, folacin, pteroylglutamic acid, or PGA)	Production of RNA, DNA and hemoglobin; maintaining health of digestive tract lining; amino acid metabolism.	400 mcg. Probable safe supplemental dose: up to 1200 mcg. (May increase need for zinc.)	Red meats, spinach, kale, beet greens, asparagus, broccoli, whole wheat, bran, Brewer's yeast, legumes, seeds.	400 mg. Large doses can cover up the presence of a Vitamin B$_{12}$ deficiency.

(table continues)

TABLE 8. VITAMINS, continued

NUTRIENT	WHAT IT DOES (MAIN FUNCTIONS)	RDIs AND PROBABLE SAFE SUPPLEMENTAL DOSES*	SOME MAJOR FOOD SOURCES**	TOXICITY LEVELS/CONCERNS
VITAMIN B₁₂ (cobalamin)	Protein metabolism; synthesis of red blood cells; maintenance of nerve cells.	6 mcg. Probable safe supplemental dose: up to 300 mcg; 500 mcg for some treatments.	Primarily animal foods such as red meat, fish, poultry, milk, yogurt, cheese, eggs. Also miso and tempeh.	No known toxicity although large doses in conjunction with large doses of vitamin C can cause nosebleeds.
BIOTIN	Energy metabolism; fat synthesis; amino acid metabolism; CHO metabolism.	300 mcg. Probable safe supplemental dose: up to 300 mcg.	Widely available in foods, especially poultry, meat, soybeans, milk, whole wheat flour, rice bran, egg yolk.	Possibly 50 mg, although largely considered to be nontoxic.
VITAMIN C (ascorbic acid)	Formation of collagen; antioxidant; increased absorption of iron; amino acid metabolism; aids wound healing.	60 mg. Probable safe supplemental dose: up to 2000 mg. 10,000 mg for some treatments.	Papaya, orange juice, cantaloupe, broccoli, peppers, berries, kale, potato, greens, parsley, cabbage, cauliflower, chives, watercress, guava.	Some people experience diarrhea with 2000 mg. Large doses can interfere with various medications. Symptoms of overdose include headache, nausea, vomiting, abdominal cramps.
VITAMIN D (calciferol, cholecalciferol)	Mineralization of bones; calcium absorption.	10 mcg (or 400 IU). Probable safe supplemental dose: up to 600 IU.	Fortified milk, eggs, sardines, herring, tuna, fortified cereal. Also synthesized in the skin by sunlight.	5000 IU, perhaps less. Can be fatal. Symptoms include headache, fatigue, calcification of soft tissues.
VITAMIN E (alpha-tocopherol)	Antioxidant; stabilization of cell membranes; protects unsaturated fats and vitamin A.	30 mg (30 IU). Probable safe supplemental dose: up to 800 IU. (The natural form of vitamin E is generally recommended.)	Cold-pressed vegetable oils, wheat germ, green and leafy vegetables, whole grains, nuts, seeds.	Possibly 1200 IU. Can be dangerous if have high blood pressure. Enhances effect of anticoagulants and can cause bleeding.
VITAMIN K (phylloquinone, naphthoquinone)	Blood clotting; regulation of blood calcium.	80 mcg. Supplements generally not recommended as deficiencies are rare.	Spinach, green cabbage, tomato, lean meat, liver, egg yolk, whole wheat, strawberries. Intestinal bacteria synthesize it also.	Possibly 10 mg. Can cause hemolytic anemia and interfere with anticlotting medication.

*RDIs (Reference Daily Intakes), formerly called U.S. RDAs, are the references used on food and supplement labels for adults and children over 4 years of age. Where no RDI is established, I used the highest RDA given for nonpregnant adults. The "probable safe supplemental doses" refers to doses sometimes recommended to adults for optimum health and/or treatment of various conditions. Much controversy surrounds vitamin/mineral therapy, so it is recommended you check with your physician or other health care practitioner before taking supplements in doses of more than 5 times the RDI.
**These foods are not specifically recommended. Some of them are high in cholesterol, saturated fat, or sodium or may otherwise be undesirable to you. Since no foods are expressly forbidden in a healthy diet, the source list is not restricted. Select foods according to your own needs.

TABLE 9. MAJOR MINERALS AND TRACE MINERALS

NUTRIENT	WHAT IT DOES	RDIs AND PROBABLE SAFE SUPPLEMENTAL DOSES*	SOME MAJOR FOOD SOURCES**	TOXICITY LEVELS/CONCERNS
BORON—not yet established as an essential nutrient	Involved in calcium metabolism and protecting mineralization of bone.	None (3 to 6 mg have been used to treat women at risk for osteoporosis).	Noncitrus fruits, leafy vegetables, nuts, and legumes.	Unknown.
CALCIUM	Formation of bones and teeth; blood clotting; nerve transmissions; secretion of hormones and neurotransmitters; essential for muscle contraction; helps regulate blood pressure.	1000 mg. Probable safe supplemental dose: up to 1500 mg. 2000 mg is used in some treatments.	Milk, cheese, yogurt, fortified soy or rice milk, canned salmon, sardines, kale, broccoli, collard greens, clams, shrimp, oysters, tofu.	12,000 mg. Long-term supplementation with 1500 mg may actually slow bone repair in people with osteoporosis.
CHLORIDE	Fluid and acid-base balance; necessary for proper digestion.	No RDI; estimated minimum requirement is 750 mg. Typically, not used as a supplement.	Salt, soy sauce, present in most unprocessed foods, very high in processed foods.	Not sure. Symptoms include weakness, vomiting, and abnormalities of acid-base and fluid balance.
CHROMIUM	Necessary for carbohydrate, protein, and energy metabolism.	No RDI; estimated safe and adequate intake is 50 to 200 mcg. Probable safe supplemental dose: up to 600 mcg.	Brewer's yeast, meats, cheese, whole-grain cereals and bread, vegetable oils.	Unknown. High sugar intake increases urinary losses of chromium.
COBALT	Is a component of vitamin B_{12}.	None. Typically not used as an over-the-counter supplement.	Beet greens, buckwheat, cabbage, figs, milk, oysters, spinach, watercress, lettuce, organ meats, some beers.	20 to 30 mg has been shown to cause thyroid and heart problems.
COPPER	Component of many enzymes, formation of the protective covering of nerves, necessary for iron absorption and function.	2 mg. None. Typically not used as an individual supplement.	Liver, shellfish, meats, nuts, legumes, whole-grain cereals, raisins, some drinking water.	10 to 15 mg can cause vomiting and diarrhea. 100 mg can be fatal. Toxicity is seen in Wilson's disease.
FLUORIDE	Component of bone and teeth.	None. Estimated safe and adequate intake is 1.5 to 4 mg. Typically not used as an over-the-counter supplement. May be prescribed as part of treatment for osteoporosis.	Drinking water, tea, coffee, seafood, rice, soybeans, spinach, gelatin, onions, lettuce.	20 mg. Symptoms include discoloration of teeth, nausea, vomiting, diarrhea, chest pain, itching.

(table continues)

TABLE 9. MAJOR MINERALS AND TRACE MINERALS, continued

NUTRIENT	WHAT IT DOES	RDIs AND PROBABLE SAFE SUPPLEMENTAL DOSES*	SOME MAJOR FOOD SOURCES**	TOXICITY LEVELS/CONCERNS
IODINE	Component of thyroxin, a hormone that regulates metabolism, growth, and development.	150 mcg. Not commonly used as an over-the-counter supplement.	Iodized salt, seafood, seaweed, can be widely distributed in plants depending on iodine content of soil.	2000 mcg. Toxicity causes enlargement of thyroid and depressed thyroid activity.
IRON	Component of hemo-globin and myoglobin; part of many enzymes involved in energy metabolism.	18 mg. Probable safe supplemental dose: up to 30 mg, perhaps more for treatment of iron-deficiency anemia.	Meat, poultry, fish, eggs, whole or enriched grains, legumes, spinach, blackstrap molasses, dried fruits.	100 mg. Perhaps less in individuals with hemosiderosis and hemochromotosis. Toxic levels affect the immune system.
MAGNESIUM	Acts as a co-enzyme; is involved in protein synthesis, bone mineral-ization, muscle contractions, nerve transmission, and energy metabolism.	400 mg. Probable safe supplemental dose: up to 750 mg, more for treatment of certain conditions.	Almonds, fish, soybeans, sunflower seeds, wheat germ, legumes, whole grains, chocolate, cocoa, blackstrap molasses.	6,000 mg. Lower levels can have a laxative effect.
MANGANESE	Component of many en-zymes; involved in fat synthesis and many other processes.	None. Estimated safe and adequate intake is 2 to 5 mg. Probable safe supplemental dose: up to 30 mg.	Widely distributed in foods, especially hazel-nuts, pecans, avocado, seaweed, whole grains.	Rare. Side effects have been reported with intakes of 700 mg.
MOLYBDENUM	Works with various en-zymes to promote normal cell function throughout the body.	None. Estimated safe and adequate intake is 75 to 250 mcg. Typically not used as a single supplement, but may be present in a multiple.	Legumes, cereal grains, organ meats, dark-green, leafy vegetables.	10 mg. Toxicity creates goutlike symptoms.
NICKEL	Functions not well under-stood in humans. Probably involved in hormone, fat, and membrane metabolism.	None.	Widely distributed in foods, especially fruits and vegetables.	Minimum toxic dose unknown, but known to be toxic in excess, caus-ing skin problems and lung cancer.
PHOSPHORUS	Essential to energy metabolism; a component of bones, teeth, and phospholipids; important in acid-base balance.	1000 mg. Generally not taken as a supplement because it is easy to obtain plenty of phosphorus from the diet.	Found in nearly all foods, especially milk products, meats, fish, carbonated soft drinks, nuts, grains, beans.	12,000 mg. Diets too high in phosphorus can cause a calcium imbal-ance, especially if dietary intake of cal-cium is low.
POTASSIUM	Involved in acid-base balance, water balance,	None. Estimated minimum requirement is	Widely distributed in whole, unprocessed	18,000 mg. Can cause muscular weakness,

TABLE 9. MAJOR MINERALS AND TRACE MINERALS

NUTRIENT	WHAT IT DOES	RDIs AND PROBABLE SAFE SUPPLEMENTAL DOSES*	SOME MAJOR FOOD SOURCES**	TOXICITY LEVELS/CONCERNS
POTASSIUM (cont.)	transmission of nerve impulses, and muscle contractions; protein synthesis.	2000 mg. Generally not necessary as a supplement, except in certain medical conditions.	foods: milk, meats, fruits, vegetables, whole grains, legumes.	irregular heartbeat, and possibly heart failure.
SELENIUM	An antioxidant that works with vitamin E.	70 mcg. Probable safe supplemental dose: up to 200 mcg. More is used in some treatments.	Seafoods, meats, whole grains.	Reports vary for minimum toxic dose from 200 mcg to 1000 mcg. Symptoms include a garlic-like odor in breath, urine, and sweat.
SODIUM	Water balance, acid-base balance, transmission of nerve impulses.	None. Estimated minimum needs is 500 mg. Generally not needed in supplemental form.	Processed foods containing sodium additives, table salt, soy sauce, pickled foods, present in moderate amounts in most whole, unprocessed foods.	Excess intakes associated with increased risk of high blood pressure and calcium imbalance. Salt tablets not recommended for athletes; they are unnecessary and potentially dangerous.
SULFUR	A component of some proteins, biotin, vitamin B_1, and insulin; aids in detoxification processes.	None. Is not used as a nutrient by itself and there are no established recommendations for intake. Typically not used as a supplement.	All protein-containing foods, such as milk, cheese, meats, poultry, fish, eggs, legumes.	No information available.
TIN	Not known if essential to humans or its specific functions in the body.	None.	Unknown. Some is ingested from canned foods. Also found in multiple vitamin and mineral supplements in very low doses, 10 mcg.	Animal data shows high doses can cause anemia. Toxicity levels are not known.
ZINC	Involved in many processes as part of enzymes; protein synthesis and metabolism; immune reactions; vitamin A metabolism; normal growth and development.	15 mg. Probable safe supplemental dose: up to 50 mg. 100 mg used in some treatments.	All protein foods, especially oysters, dark meat poultry, meats, eggs, fish, legumes, and whole grains.	Adverse effects have been reported with intakes over 100 mg. High doses may, over time, interfere with copper status and can cause LDL (bad) cholesterol levels to rise.

*RDIs (Reference Daily Intakes), formerly called U.S. RDAs, are the references used on food and supplement labels for adults and children over 4 years of age. Where no RDI is established, I used the highest RDA given for nonpregnant adults. The "probable safe supplemental doses" refers to doses sometimes recommended to adults for optimum health and/or treatment of various conditions. Much controversy surrounds vitamin/mineral therapy, so it is recommended you check with your physician or other health care practitioner before taking supplements in doses of more than 5 times the RDI.
**These foods are not specifically recommended. Some of them are high in cholesterol, saturated fat, or sodium or may otherwise be undesirable to you. Since no foods are expressly forbidden in a healthy diet, the source list is not restricted. Select foods according to your own needs.

TABLE 10. COFACTORS AND QUASI-NUTRIENTS

The following are not considered essential nutrients that must be supplied by diet or supplements. They are all present in the body and have a role in health. They are often found as part of a multiple vitamin or mineral supplement. Some of them are sold as single supplements.

COFACTOR	WHAT IT DOES (KNOWN OR SUSPECTED FUNCTIONS)	PROBABLE SAFE SUPPLEMENTAL DOSES*	SOME MAJOR FOOD SOURCES**	TOXICITY LEVELS/CONCERNS
BIOFLAVINOIDS (also called hesperidin and rutin)	Antioxidant, increase absorption of vitamin C, strengthen capillary walls.	Up to 5000 mg. More is used in some treatments.	Citrus fruit, green peppers, apricots, cherries, grapes, papaya, tomatoes, broccoli.	Information not available. No adverse side effects expected.
CHOLINE	Involved in fat metabolism; component of acetylcholine, a neurotransmitter in the brain; component of compound in cell membranes.	Up to 300 mg.	Egg yolk, meats, legumes, cabbage, cauliflower, green beans, whole grains.	Toxicities have been reported with symptoms including dizziness, nausea, diarrhea, depression, and a fishy odor. No information available about minimum toxic dose.
COENZYME Q10 (also called ubiquinone)	Involved in energy metabolism.	Up to 300 mg.	Beef, sardines, spinach, peanuts.	Minimum toxic dose not known. Not recommended if you have heart disease. See more information under sports nutrition supplements later in this section.
INOSITOL (also called myo-inositol)	Is a coenzyme in metabolism; may be involved in the synthesis of phospholipids (compounds essential for the digestion and absorption of fats).	Up to 300 mg.	Beans, peas, cantaloupe, oranges, nuts, oats, rice, pork, wheat germ, whole grains.	Minimum toxic dose not known. If diabetic, use under medical supervision. High intakes of caffeine may interfere with adequate inositol levels in the body.
LIPOIC ACID	Works with vitamin B_1 in energy metabolism.	Up to 200 mg.	Liver, brewer's yeast.	Unable to find toxicity information.
PARA-AMINOBENZOIC ACID (PABA)	May be involved in protein metabolism. Increases effectiveness of B vitamins and vitamin C.	Up to 300 mg.	Bran, brown rice, organ meats, molasses, sunflower seeds, wheat germ, whole grains, yogurt.	Has been shown to be toxic to the liver in doses of 8000 mg. May interfere with antibiotics and sulfa drugs.

*RDIs (Reference Daily Intakes), formerly called U.S. RDAs, are the references used on food and supplement labels for adults and children over 4 years of age. Where no RDI is established, I used the highest RDA given for nonpregnant adults. The "probable safe supplemental doses" refers to doses sometimes recommended to adults for optimum health and/or treatment of various conditions. Much controversy surrounds vitamin/mineral therapy, so it is recommended you check with your physician or other health care practitioner before taking supplements in doses of more than 5 times the RDI.
**These foods are not specifically recommended. Some of them are high in cholesterol, saturated fat, or sodium or may otherwise be undesirable to you. Since no foods are expressly forbidden in a healthy diet, the source list is not restricted. Select foods according to your own needs.

sodium per day. That's just about the amount in 1 teaspoon of salt. Average sodium intakes are estimated to be 3000 to 7000 milligrams in the United States.

The need for everyone to cut sodium intake is not supported by all researchers of HBP and heart disease. High-sodium diets do not cause or improve all cases of HBP. There are probably other dietary factors involved too, such as too little calcium, potassium, and magnesium in the diet. Perhaps we eat too much sodium *in relation* to these other minerals. This is an easy thing to do when one relies primarily on processed foods.

Sodium is widely used in the processing of foods, such as baked goods, frozen dinners, canned or dry soups, rice mixes, cured meats, and pickled foods. One cup of canned chicken noodle soup contains 1107 milligrams of sodium! An estimated 75 percent of our sodium intake comes from processed foods. At the same time, processing often causes losses in other minerals, resulting in a disproportionately high sodium content.

HBP and mineral imbalances are dangerous enough to warrant using sodium in moderation, even if your blood pressure is normal now. Begin by using fewer processed foods high in sodium. Look for low-salt soups and throw away the seasoning packets in packaged foods. Use herbs and spice blends, such as Mrs. Dash, for seasoning. Read food labels to become aware of sodium levels in foods. And don't salt your food until you've tasted it!

Maximizing Workouts: What to Eat Before, During, and After Exercise

What you eat and when you eat it in relation to your workouts can make a big difference in how an exercise session goes. When exercising, your body shifts blood flow away from the digestive tract to the working muscles. Food digestion takes a backseat and you will want to time your meals accordingly.

FOOD BEFORE EXERCISE

Most of the energy used during a workout comes from your stores of glycogen and fat. However, if you exercise longer than one hour, a preexercise meal can contribute necessary glucose for long workouts. If you decide to take a run first thing in the morning, you will be low on glycogen stores from your overnight fast. A light, high-carbohydrate snack, perhaps a bagel with jam one hour before, will help abate hunger and prevent low blood sugar. If exercising at low to moderate intensity, you will probably feel fine on an empty stomach, provided you ate a high-carbohydrate meal the night before.

We used to think overweight people would burn more calories if they ate after, not before, exercising, due to an increased TEF (thermal effect) for the postexercise meal. More recent research indicates this is not true. However, exercise may decrease hunger for the following meal.

The shorter the time period between food intake and exercise, the smaller and lighter the meal should be. You will want to minimize fat *and* fiber if eating less than three hours preexercise to avoid bloating and discomfort. Experiment to see what works best for you. Some guidelines to follow for preexercise meals:

- If eating less than one hour before exercising, choose a small snack, such as half a bagel, one slice of toast with jam, or a glass of skim or low-fat milk.
- If eating one to two hours before exercising, choose a liquid meal to provide calories in an easily digestible form. Liquids leave the stomach sooner than solids. A fruit-and-yogurt smoothie with a little cereal or wheat germ added should be enough.
- If eating two to three hours before exercising, choose a small meal, such as a small bowl of cereal with low-fat milk, toast with jam, and juice.
- If eating three to four hours before exercising, choose a larger meal, consisting of foods that have a low G-I (see Table 8)—for example, a bowl of hearty bean soup with RyKrisp crackers, skim or low-fat milk, and an orange.

Remember, eat a high-carbohydrate diet *regularly* to maintain glycogen stores.

Carbohydrates During Exercise: Exercise lasting longer than 1½ hours can be enhanced by consuming carbohydrates with a high G-I throughout the exercise session. Small amounts of sugar help prolong exercise by providing a ready source of energy to the muscles and by maintaining blood-sugar levels. Most sports drinks, candy, bananas, and raisins are all high G-I foods.

About Sports Drinks: Sports drinks vary in their source of carbohydrate, glucose, sucrose, fructose, glucose polymers, or maltodextrins. But, more important, is the *amount* of carbohydrate—ideally a 6 to 8 percent concentration or 14 to 19 grams per cup.

Is one source of CHO better than another? Fructose has a low G-I, so fructose-based beverages (e.g., ReHydrate) may not be as useful during exercise as a sucrose-based beverage (Gatorade). Glucose polymers (Exceed brand) may cause less stomach discomfort than other sugars. Cytomax claims to be the best because, in addition to CHO, it contains polylactate. The makers of Cytomax claim the polylactate lowers lactic acid during and after training so you have less muscle burn and soreness. They also claim Cytomax will make you feel less fatigued. Theoretically, the idea of adding lactate is sound. Practically, it doesn't work,

PACKING YOUR PANTRY

QUICK BREAKFAST FOODS TO KEEP ON HAND

A variety of dry cereals—shredded wheat, bran flakes, low-fat granola, Muesli, Grape-Nuts, etc.
Skim or 1% milk
Nonfat or low-fat yogurt, plain and fruited
Frozen, unsweetened fruit
Bagels
Cottage cheese
Fat-free cream cheese
Health Valley Fat Free Granola Bars
Fantastic Foods brand Hot Cereal cups
Health Valley Fat Free Muffins
Fresh fruit
Frozen juices
Wholesome & Hearty Garden Sausage (frozen patties)
Small cans or boxes of 100% fruit juice, such as Minute Maid
Frozen egg substitute (thaws quickly in microwave)
Nutri-Grain Waffles by Eggo
Pancake mix, such as Aunt Jemima Complete Pancake & Waffle Mix
Pure maple syrup
Raisins and other dried fruits
Whole grain bread

CONVENIENT PACKABLES FOR LUNCH AND SNACKS

Light 'n Tangy V-8 Juice
Sparkling fruit juice and water—Sundance, Everfresh, Fruit TeaZer
Instant bean and lentil soups—Nile Spice or Fantastic Foods
Fat-free bean dip—Bearitos or Guiltless Gourmet
Fat-free tortilla chips—Amazing Bakes, Guiltless Gourmet, Slim Chips, etc.
Nonfat or low-fat cheese
Peanut butter, the natural kind
Whole-grain crackers—Kavli, Wasa, RyVita
Low-fat crackers—saltines, Snackwell's, Health Valley
Pretzels, preferably low-salt
Rice cakes
Carrots, prewashed
Pocket bread (fill with veggies, hummus, etc.)
Sports bars—Clif Bar, Power Bar, X-TRNR, etc.
Meal-replacement bars—Great Cakes, Bear Valley MealPack
Fruit cups, fruit canned in juice or unsweetened applesauce
Tuna, small pop-top cans

EASY-TO-PREPARE FOODS TO KEEP ON HAND

Boca Burgers (a pre-shaped vegetarian burger)
Bean Cuisine Creative Dishes
Butterball seasoned, skinless chicken breasts
One-Step Gourmet Rice & Lentils by Lundberg Farms
Fantastic Foods Tabouli Salad Mix (use half the oil)
Prewashed spinach
Frozen vegetables, plain
Canned beans—black, garbanzo, etc.
Refried beans—fat-free or vegetarian refried
Tortillas (serve with beans)
Fresh veggies that store well—carrots, onions, potatoes
Chinese noodles (cook in three minutes)
Variety of noodles/pasta
Couscous
Marinara pasta sauce
Swanson's canned chicken, premium white
Uncle Ben's Country Inn Recipes
Uncle Ben's Long Grain & Wild Rice mix
Low-fat frozen meals—Healthy Choice, Lean Cuisine, Tyson's, etc.
Popcorn, microwave—Orville Redenbacher's Smart Pop, Jolly Time Light

according to the research. And high levels of lactate can cause diarrhea. Cytomax is an effective sports drink because of its carbohydrate and sodium content. But it doesn't appear to be better than other drinks of similar CHO content.

You can make your own sports drink by adding 5 to 6 tablespoons of sugar and ⅓ teaspoon salt to one quart water. It will cost you only one-tenth as much as commercial brands, though the flavor may not be as enticing.

Individual tolerance is the critical factor in choosing a sports drink. Use these drinks when and if you really need them; otherwise they contribute unnecessary calories along with the water you definitely need. Remember, no amount of sports drink will enhance your exercise much if you have low glycogen stores to begin with.

EATING AFTER EXERCISE

This is the time to feed your muscle cells, and they like mostly carbs with a little protein! The first two hours after heavy exercise is the best time to replenish glycogen stores. The muscle cells are ravenous as well as thirsty, if you have worked long and hard. The first meal following exercise should be primarily carbohydrates, especially the high G-I variety. Eat a baked potato or rice with rolls and some grapes, for example, instead of a fatty cheeseburger and fries. Also, if you want a sugar fix, a soda or candy bar, this is the time to have it. All that sugar will be gobbled up by your muscle cells. Drinking fruit juice, a soda, or even a special *recovery* drink after exercise will replace needed water *and* carbs.

Carbohydrate Recovery: If you are an endurance athlete or bodybuilder, eating carbs *immediately,* within 30 minutes after exercise lasting more than 90 minutes, is critical to maximizing and maintaining your glycogen stores. This is known as *carbohydrate recovery.* Eat or drink 100 grams CHO within 30 minutes post-workout. Then continue to eat high-carbohydrate meals throughout the day. Current research shows that adding a little protein, 5 to 10 grams, to your recovery meal enhances the rate of glycogen replacement and aids muscle growth.

Since timing is so important in recovery, using a liquid meal right after exercise tends to work best. There are now several recovery drinks on the market, such as Carbo Fuel, Carb Xcelerator, Cytomax, and Ultra Fuel. Most of these contain only CHO. Others, such as Opti-Fuel and ProAmmo, also contain protein, but the CHO-to-protein ratio is not optimal. The liquid version of TwinLab's NitroFuel looks pretty good at 100 grams CHO and 15 grams protein. It also contains chromium, so be careful if you are taking other chromium supplements. Again, an alternative to these expensive formulas is to make your own. See my recipe for a "Recovery Smoothie."

RECOVERY SMOOTHIE

1 cup apple juice
1 banana
1 cup fresh or frozen blueberries, unsweetened
8 ounces fat-free vanilla yogurt

Mix all ingredients together in a blender. Add 4 ice cubes if using fresh berries instead of frozen. Blend until smooth. Provides 111 grams CHO and 13 grams protein (13,000 aminos!).

The average exerciser, working out less than 90 minutes, probably doesn't run out of glycogen in a typical exercise session. But it is always a good idea to *think carbs* the next time you are hungry after a workout anyway.

Planning Tips

Healthy meals don't just happen unless you think *nutrition* when you think about food. Planning menus ahead is an invaluable tool in helping you stay on track with the Power Nutrition Plan. You may shy away from planning because of the time involved, but I spend less than one hour a week planning menus. That hour saves me time later in trying to figure out what to cook. Also, if I am tired at the end of the day and haven't pre-planned dinner, I am more likely to opt for a quick dinner out or a frozen pizza. Here are some simple strategies for planning and preparing healthy menus:

- Look through cookbooks to select recipes and dishes. Select four or five dinner meals for the week.
- Shop according to the recipes so that you have everything you need on hand.
- Prepare extra amounts of foods that are called for in more than one dish. For example, you could have baked chicken with rice and then use the leftovers to make a vegetable-chicken stir-fry.
- Always cook enough for leftovers. Use these for the next day's lunch whenever possible. Freeze the rest for an easy meal later. You can even make your own TV dinners by freezing individual meals on divided plates.
- Keep plenty of quick breakfast and lunch items on hand to fill in when there are no leftovers. See Packing Your Pantry on page 78.

SURVIVING THE GROCERY STORE

I actually *enjoy* going to the grocery store, checking out the new products, and selecting healthy, delicious foods. But I know a lot of people lose their imagination when it comes to food. Grocery shopping becomes a tedious chore they try to get through as quickly as possible. They buy the same foods over and over, only to find themselves bored with the task of putting food on the table. It doesn't have to be that way! The next time you go grocery shopping:

- Go when you are not already exhausted.
- Have a shopping list to ease the trauma of decision making. This is especially helpful if do you end up at the store feeling tired.
- Allow yourself plenty of time. Read a few food labels and get acquainted with new products. Comparison shop on the basis of ingredients and fat grams in addition to price. For example, if you are looking for a granola bar, choose one that lists a real food as the first ingredient—fruit or whole grain—as opposed to a sugar. Then check the fat grams before deciding which brand to buy.
- Plan to purchase one new food each week—a new vegetable or low-fat item, for example. The *natural foods* aisle or a natural foods store is a great place to explore. You will find unusual grains, as well as some healthy convenience foods.

- Leave the kids at home, unless they are old enough to be helpful.
- Don't go with a ravenous appetite or an overly full belly. If you arrive at the store hungry, take the time to get a snack before you start shopping.

THINGS TO CONSIDER ON A FOOD LABEL

Recent changes in food labeling laws make it easier to understand the nutritional value of foods. Here are some basics to know:

- **Ingredients are listed in descending order by weight.** The item listed first is present in the largest amount, based on weight, not volume or calories. The further down the list, the less there is of that item.
- **The bold print is marketing.** Even though health claims are regulated by law, food companies take as much liberty as possible in promoting their products. Read the nutritional information before deciding if the product meets your standards.
- **Pay attention to serving size.** It is the amount of food that corresponds to the nutrition facts presented. Under the new regulations, serving sizes are now standardized for similar products, making it easier to compare brands.
- **Nutrition Information.** Now called "Nutrition Facts" on food labels, this information has been updated to provide data more pertinent to health issues today. Calories from fat are given in addition to total calories. Also new is the requirement to list grams of sugar and dietary fiber, along with the total amount of carbohydrate present.

   Since deficiency of B vitamins is no longer a major health concern in the United States, they are no longer listed. Now only vitamins A and C, calcium, and iron are required. Of course, sodium, protein, saturated fat, cholesterol, and total fat grams are still listed.
- **% Daily Value.** This refers to the amount of nutrients present compared to the amounts recommended in a 2000-calorie diet. The 2000-calorie reference diet is based on average needs for women, children, and men over age 50.

- **Daily Values Footnote.** A list of the daily values (not percentage) for fat, saturated fat, cholesterol, sodium, carbohydrate, and dietary fiber in the 2000-calorie reference diet. Some labels will also give daily values for a 2500-calorie diet, an average amount needed by teenage boys, men under 50, and very active people.
- **When the bold print says *93% fat free, 7% fat.*** It is usually referring to fat by weight, not by calories. You will often see this on meat products. The fat by calories could be way over 30 percent. Check the fat grams and calories per serving to decide if it is a low-fat product.
- **Easy guideline.** Any food with three or fewer fat grams per 100 calories is a low-fat food. You don't have to eat low-fat foods exclusively—it is your total fat intake that counts—but it is helpful to compare the fat content of different brands of the same food.
- **Fat-free foods.** There are literally hundreds on the market now. Some are useful and others are just fat-free junk foods. Be aware that many low-fat products have traded the fat for sugar and additives. Just because a food is fat-free doesn't make it healthy.

COOKING TIPS THAT REALLY WORK

Preparing healthy foods is not difficult. Here are some suggestions for improving the nutritional value of prepared foods.

- Always read a recipe entirely before beginning to prepare it. Get out all the necessary ingredients before you begin; this will save time later on.
- Invest in some good nonstick cookware and the utensils that won't scratch them.
- Canned products are usually cheaper than the same product in jars.
- Use nonfat yogurt or blended cottage cheese instead of sour cream.
- Sauté or stir-fry vegetables in water or broth instead of oil. Or, if using a nonstick skillet, coat it with a cooking spray or pump first. Then you can get by with using only 1 teaspoon of oil for cooking.
- Use 2 egg whites in place of 1 whole egg to cut fat and cholesterol. Separating the eggs yourself is less expensive than buying egg substitutes.

- To substitute liquid oil for solid fats, use one-quarter less oil than the recipe calls for. Example, use 3 tablespoons oil instead of 4 tablespoons shortening. You will have to experiment with this method in baked goods to get the right consistency.
- Cut the sugar by one-quarter to one-half in baked goods and desserts. Add extra spice or flavoring, such as orange peel, to enhance the impression of sweetness.
- Substitute nonfat dry milk for part of the sugar in cookies and loaf breads to increase calcium and protein.
- You can safely cut the salt by half in most recipes without altering flavor.
- Experiment with herbs and spices to replace both salt and added fat in recipes. Dry fresh herbs in the microwave for 10 to 15 seconds, on low.
- Increase the fiber in baked goods by using whole-grain flour for half of the total flour called for. If you choose to use all whole-grain flour, use 2 tablespoons *less* per cup.
- Add oat bran or wheat germ when cooking hot cereals to increase fiber and nutrients.
- Add more fruit or vegetables than called for in casseroles or other recipes.
- Add grated carrots or zucchini to meat loaf.
- Cook with a mixture of fat-free cheese and low-fat cheese instead of regular cheese. This works well in casseroles, on pizza, or in other dishes with baked cheese.
- Omit the oil and salt in the cooking water for rice or pasta. They aren't necessary. Rinse cooked pasta with cool water immediately after cooking to keep it from being sticky.
- To enhance the flavor of beans without fat, use chilies, coriander, cumin, turmeric, oregano, thyme, or savory.
- To reduce gas formation from beans, boil the beans in water for 3 minutes and let them soak for 8 hours or so. Add one or two strips of kombu seaweed (found in the natural foods department) during cooking. You can remove the seaweed before serving, if desired; it does not flavor the beans.
- Do not soak fresh produce to clean it. This leaches out water-soluble nutrients.

- Fresh vegetables are superior in nutrition to canned and frozen ones only if they are handled properly. Cook them with as little water as possible, cover while cooking, and cook only until tender. Use steaming, stir-frying, or pressure cookers instead of boiling. Do not overtrim or overchop vegetables, as this causes more nutrients to be lost.
- Use glass containers in the microwave whenever possible. Chemical compounds in plastic containers can migrate into fatty foods (another good reason to cut the fat!).

WHEN IN RESTAURANTS

- Initially, choose restaurants that you are familiar with. Before you get there, plan what you will order. (Save room during the day for a little extra fat from the restaurant meal.) Look at the menu to confirm your choice by evaluating how it is prepared.
- Request sauces be brought on the side or eliminated. *Be assertive; after all, you are the paying customer!*
- Ask questions about how foods are prepared: "Are the vegetables seasoned with butter or some other source of fat?"
- Don't be shy about making special requests: "Please substitute a baked potato for the french fries and bring the sour cream on the side." Some waiters will act as if it can't be done or be miffed that you are making their job more difficult. *Too bad!* They are there to serve you. You are paying them to do it and it is your right to get what you want if at all possible. You may have to gently, but firmly, remind your waiter of that.
- Choose items that are *steamed, poached, grilled, or barbecued* instead of *fried, deep-fried, topped with cheese, or in cream sauce.*
- Look for items that are marked as *heart healthy* or *low fat.* Many restaurants now offer such items.
- It is entirely possible to follow the Power Nutrition Plan while eating out. Remember, there are no forbidden foods. By knowing your daily fat gram allotment, you can eat whatever you want and still stay within your fat budget.
- Instead of viewing restaurant meals as opportunities to splurge, focus on the benefits of eating out: not having to cook or clean up, being waited on, pleasant atmosphere, etc.
- If you eat out frequently, pick up a copy of *The Restaurant Companion* by Hope Warshaw (Chicago: Surrey Books, 1990).

Sports Nutrition Supplements— Do They Really Work?

The shelves of every drugstore and natural foods store are filled with nutrition products for fitness enthusiasts and people concerned with losing or gaining weight. Some of these supplements are beneficial; others are safe, but may or may not be effective; and still others are utterly ridiculous. Nutritional science has only recently begun to explore the benefits of nutritional supplements for fitness. We have a lot to learn. Unfortunately, the supplement industry does not have to prove products work before they sell them. It is easier (and cheaper) to make a product based on theory or slim evidence than to actually determine its effectiveness in well-controlled scientific studies.

My best advice when buying supplements is *caveat emptor,* buyer beware. Beware of the hype, impressive buzzwords, and photos that accompany supplements. Read the fine print and the ingredients list to bypass the marketing and get to the facts. One of my favorite examples is the print ads for Cybergenics products seen in popular fitness magazines. The before-and-after pictures are impressive. But the fine print tells you the truth, that results seen in the pictures are not "what the typical user might expect to experience" and the components "do not promote faster muscular gains or fat loss."

Another example is the print ads for Victory Super Mega Mass 2000, a Weider product for weight gain. The ads claim the pictures are of real people with real achievements. I don't question that. But what the ad doesn't tell you is this: The reason the guys gained weight is that they consumed 2000 extra calories a day while performing weight training exercise. The product itself is nothing magical. Any 2000 low-fat, extra calories, combined with the right exercise, would produce the same results. But Weider is so impressed with the product, Mega Mass is offering $25,000 to any company that can prove to have a more effective product. Good marketing!

When considering nutritional supplements, remember the power of the *placebo effect*. The placebo effect refers to the benefits received from the belief that the product will help, rather than from the product itself. The benefits are real and measurable, proving that the mind can indeed have tremendous power over the body. Using top athletes and scientific buzzwords to sell products enhances the placebo effect by convincing consumers they work. As long as the products are not harmful, all you have to lose with a bogus product is your money.

SUPPLEMENT BUZZWORDS

Apparently, the billion-dollar supplement industry is getting more and more competitive. One strategy used for selling products is to use nutritional buzzwords that grab attention. Names like "fat burners," Turbo Charge, and "thermogenic" are particularly popular these days. These words conjure up images of being that lean, mean, fighting machine you fantasize about. To help you sort fact from fiction, here is a list of some common terms used on supplement labels or in ads and what they mean.

Aminos (amino acids): Amino acids are simply the building blocks of protein. They exist in all protein-containing foods. Many amino acid supplements are actually very low in amino acids compared to the levels found in common foods. If a label claims "1000 aminos," for example, the product provides 1000 milligram's (1 gram's) worth of amino acids per serving. Compare that to a chicken breast that provides, on average, 28,000 milligrams (28 grams) of amino acids! Most of these products contain all the essential amino acids as well as others, just as food does. These are perhaps the worst offenders in the "bogus supplement" department because they are very expensive for what you get: a ridiculously low-dose protein supplement.

Anabolic: Refers to chemical processes that build tissue in the body. Often used interchangeably with the term *anti-catabolic*. (Catabolism is the chemical process that breaks down body tissue for the release of energy.) The term is often used on products containing amino acids (protein). Used in conjunction with the term *steroid-free*, it implies that the product offers a response similar to, but safer than, steroids.

ATP (adenosine triphosphate): ATP is the actual energy-containing compound in the body. CHO, fat, and protein yield ATP when metabolized for energy. ATP may be referred to on a supplement label to indicate the product gives you more energy. But the determining factor of how much energy (ATP) you get is the CHO, fat, and protein content of the product.

Bioavailability: A term found on protein supplements, *bioavailability* refers to how well nutrients are absorbed. Protein supplements compete with each other by claiming to have greater bioavailability with the type of protein provided.

Electrolytes: These minerals carry an electrical charge when dissolved in water. They are critical to muscle contraction and to maintaining fluid balance and acid-base balance in the body. Potassium, sodium, chloride, and magnesium are the electrolytes generally referred to in sports nutrition supplements. Typically, exercisers can replace their electrolyte needs through ordinary fluids, such as water and fruit juices, and moderate use of table salt. Check out the Power Nutrition Recipes in the back of this chapter. You may be surprised at the potassium you get in these ordinary foods.

Ergogenic: Literally, *ergogenic* means "making energy." Use of this term implies that the product will increase your energy level or sports performance beyond that of a healthy sports diet and proper training.

Fat burners: These are ingredients that will, supposedly, increase your body's ability to burn stored body fat. Often-included ingredients are L-carnitine, chromium picolinate, inositol, choline, B_6, methionine, and various herbs. Some of these ingredients are discussed individually in the supplement table that follows or in the nutrient tables presented in the Vitamin,

Mineral, and Cofactors section of this chapter. Frankly, there is *no* formula known to burn fat or enhance fat loss to a greater extent than the age-old combination of eating less and exercising more.

Krebs cycle complex: These are usually minerals attached to compounds, such as citric acid, fumaric acid, and succinic acid, found in the Krebs cycle. The Krebs cycle is the energy cycle within the mitochondria of cells. Products claim this mineral complex "increases solubility and sustains balanced energy." I've seen no evidence to support these claims.

Lipotropic: Meaning "to have an affinity for lipids [fats]," such products are meant to prevent the accumulation of fat in the body. They are similar to "fat burners," described above.

MCT oil: Found in some sports bars, such as Hard Body, or as a separate supplement, MCT oil is promoted to bodybuilders as an alternative fuel source on a low-CHO diet. MCT, which stands for medium-chain triglyceride, is sometimes referred to as the "fatless fat." Because MCTs are absorbed and metabolized differently from other fats, they do not require carnitine for metabolism and they are not readily stored as body fat. They are a high-density-calorie fuel, however, at 8.4 calories per gram and 115 calories per tablespoon. See more about MCTs in Table 12.

Metabolic: *Metabolism* means the sum total of all chemical processes in the body. The term *metabolic* is used to imply that the product will enhance your metabolism by burning off calories and/or building lean mass. Also used to imply that the product is used directly in the body's metabolic processes, and therefore is effective.

Predigested: Usually used on amino acid (protein) supplements containing single amino acids or paired amino acids (dipeptides). The implication is that because the protein is already broken down (digested), it will be easier to absorb. The value of predigested protein is questionable in healthy people with a working digestive tract.

Stacking: The term refers to the practice of taking more than one supplement at a time to improve performance. It is used mostly in the world of bodybuilding and comes from the practice of taking multiple kinds of steroids.

Thermogenic: Literally, "making heat," the term is used on products marketed for energy or weight loss, implying that the ingredients will increase your metabolism so you can have more energy or burn off more calories than normal. Most of these products contain an herbal blend of ma huang (which contains the stimulant ephedra), guarana or kola nut (containing caffeine), white willow bark, and kelp (to "normalize" the thyroid gland). The combination is supposed to act as a mild appetite suppressant and mood elevator. Ephedra has drawn a lot of attention lately because it can have serious side effects when abused. It is especially dangerous if you have any of the following medical problems: heart or thyroid problems, high blood pressure, diabetes, asthma.

Selecting Supplements That Are Right for You: Because vitamins and minerals are essential to health, people sometimes assume "more is better." This is a potentially dangerous assumption. With vitamin and mineral intake, more is better only up to a point and then more is either neutral in its effect or toxic. Whether or not athletes require more vitamins and minerals than nonathletes is an interesting topic. There is a higher need for some nutrients whose requirement level is tied to energy expenditure—vitamins B_1 and B_2, for example. But exercisers usually eat enough food to meet this increased need, unless they maintain a low body weight or make poor food choices. The bulk of scientific data does not seem to support the idea that athletes' nutritional needs are significantly greater than those of others. Table 11 compares two diets, to illustrate how easy it is to meet nutritional needs with food.

If you are like most Americans eating a less-than-spectacular diet, you may want to consider taking a multiple vitamin and mineral supplement. It is cheap insurance for nutritional health. I make that suggestion with one caveat, however. In my experience as a nutri-

TABLE 11. NUTRIENT COMPARISON OF TWO DIETS

EATS WELL	EATS POORLY
1 cup orange juice	½ cup orange juice
1 cup skim milk with 2 oz. organic raisin bran cereal	1 cup 2% milk with 1 cup Apple Jacks cereal
1 slice multigrain toast with 1 tsp. low-fat margarine	
1 banana	1 glazed yeast doughnut
1 nonfat fruited yogurt	12 oz. Diet Coke
6 oz. bean soup	large tossed salad with 2 Tbsp. regular blue
large tossed salad with 3 oz. raw broccoli	cheese dressing
and 2 Tbsp. low-fat French dressing	10 cheddar cheese snack crackers
small can V-8 juice	sweetened iced tea
1 whole wheat roll	
2 brown rice cakes (sesame)	6 saltine crackers
1 Tbsp. almond butter	1 oz. American cheese
1 cup apple cider	12 oz. Diet Coke
2 cups brown rice with 6 oz. tofu	1 Big Mac
½ cup carrots and ½ cup podded peas,	1 small order french fries
cooked with ½ Tbsp. sesame oil	sweetened iced tea
1 cup steamed kale	
2 Fig Newtons	½ cup vanilla ice cream
1 cup skim milk	2 Tbsp. chocolate syrup

ANALYSIS	ANALYSIS
2190 calories	2205 calories
15% protein (83 grams)	11% protein (61 grams)
70% CHO (389 grams)	50% CHO (281 grams)
16% fat (39 grams)	39% fat (97 grams)
Percent of RDI	*Percent of RDI*
vitamin A: 643%	vitamin A: 116%
vitamin E: 275% (22 mg)	vitamin E: 50% (4 mg)
thiamine: 166%	thiamine: 218%
riboflavin: 169%	riboflavin: 134%
niacin: 168%	niacin: 106%
B_6: 199%	B_6: 84%
folate: 470%	folate: 191%
B_{12}: 112%	B_{12}: 168%
vitamin C: 696% (418 mg)	vitamin C: 260% (156 mg)
potassium: 293%	potassium: 125%
iron: 141%	iron: 116%
calcium: 1328 mg	calcium: 961 mg
magnesium: 502%	magnesium: 84%
phosphorus: 256%	phosphorus: 168%
zinc: 96%	zinc: 79%

tion counselor, if most people put as much time and money into their food intake as they do searching for a miracle pill, they would be further ahead in the fitness game. Supplements are in no way a substitute for healthy, wholesome foods. They cannot replace whole grains and vegetables in your diet, because foods are much more than their vitamin and mineral content. So put some energy into eating well first. Then consider how you may benefit from a supplement.

Table 12 highlights 15 popular sports and weight-loss supplements. You can judge for yourself if they are mostly hype or potentially helpful. Some other commonly used supplements, such as antioxidants and protein powders, are also reviewed below.

Choosing a Multiple Vitamin/Mineral Supplement: Dozens of supplements line the shelves of most grocery stores, drugstores, and natural foods stores. How do you know which one to choose? I divide the multiple supplements by dosage: low or high. Low-dose supplements are those that provide about 100 percent of the RDI for most vitamins and several minerals. They usually do not contain much calcium because calcium is very bulky and takes up too much room. The low-dose supplements usually are of the "one-a-day" variety, such as Centrum brand. They may contain some artificial colors and flavors. If that is not a problem for you, these low-dose pills are inexpensive, less than 50 cents a day. If you have no health problems, a low-dose supplement is probably adequate and certainly safe. By the way, the so-called timed-release or slow-release supplements are usually more expensive, and there is no evidence that they are better.

High-dose multiple supplements often provide several hundred or thousand percent of the RDI for vitamins, especially B vitamins. The mineral content is usually closer to the RDI. Again, calcium is often not present in large amounts, but can be. Many of these supplements also contain ingredients such as herbs, seaweed, quasi-nutrients, and amino acids that make these products substantially more expensive, one to two dollars a day. In my estimation, the benefit of these additional substances is questionable because the doses are usually quite small. You will have to take three to six pills a day to get the dose listed on the label. If you have some health problems that might benefit from higher supplemental doses of vitamins or minerals, I suggest you talk to your physician or nutrition counselor about your needs. Review the vitamin and mineral charts presented earlier in this chapter regarding safety of high-dose supplementation.

About Antioxidants: Antioxidant nutrients (beta-carotene, vitamin C, vitamin E, and selenium) have stolen the nutritional limelight in recent years because of their effects on aging and in disease prevention. Antioxidants serve a major protective function in the body, by reducing the damage done to cells by *free radicals*—the by-product of normal metabolic processes and environmental pollutants. Intense exercise, such as in endurance sports, causes increased levels of these harmful compounds because of the increased utilization of oxygen, leading to muscle damage and reduced immunity. Though results are equivocal, many researchers in the field of antioxidants recommend supplementation, for both exercisers and nonexercisers. The benefits to exercisers, especially those doing a lot of intense exercise, may include reduced muscle damage, reduced muscle soreness, and improved immune function. Recommendations vary, but commonly include 8 to 30 milligrams beta-carotene (equivalent to 13,000 to 50,000 IU vitamin A activity), 500 to 3000 milligrams vitamin C, 400 to 800 IU vitamin E, and 200 mcg selenium. If you make healthy food choices, you can easily meet the minimum recommendations for beta-carotene and possibly vitamin C (see the diet comparison in Table 11). The content of selenium foods is dependent on soil content, and vitamin E would be impossible to obtain in the above levels through food. Refer to the vitamin and mineral tables presented earlier in this chapter for food sources of the antioxidant nutrients.

Other antioxidants making their debut in the supplement market in recent years are pycnogenol, grape seed extract, and N-acetyl cysteine (a form of the amino acid cysteine). These products are generally quite expensive compared to the nutrients discussed above. There is little scientific information available about them, at least in the mainstream nutrition and health literature.

TABLE 12. FACTS ABOUT 15 CONTROVERSIAL BUT POPULAR SPORTS SUPPLEMENTS

NAME	CLAIMS FOR EXERCISERS	FACTS	SAFETY/COMMENTS
AKG (alpha-ketoglutarate)—The ammonia-free carbon skeleton of the amino acid glutamine. An intermediary in energy metabolism.	Stimulates growth hormone. Replaces glutamine lost during intense exercise.	Unknown. Found no research specific to athletes, except in combination with vitamin B_6. See About B Vitamins (page 89) for more detail.	Unable to find this information. Critics of amino acid supplements are concerned with upsetting the overall amino acid balance in the body, thereby compromising protein metabolism in various ways.
BCAA—The essential branched chain amino acids isoleucine, leucine, and valine.	Improves endurance, stimulates growth hormone, and increases muscle mass through better nitrogen retention.	Are known to be burned as fuel during endurance exercise. Research in athletes is limited. Recommendations are mostly theorized from work in various disease conditions. One small study using 14 grams for 2 weeks showed improved performance in endurance athletes.	Safety of long-term use is unknown. Critics cite concerns over upsetting overall amino acid balance. It is easy to meet increased needs for these amino acids through animal protein foods.
L-CARNITINE—Facilitates transport of fatty acids and BCAA into the energy cycle. Facilitates glucose metabolism. Made in the body by two essential amino acids: methionine and lysine.	Improves VO2 max and endurance. Decreases lactic acid buildup during anaerobic exercise.	Use of 4000 mg per day for 2 weeks increased VO2 max by 6 percent in endurance-trained athletes. Research is limited, however.	L-carnitine has shown no toxicity over 3 weeks of daily intake. Long-term use is not well researched. The DL-form may be toxic.
CHROMIUM PICOLINATE—Chromium is a mineral essential to carbohydrate metabolism. The picolinate form is considered well absorbed and biologically active.	Decreases body fat and increases muscle mass. Safe alternative to steroids.	Research results are mixed. Benefits depend on the chromium status of the individual. Will not replace training, which yields the biggest benefits.	Very low toxicity. Considered safe in doses up to at least 600 mcg daily. Large doses may interfere with absorption of zinc and iron.
COENZYME Q10—also known as ubiquinone. A key component in the body's energy cycle. Not considered an essential nutrient.	Improves endurance.	Some studies have shown significant improvement in performance of endurance athletes. However, research results are mixed.	Appears safe with doses up to 100 mg taken daily for 4 years. Toxicity levels are not known.
CREATINE (creatine monohydrate)—A part of the high-energy molecule phosphocreatine.	Increases ATP production; delays fatigue.	Research using 5 grams, 4 times a day, for 1 week precompetition showed increased ATP generation. Effectiveness may be partly due to low protein intakes.	Current research is investigating whether or not a daily maintenance dose is appropriate. A daily dose of 2 to 5 grams appears to be safe.

(table continues)

TABLE 12. FACTS ABOUT 15 CONTROVERSIAL BUT POPULAR SPORTS SUPPLEMENTS, continued

NAME	CLAIMS FOR EXERCISERS	FACTS	SAFETY/COMMENTS
GAMMA ORYZANOL— A mixture of plant sterols and ferulic acid, extracted from rice bran oil.	Marketed as an alternative to steroids. Promotes muscle growth by increasing testosterone and growth hormone. Improves recovery time.	No human research using appropriate scientific methods has been performed. Animal data shows negative effects on various hormones. Humans cannot absorb it well.	Probably low toxicity because it is poorly absorbed, except in people with abnormal absorption. Some research indicates that some phytoserols may suppress the immune system.
GARCINA CAMBOGIA (Citrimax)—The active ingredient is (-)-hydroxycitrate.	Suppresses appetite. Prevents conversion of CHO to fat stores. Preserves muscle tissue during weight loss.	No objective information available.	Unknown. Long-term usage is questionable for safety.
GINSENG (Panax ginseng)— An herb. Active ingredients are ginsenogides. Used in Oriental cultures to decrease fatigue.	Increases endurance; decreases fatigue.	Most of research is in animals. At least one study using 200 mg/day for 12 weeks, combined with training, of standardized ginseng extract showed increased muscle strength.	Long-term use can result in "ginseng abuse syndrome," which includes nervousness, insomnia, and depression. Ginsengs vary significantly in amount of active ingredients present.
MCT OIL (medium chain triglyceride oil)—A fat, but it is metabolized more like a CHO. Provides no essential fatty acids. (Also reviewed in the section on buzzwords.)	Marketed to bodybuilders primarily. Not stored as body fat. Can spare muscle protein from being burned as fuel when on a low-CHO diet.	One study using MCT for 50 percent of total calories found that it is burned preferentially over protein. Another study found that a combination of MCI oil and carbohydrates improves performance in endurance cycling over that of carbohydrates alone. Not useful in short-term, high-intensity exercise.	Not recommended for long-term use. Not recommended if you have diabetes, liver disease, or chronic obstructive pulmonary disease.
OKG (ornithine alpha-ketoglutarate)—A form of the amino acid ornithine.	Reduces exercise-induced ammonia. Stimulates growth hormone. Preserves muscle, especially if overtraining.	Most of research on anabolic effects was not performed in athletes, but in patients recovering from traumas. Research in weight lifters has shown no anabolic effect in doses generally recommended by product manufacturers.	Unable to find this information.
PHOSPHATES—Phosphate bonds carry energy in ATP molecules and phosphocreatine. Phosphorus is an essential mineral.	Buffer muscle acid; increase oxygenation of muscles; increase use of glycogen during exercise.	Some studies in trained athletes using 4 grams of phosphates for 3 days have shown increases in VO2 max. Others have shown no effect. Data is inconclusive.	Short-term use appears safe, typically around 4 grams for 3 days prior to an athletic event. Toxicity is possible with high doses over time. Also, chronic use may interfere with calcium balance.

TABLE 12. FACTS ABOUT 15 CONTROVERSIAL BUT POPULAR SPORTS SUPPLEMENTS

NAME	CLAIMS FOR EXERCISERS	FACTS	SAFETY/COMMENTS
SUCCINATES—Intermediaries of the Krebs cycle (energy cycle).	Speed up aerobic metabolism.	Rate of aerobic metabolism is controlled by enzymes in the pathway, not succinates. Has no ergogenic benefit.	No information available.
VANADYL SULFATE (also BMOV, or bis[maltolato] oxovanadium)—forms of the mineral vanadium.	Improves efficiency of insulin and is therefore anabolic. Improves carbohydrate metabolism. Sometimes referred to as a glycemic factor.	Benefits theorized from research on diabetic rats. No evidence of ergogenic benefits in humans.	Reports on toxicity are conflicting. However, it may be toxic to liver and kidneys in doses that would affect carbohydrate metabolism. May interfere with chromium.
YOHIMBE—The bark of the yohimbe tree; active compound is yohimbine.	Promotes muscle building and endurance.	No research to support claims.	Can be toxic, especially to children and adults over age 55. Symptoms can include muscular paralysis, weakness, high blood pressure, and fatigue.

About B Vitamins: B vitamins are intricately involved in energy metabolism. Because of this, they are of much interest in the sports nutrition world. Do B vitamin supplements improve exercise performance? One big hindrance to finding this out is the difficulty in isolating any positive effects from those of the exercise training performed during research. So far, the research indicates that vitamins B_1, B_2, B_{12}, and pantothenic acid have no impact on performance when given individually. Vitamin B_6, when combined with alpha-ketoglutarate, was found in one study to increase maximum aerobic power by 6 percent and decrease lactate accumulation in trained volunteers. The dose used was 30 milligrams of the complex per kilogram body weight, given daily for 30 days. Neither B_6 nor the alpha-ketoglutarate had this effect when given separately.

Another study showed that a complex of vitamins B_1, B_6, and B_{12} may increase sensory motor control, which could be useful in some sports, such as shooting. B complexes may also reduce fatigue in hot climates. But no boost in endurance has been found in most studies. Niacin supplementation may inhibit performance in endurance sports by decreasing free fatty acids available for fuel during exercise.

About Calcium: Calcium is a concern in this country because of the high incidence of osteoporosis, especially in women. Food intake studies indicate American women do not consume enough calcium during adolescence and early adulthood, which can compromise bone health in later life. Women who diet or maintain a very low body weight are also at risk for poor calcium status, especially if menses has stopped. Menopause causes calcium loss from bones, so women who enter menopause with suboptimal calcium status are at increased risk for fractures due to osteoporosis.

Most multiple vitamin/mineral supplements do not contain substantial amounts of calcium, because it is quite bulky and won't fit in a typical one-a-day type supplement. If you do not consume dairy products or calcium-enriched soy and rice milks, you may want to consider a calcium supplement. Recommended intakes range from 500 milligrams to 1200 milligrams, depending on diet, age, and risk for osteoporosis. Calcium carbonate supplements give you the most calcium per pill, are relatively inexpensive, and are well absorbed by most people. Calcium citrate seems to be better absorbed by people with low stomach acid, such as the elderly. It is a good idea to choose a supplement with some vitamin D to enhance the absorption of the calcium. A couple of cautionary notes about calcium supplements: Do not take them with supplements containing iron if you are at risk for iron deficiency; calcium will reduce iron absorption. And if you take other supplements containing vitamin D, be sure your combined intake of vitamin D is not over 600 IU.

About Protein Powders: There are dozens of these products on the market. They vary in protein and calorie content, vitamin/mineral fortification level, and source of protein. Do you need any of them? If so, which one do you choose?

Let's talk about protein content first. In terms of total protein, first evaluate if you need the extra protein provided in a supplement or if you are already getting enough through your foods. Protein powders are generally very expensive, and protein is not all that difficult to get in food. On the other hand, if you have high protein requirements due to your exercise needs and body size, using a protein powder may be helpful. It can be more convenient than food for busy athletes, especially those who don't cook.

What about protein source? You can choose between egg, milk, soy, whey, casein, or hydrolyzed animal collagen. Proteins do vary in their quality, which is measured by biological value and protein efficiency ratio (PER). Proteins are rated for quality based on the presence of essential amino acids, the ratio of amino acids, and how well the protein supports nitrogen retention and growth. These are important considerations if you live on a formula of some sort with only one source of protein, as do infants or people being fed artificially in the hospital. If you eat a balance of foods, using a protein powder only to boost total protein intake, the source is probably less important. Still, if you are going to pay through the nose for protein, you might as well get the best. The body utilizes whole protein better than single amino acids. Egg is the protein by which all others are judged. It is very high quality, with a PER of 4.0. Milk is also a high-quality protein, though rated lower than egg (PER = 3.1). Casein and whey are both proteins found naturally in milk. Some athletes prefer whey because it has been suggested that whey has a positive effect on the body's immune system. Whey is also high in the BCAAs.

For vegetarians or people with milk and egg allergies, soy protein isolates offer a good alternative source of protein. Soy is rated about the same as milk in terms of quality. Other vegetarian formulas are available without soy. Some brands are fortified with appropriate amino acids to raise the protein's quality and can claim "the PER exceeds the U.S. government standard for high-quality protein."

On a recent trip to a local supplement shop, I found some protein supplements that are made from hydrolyzed collagen (essentially, gelatin). Collagen is a component of connective tissue in humans and animals. However, nutritionally speaking, it is not a high-quality protein. When you digest the collagen, it becomes a supply of amino acids, just as any other protein. It will not directly affect your collagen status. I can't see any benefit from using collagen. It would be my last choice.

Many protein powders supply more than protein. They may contain calories from carbohydrate, a little fat, and varying levels of vitamins and minerals. If you want a powder that can replace meals, you will need these extras. If you just want the protein, then the extra carbs and fat are simply extra calories you may not want. If you are taking vitamin and mineral pills, in addition to a fortified protein powder, be sure you aren't inadvertently overdoing it.

What Are Engineered Foods Also called *biodesigned,* in the world of sports nutrition, engineered foods are products that claim to be specially formulated for athletes to exert a specific metabolic effect on the body. In the case of MET-Rx, the protein used, according to product literature, is one specifically created to limit the breakdown of muscle cells during intense exercise. A review of the product by Janine Baer, Ph.D., R.D., a sports nutrition researcher, reveals the MET-Rx protein is a blend of casein, whey, and egg whites, similar to that found in many high-protein supplements.

Obviously, there is disagreement among supplement manufacturers as to what is the best nutrient mix for athletes. RxFuel, by Twinlab, claims to be superior to MET-Rx due to different levels of various nutrients. MetaForm, so-called technically advanced nutrition, makes the same claims. I have seen no research on these products to back up their claims.

Historically, formulas scientifically engineered to provide total nutrition have been created for people who could not eat real food. The sports formulas are not. They are just supplements made with the assumption that the user also eats a variety of real food. So, the "specialness" of their formulas is going to be diluted by the other foods that will alter the total composition of the diet. In my mind, and in the absence of research backing up their claims, this reduces them to high-protein supplements that simply cost more than other protein powders.

What About Sports Bars? Not the kind where you drink beer, watch big-screen TV, and vicariously live the life of a sports legend. I'm referring to the ever increasing number of food bars marketed to exercisers, such as Power Bar, Hard Body, Clif Bar, etc. Sports bars make convenient snacks to carry on long bike rides or hikes. They can be useful as part of a recovery meal because they are usually high in carbohydrate, low in fat, and supply a moderate amount of protein. They vary in vitamin/mineral fortification.

Again, when choosing a sports bar, bypass the hyperbole and go to the Nutrition Facts on the label. There is no magic in these bars, they are simply options for fuel and sometimes more convenient than regular food. Typically, they are high in carbohydrate and low in fat and fiber, making them an easily digested source of fuel to use before or during exercise. After a workout, consider your needs for a recovery meal as detailed earlier in this chapter. One sports bar, such as Stoker or Edge Bar, contains 40 to 50 grams of carbohydrate and around 10 grams of protein. Add 12 or 16 ounces of fruit juice and you have a recovery meal that requires no preparation. You can eat it in the locker room while cleaning up.

What Are Phytochemicals? Phytochemicals, sometimes called *phytonutrients* on supplement labels, are the latest find in the connection between food and health. Part of the reason why a diet high in fruits and vegetables is protective from various diseases, is the presence of phytochemicals in these foods. Phytochemicals, which simply means "plant chemicals," are not nutrients, but they do have biological activity. For example, lycopene, a phytochemical found in tomatoes, has been associated with lower risk of prostate cancer. Genistein, from soybeans, may be protective against heart disease, osteoporosis, and cancer. Phytochemicals hold a lot of promise for disease prevention and are the focus of a lot of research.

The supplement industry has jumped on the phytochemical band wagon. You can now buy phytochemicals in a capsule, supposedly in amounts equivalent to those found in several servings of fresh vegetables and fruits. I don't know if phytochemicals hold up to whatever processing is needed to convert whole food to pills. It's hard to get that kind of information from the manufacturers. At any rate, don't give up eating real food yet. Science continues to verify that whole foods are key to health. It is very difficult to translate information learned from research on food to claims made for these supplements.

Are You a Supplement Junkie? You might be, if:

You are taking products without knowing why. Will you take just about anything if it promises to make you leaner, stronger, or younger? In my work as a consultant to a natural foods store, I run into people all the time who cannot tell me why they are taking this product or that. They simply "heard from a friend that it was good." If that is all you base your choice of supplements on, then perhaps you are looking for miracles that will turn you into something you want without the hard work required to achieve it. If that's the case, you are not alone, just deluded.

You do not know the amounts of various nutrients you take. Unfortunately, this is very common. When taking a nutrition history, I always ask what supplements and how much a client is taking. More often than not, the client can rattle off a number of products, but has no idea how much they are taking or even the ingredients. That is understandable to a point, but you really ought to know what and how much you are consuming. Frequently, I find consumers who are unknowingly getting the same nutrient in several different products. At best, this is just a waste of money, but it can be dangerous. It is quite easy to get potentially harmful doses of nutrients this way, especially vitamins A, B_6, and D. This is especially true for people who frequently use sports bars, protein powders, and fortified breakfast cereals *and* take vitamin/mineral supplements daily. They have no idea that they are overloading on supplements. Remember, more is not necessarily better. It could be toxic! Most reports of health problems associated with supplement use involve people who forgot this fact.

You forego buying high-quality, wholesome foods because of the cost, yet you spend a small fortune on supplements. People balk at the cost of fresh strawberries or leaf lettuce, but will pay 40 dollars for a supplement if they think it will make them slimmer, firmer, or more beautiful. There is no product on the market that can replace food as your primary source of fuel and nutrition. As sophisticated as the supplement industry is, food still works best for optimum health and sports performance.

You are looking for supplements that will take the place of food, sleep, or exercise. People never cease to amaze me—myself included, of course. I am frequently asked to recommend a product that will "give me more energy." With just a few questions, it is obvious that the request is coming from someone who is overworked, underexercised, and sleep-deprived. When I start making suggestions about how he or she might change his or her lifestyle, I see eyes glaze over and an "I don't want to hear it" expression on the face. You can try ginseng, caffeine, or any other stimulant, but feeling truly energetic comes from good self-care. If you do not have enough food, sleep, or exercise, eventually the body will start to fight you. Stimulants are not a long-term solution. Vitamins, minerals, and herbs may help some, but they can't fix a chronically run-down body.

Fitness Versus Fanaticism

Has your quest for fitness become an obsession with thinness? If you come unglued when you have to miss a workout or when you gain one pound, perhaps you have lost sight of what fitness means. Fitness is having a strong cardiovascular system, muscle endurance and a strong cardiovascular system, muscle endurance and strength, and flexibility to support daily activities and play. As we age, the importance of physical fitness becomes more obvious in how well we get around and whether or not we can do the things we want to do without injury.

Weight is only one measure of health, and the number on the scale is the least effective way to evaluate weight. Body mass index (BMI) and body fat are more important. Maintaining a BMI of 19 to 25 is associated with lowest health risk due to weight. This means, if you are 5 feet, 6 inches, ideally your weight should fall between 117 and 154 pounds. The formula for BMI is given in Table 13.

TABLE 13. BMI FORMULA
$$BMI = \frac{weight\ (pounds)}{height\ (inches)^2} \times 705$$

BMI alone is not enough to assess body weight because it does not distinguish between lean weight and fat weight. Someone can have a high BMI, yet be very lean—a football player or bodybuilder, for example. So it is important also to know your body fat percentage (BF%). Although estimates vary, men probably require a minimum of 5 percent fat weight and women require 12 to 15 percent body fat to sustain life and good health. Optimum fitness is likely achieved with body fat levels higher than the minimum, 10 to 25 percent for men and 15 to 30 percent for women. These may seem like pretty liberal ranges. However, people vary greatly in how healthy they are at certain body weights and body fats. We tend to forget this fact in our fat-phobic society. I have known exercisers who feel too lethargic and get sick more often when their body fat gets lower than optimum for them. As you work to achieve the look you want, pay attention to how your body feels. You may be more comfortable at a slightly higher body fat than shooting for the lowest level you can achieve.

The best way to determine your BF% is to seek out someone with the knowledge and expertise to measure it accurately. Registered dietitians, exercise physiologists, personal trainers, and even some physicians measure BF% using the skinfolds method or electrical impedance. Health clubs and universities usually have someone on staff who can measure BF%. They might even offer the underwater weighing method, the gold standard of body fat measurements.

Waist-to-Hip Ratio (WHR) is another way to assess health risk due to body fat. Fat around the abdomen is considered a greater health risk than fat in the hips and thighs. Using a tape measure, measure your waist (in the area of your navel) and your hips (at the hip bone). Divide the waist measurement by the hip measurement. For example, if your waist measurement is 32 inches and your hip measures 38 inches, your WHR would be 32/38, or 0.8. Lowest risk is associated with a WHR of less than 0.8 in women and less than 0.95 in men.

DO YOU HAVE A FAT BODY OR A FAT BRAIN?

If your weight checks out fine, but you still want to be thinner, perhaps you see yourself as fatter than you really are. Maybe you don't have the body of a model, but how thin is thin enough? Thin enough for what? If we are talking about fitness, you can determine that with the above measurements. If we are talking about society's notion of *ideal*, then one can never be too thin. Of course, society is wrong about that. People can become too thin, jeopardizing their health and quality of life, by undereating and overexercising.

A healthy body is one you can live in. You should be able to eat a variety of foods, including dessert. You should be able to maintain a healthy body weight with a reasonable commitment to exercise. Exercise and food do not have to rule your life.

If you cannot be what society calls "thin" without being obsessive about your behavior, it is time to accept your body as it is. You can't entirely control the parts of you shaped by genetics. If you were born with Aunt Thelma's thighs, you will always have Aunt Thelma's thighs (or some version of them), no matter how hard you try to change them. Learn when to quit trying to look like someone else. Instead, focus on how it *feels* to be fit rather than how it *looks* to be "thin." Instead of criticizing your body for not being "perfect," appreciate it for the wonderful things it does for you— it takes you dancing, it gets you to work in the morning,

it allows you to play with your children or your dog, it lets you do the physical activities you enjoy. A "thin" body doesn't do these things for you, a fit body does. And fitness comes in a variety of shapes and sizes.

ALL FOODS ARE MORALLY NEUTRAL

Believe it or not, it isn't necessary to feel guilty about eating things like "real" chips or regular ice cream or chocolate. Every food contributes something to a healthy diet, even if it's just calories for fuel. Sure, if you choose all junk food with few vitamins and minerals, your total diet will be unhealthy. But chocolate isn't going to hurt you, a nutrient-poor diet will.

It is important to eat food that tastes good and is satisfying. If you get a craving for chocolate, by all means eat it! When people deny themselves for too long, they tend to overindulge when they finally give in. It's like holding your breath. You can't do it for very long. If you treat all food as morally neutral, and morally equal, then you can decide what to eat based on what your body needs at that moment. Sometimes you want french fries and sometimes you want a salad. If you really pay attention to your body, you will find that a fit body wants mostly healthy foods. You won't feel satisfied or energetic living on a junk food diet for very long. You end up wanting more of what you need! So, *enjoy eating* and forget the guilt.

TIPS FOR WEIGHT LOSS

If you really do need to lose weight for optimum health, follow these strategies, in addition to exercising regularly.

1. Eat when you are hungry and stop when you are satisfied. What a concept! This is the most natural way to eat, but many people seem to have forgotten it. If you aren't hungry, save the food for later or toss it out.

2. Set a realistic weight goal and plan to lose slowly, no more than ½ to 2 pounds a week. In addition to eating a low-fat diet, cut your calorie intake by no more than 200 to 500 calories a day.

3. Weigh yourself only once a week, at most! Better yet, rely on how you feel and how your

clothes fit to determine if you are making progress. It makes more sense to focus on your behavior than on your weight. The behaviors of exercising, eating in accordance with hunger and satiety cues, and cutting out excess fat are what get you thin *and* keep you thin.

4. Don't deprive yourself of foods you really want. Eat them in reasonable portions and when you are hungry. Remember, there are no forbidden foods.

5. Drink plenty of water, 8 or more glasses a day.

6. Keep a daily record of food intake and exercise. Record keeping helps you stay focused on what you are doing. Use the Goals/Affirmation Sheet in the back of this chapter.

7. Do not expect yourself to be perfect. Forgive yourself when you overeat or underexercise. A setback does not have to spell disaster unless you let it. And you don't have to wait until tomorrow, or next Monday, to get back on track. Do it now.

8. Celebrate your successes! Reward yourself for healthy behaviors—eating healthy and exercising—not for losing weight. Remember, it is the behaviors that must be firmly established in order to maintain weight losses. Do not, however, use food as the reward!

9. Wear clothes that fit and look nice on you now. Get rid of your fat clothes, along with any skinny clothes you purchased after your last starvation diet. If you cannot realistically maintain that skinny body, having clothes around that don't fit will just make you feel bad.

10. Live today as though you had already reached your goal weight. The things in life that make it wonderful can be had at any weight. Everyone wants to be attractive, but life is about more than being thin. If you learn to enjoy yourself now, losing weight and keeping it off will be much easier.

COMMON QUESTIONS ABOUT SPORTS NUTRITION

Can I Build Mass on a Vegetarian Diet? Absolutely! As mentioned in the section about protein, a vegetarian diet can provide plenty of high-quality protein, especially if you combine foods to insure intake of all the essential amino acids. Follow all the other guidelines for amounts of carbohydrate, protein, and fat to eat. If you eat no animal products at all, you may find it a challenge to meet your protein needs. There are a number of vegetarian protein powders and sports bars available.

I'm Eating Hardly Any Fat and I Still Can't Lose Weight. What's Wrong? Perhaps you are not eating enough fat! Remember, you have to eat some fat to get adequate amounts of essential fatty acids and to feel satisfied after meals. When you cut fat intake too low, you may end up eating too many calories in order to get full. A lot of fat-free foods are high-sugar foods, which are not particularly filling. If you can eat a whole pint of fat-free yogurt and still not feel satisfied, this may be your problem.

It is also possible that you have carbohydrate sensitivity and are not metabolizing carbohydrate normally. Visit a qualified sports nutritionist or physician for an evaluation. Also, be sure you are being realistic about your expectations. Could it be that you were expecting to lose more quickly than you can? Or maybe you are building lean body mass while burning off fat mass. If so, the number on the scale won't change immediately, though you should notice a change in how your clothes fit.

Is It True That Carbonated Beverages Are Not Good for Athletes? There has been some concern that carbonation, carbon dioxide, would interfere with exercise by affecting oxygen in the body. Not true. By the time the liquid is absorbed, most of the CO_2 has dissipated. However, carbonation may cause stomach upset in some athletes. Also, it is harder to drink the amount of water you need during and after exercise from carbonated liquids because they cause bloating. On the other hand, some athletes prefer the lightly carbonated sports drinks, such as All Sport. Again, the important thing is getting enough water and having some carbohydrate during endurance activities. If carbonated liquids help you meet those needs, then use them. Just try to avoid sodas with caffeine when rehydrating after exercise.

I Have Been Skinny All My Life. What Can I Do to Gain Weight? People who have a hard time gaining weight have to work as hard at putting pounds on as overweight people have to work at losing them. You have to shift your energy balance so that you are eating more calories than you burn. That requires eating more and not doing too much aerobic activity. Weight training will help you gain lean weight, instead of fat weight. Expect to gain ½ to 1 pound per week. Try these tips:

1. DO NOT SKIP MEALS! You will need at least three meals per day. Eat larger portions of the high-carbohydrate foods, such as grains, breads, cereals, starchy vegetables, and fruits. Don't pile on the fat, but don't skip it either. Use the form "How Much Fat Can I Eat?" presented earlier in this chapter. Figure your daily fat gram allotment at 30 percent of total calories.
2. Eat snacks as often as you are hungry. Snacks need to consist of healthy foods and not be so large that they curb your appetite for meals.
3. Drink high-calorie liquids such as fruit juice and milk instead of iced tea or coffee with meals. You do need to drink some plain water, also, but at least half your liquids should contain calories.
5. Surprisingly, your need for increased protein while gaining weight can easily be met through food. You do not need to purchase expensive protein supplements. In fact, getting too much protein is not healthy. If you believe you cannot eat enough protein in your diet, talk with a sports nutritionist before spending money on a product that may be unnecessary and even detrimental.
6. A high-calorie, weight-gain supplement may come in handy if you have a hard time eating

TABLE 14. LOW-CALORIE VERSUS HIGH-CALORIE FOOD CHOICES	
LOW-CALORIE CHOICES	HIGH-CALORIE CHOICES
Orange juice	Grape juice
Grapefruit juice	Apple juice
Applesauce	Dried fruit
Rice Krispies	Granola
Cheerios	Grape-Nuts
Vegetable soup	Split pea soup
Green beans	Corn
Summer squash	Winter squash

enough food to meet your increased calorie needs.
7. Learn to choose the higher-calorie foods within each food group. Some examples are listed in Table 14.
8. Weight training is critical to your ability to gain muscle instead of fat. If you do not already lift weights, seek out a trainer who is experienced in this area of fitness.

Is It True That Caffeine Burns Fat? Well, not exactly. Caffeine causes free fatty acids to be released into the blood. The body can use these fatty acids as fuel. Caffeine may increase exercise endurance for this reason, although it is not really very effective for many athletes because of unpleasant side effects. And research shows that caffeine gives no benefit to athletes over eating a high CHO diet, which you need anyway.

Using coffee or diet sodas to avoid eating is a common dieting strategy. You get a kick from the caffeine and the diet soda will fill you up, for a while, anyway. Caffeine is a stimulant, but it has no significant direct effect on overall fat burning or weight loss.

Why Am I Hungry All the Time? I Thought Exercise Decreased Appetite. That depends on how much exercise you are doing. Exercise can suppress appetite by increasing internal body temperature and causing the release of various brain chemicals, such as endorphins. The extent of the effect depends on the intensity and duration of the exercise.

Exercise lasting less than 30 minutes or longer than 90 minutes may not decrease appetite at all. Your body will be driven to eat back the calories you burned off to maintain energy balance. If you don't need to lose weight, then this is as it should be. If weight loss is your goal, try exercising at a moderate pace for one hour. This level of exercise has been reported to offer the best overall reduction in calorie intake, although you won't notice a dramatic loss of appetite. The most important thing is to work out an exercise regimen that works for you—one that you can do consistently without injury and that you enjoy.

I've Been Told Gatorade Is Not a Good Sports Drink Because It Is High in Sodium. Is This True? No. Gatorade does contain some sodium, 110 milligrams per cup, but that doesn't mean it is not a good sports drink. In fact, having some sodium in your sports beverage will help you absorb water better. If you are exercising hard enough to need a sports drink, you are probably exercising hard enough to be sweating. The sodium in Gatorade will help you replace the sodium lost in sweat. At 110 milligrams per cup, I wouldn't rate Gatorade as "high" in sodium. It can be a very effective sports drink. Of course, there are plenty of other ones on the market to choose from.

When looking for a sports drink, the most important consideration is carbohydrate concentration. Ideally, you want a beverage with a 6 to 8 percent CHO solution, which is 14 to 19 grams of carbohydrate per cup. Most commercial beverages meet these guidelines. The source of carbohydrate may also be important. See the section on carbohydrates during exercise, earlier in this chapter, for more information.

Should Athletes Avoid Milk? I've Heard It Causes Your Nose to Get Stuffy If You Drink It Before Working Out. Some athletes do not drink milk for that reason, but milk does not cause problems with mucous production in everyone. People with an allergy to milk may suffer a chronically stuffy nose if they drink it regularly; that would certainly make exercise uncomfortable. On the other hand, milk, especially nonfat milk, is a nutrient-dense food providing high-quality protein, calcium, vitamin D, riboflavin, and vitamin B_{12}. So, if you tolerate milk, it can be a useful food for athletes. Milk is not an essential part of a sports diet. The nutrients it contains are. If you choose not to drink milk or eat other dairy products, be sure to obtain its nutrients elsewhere, especially calcium. In the Power Nutrition food groups, nondairy sources of calcium are indicated by **.

Some of My Friends Take Diuretics to Look More Muscular. Are They Safe? Many bodybuilders use diuretics to enhance the *cut* of their muscles before a competition or photo session. Diuretics force the kidneys to excrete water that is normally found in muscles and other parts of the body. They do temporarily make you look thinner or more muscular. However, the body does not function well in a dehydrated state. It can be very dangerous to take diuretics on a regular basis. Waste products build up in the body, causing damage to various organs. The only reason you should take a diuretic is if you have an *abnormal* buildup of fluid. Even the mild nonprescription diuretics can be dangerous if abused. Your healthiest bet is to stay away from them unless recommended by your physician.

Is There a Supplement That Will Prevent Cramping from Exercise? Surprisingly, we really don't know for sure what causes muscle cramps. Changes in electrolytes, mainly potassium and sodium, during exercise seem to be the same in all athletes, yet some athletes get cramps and others don't. The prevailing opinion is that muscle cramps are primarily related to hydration. So instead of a supplement, try drinking more water. Follow the fluid guidelines found earlier in this chapter. Never exercise without water!

Power Nutrition Recipes

APPLE-RAISIN OATMEAL

Makes 1 large serving

1 cup apple juice
2 tablespoons raisins
½ cup rolled oats

In a small saucepan, bring the apple juice and raisins to a boil. Stir in the oats. Cook, stirring often, until the oats are done, 3 to 5 minutes.

Nutritional information per serving: 325 calories, 7 gm protein, 70 gm CHO, 3 gm fat, 11 mg sodium, 571 mg potassium, 47 mg calcium, 5 gm dietary fiber. Count as 3 fruit and 2 grain.

BAKED APPLE

Makes 2 servings

This recipe was modified from one in Joy of Cooking by Irma Rombauer and Marion Becker (Bobbs-Merrill Company, 1975).

2 large McIntosh or Jonathan apples
2 tablespoons sugar
½ teaspoon cinnamon
1 to 2 teaspoons low-fat margarine (I Can't Believe It's Not Butter Light works well)
4 tablespoons fat-free or low-fat granola

Preheat the oven to 375°. Wash the apples and remove each core to ½ inch from the bottom. Remove the seeds. Combine the sugar and cinnamon. Fill the apple centers with the mixture. Dot the tops with low-fat margarine. Place the apples in a baking dish with ¾ cup boiling water. Bake for 30 minutes or until tender but not mushy. Top each apple with 2 tablespoons granola. Serve immediately.

Nutritional information per serving: 237 calories, 1.6 gm protein, 55 gm CHO, 3 gm fat, 68 mg sodium, 284 mg potassium, 23 mg calcium, 5 gm dietary fiber. Each serving counts as 2 fruit, ½ grain, and 1 sweet/sugar.

BLACK BEANS AND RICE

Makes 6 servings

This recipe was adapted from a recipe in New Recipes from Moosewood Restaurant (Ten Speed Press, 1987).

2 cups brown rice (yields 6 cups cooked)
Vegetable oil spray
1 tablespoon olive oil
1 medium onion, chopped
3 cloves garlic, minced
1 medium carrot, chopped
½ green bell pepper, chopped
½ teaspoon cumin
½ teaspoon coriander
1 tablespoon dried parsley
1 14.5-ounce can stewed tomatoes
Salt and pepper
2 15-ounce cans black beans, drained
Fat-free sour cream or yogurt

Begin cooking the rice. Meanwhile, coat a large skillet with vegetable oil spray. Add the olive oil and sauté the onion and garlic for 3 minutes. Add the carrot and continue cooking for 3 minutes. Add the green pepper and sauté 5 minutes more. Add the spices, tomatoes (with juice), and salt and pepper to taste. Simmer until the vegetables are tender. Add the beans. Simmer 10 minutes more. Serve over the brown rice with fat-free sour cream or yogurt.

Nutritional information per serving (1 cup beans over 1 cup rice without sour cream): 376 calories, 13 gm protein, 72 gm carbohydrate, 4.6 gm fat, 120 mg sodium, 704 mg potassium, 77 mg calcium, 8 gm dietary fiber. Count as 2 ounces protein and 3 grain servings.

BREAKFAST BURRITO

Makes 1 large serving (or 2 small servings)

Vegetable oil spray
1 teaspoon canola oil
1 teaspoon minced garlic
¼ cup chopped onion
1 small potato, cut into small chunks (about 1 cup)
¾ cup egg substitute
1 tablespoon fresh cilantro (or ½ tablespoon dried)
¼ cup grated fat-free cheese
¼ cup chunky salsa or Pico de Gallo (page 101)
2 flour tortillas
Salt and pepper

Spray a nonstick skillet with vegetable oil spray. Heat the canola oil and garlic over medium heat. Add the onion and potato. Cook, covered, over low to medium heat, turning occasionally, until potatoes are brown and tender. Pour the egg substitute over the potato mixture and continue to cook, stirring occasionally to break up the egg. When the egg is cooked, stir in the cilantro and cheese. Salt and pepper to taste. Top with salsa and serve with tortillas.

Nutritional information per recipe: 626 calories, 38 gm protein, 83 gm CHO, 16 gm fat, 1290 mg sodium, 1440 mg potassium, 417 mg calcium, 5 gm dietary fiber. Count entire recipe, including tortillas, as 2 grain, 2 high CHO vegetable, 1 low CHO vegetable, 4 protein, and 1 fat.

"BETTER THAN EGG-A-MUFFIN"

Makes 1 serving

Vegetable oil spray
1 piece Wholesome and Hearty Garden Sausage (found in natural foods section)
1 egg
1 large bagel, toasted
1 tablespoon low-fat mayonnaise
2 large tomato slices
Salt and pepper

Spray a nonstick skillet with vegetable oil spray. Over medium heat, begin heating the sausage. After a couple of minutes, break the egg into the pan. Break the yolk. Cook the egg and sausage on both sides until done, about 5 minutes total. Spread the bagel with mayonnaise and make a sandwich using the sausage, egg, and tomato slices. Sprinkle with salt and pepper to taste.

Nutritional information per recipe: 448 calories, 19.5 gm protein, 68 mg CHO, 10 mg fat, 661 mg sodium, 236 mg potassium, 239 mg calcium, 6 gm dietary fiber. Count as 4 grain, 1 protein, 1 low CHO vegetable, and 1 fat.

EASY MICROWAVE FISH

Makes 5 portions, about 3.5 ounces each

1 pound fish fillets (orange roughy is especially good, or try sole)
½ teaspoon salt
¼ teaspoon dill weed
⅛ teaspoon pepper (or to taste)
1 tablespoon chopped fresh parsley (or 1 teaspoon dried)
2 tablespoons lemon juice
1 tablespoon light margarine or light butter

Place the fish in a glass baking dish. Sprinkle the spices and lemon juice over the fish. Dot the fish with the margarine. Cover it with waxed paper and cook on high for 5 minutes or until the fish flakes with a fork. Let stand for 4 minutes before serving.

Nutritional information per 3.5 ounces: 95 calories, 17 gm protein, <1 gm CHO, 2 gm fat, 302 mg sodium, 363 mg potassium, 38 mg calcium, 0 gm dietary fiber. Count each serving as 3 protein.

BLUEBERRY/STRAWBERRY CRUNCHY "MILK SHAKE"

Makes 1 large serving, about 2¾ cups
Makes a good recovery meal.

6 ounces plain fat-free yogurt
1 cup apple juice
¾ cup frozen or fresh blueberries
¾ cup frozen or fresh strawberries
1 to 2 tablespoons maple syrup
2 tablespoons low-fat granola

Blend all the ingredients together. Use half of the fruit frozen to make it cold and "milk-shake-like."

Nutritional information per recipe: 409 calories, 13 gm protein, 88 gm CHO, 2.5 gm fat, 175 mg sodium, 1082 mg potassium, 421 mg calcium, 6 gm dietary fiber. Count as ½ grain, 4 fruit, 1 milk/yogurt, and 1 sweet/sugar.

BREAKFAST BEANS

Makes 2 servings

1 can plain black beans
4 whole eggs
½ cup Pico de Gallo (page 101)
4 flour tortillas

Pour the beans, including juice, into a nonstick skillet. When the beans are slightly warm, carefully break the eggs over the top of the beans. Cover and cook on low-medium until the eggs are poached. Carefully scoop out half of the beans with 2 eggs on top. Top with half the Pico de Gallo and serve with warm tortillas.

Nutritional information per serving: 635 calories, 33 gm protein, 86 gm carbohydrate, 18 gm fat, 1509 mg sodium, 691 mg potassium, 125 mg calcium, 13 gm dietary fiber. Count half the recipe as 2 high CHO vegetable, 1 low CHO vegetable, 2 protein, and 2 grain.

EASY AND YUMMY BEANS

Makes about 4½ cups

1 pound dried beans (pinto or Anasazi are my favorites)
1 can Rotel tomatoes
2 canned or 1 fresh jalapeño pepper, cut into very small pieces
Fresh garlic or garlic powder to taste
⅛ cup chili powder (or more if you like)
Salt

Boil the beans in water for 3 minutes and let them soak for 8 hours or so. (This method of soaking will help reduce flatulence.) Drain and add fresh water to about 2 inches above the top of the beans. Add all remaining ingredients. Bring the mixture to a boil and then let simmer, covered, until done—usually takes 3 to 4 hours. Stir every so often and check the water level. Keep just enough water to keep the beans from burning. Add a little salt, if needed, after the beans are cooked.

Nutritional information per ½ cup: 85 calories, 5 gm protein, 17 gm CHO, <1 gm fat, 124 mg sodium, 352 mg potassium, 40 mg calcium, 5 gm fiber. Count ½ cup as 1 plant protein *or* 1 high CHO vegetable.

PUMPKIN YOGURT

Makes 1¼ cups

8 ounces vanilla fat-free yogurt
½ cup canned pumpkin

Combine ingredients.

Nutritional information per recipe: 203 calories, 9.4 gm protein, 42 gm CHO, 0 gm fat, 111 mg sodium, 608 mg potassium, 283 mg calcium, 4 gm dietary fiber. Count entire recipe as 1 high CHO vegetable, 1 milk/yogurt, and 1 sweet/sugar.

JICAMA STICKS

Makes 8 servings

This recipe, slightly modified, was discovered in the Cuisine of the American Southwest *by Anne Lindsay Greer, Harper & Row, 1983.*

1 small-medium jicama
Several fresh limes
½ teaspoon chili powder (or paprika)
1 to 2 tablespoons fresh cilantro, chopped

Peel the jicama with a sharp knife and remove the fibrous, inner layer. Slice the white meat of the jicama into strips. Squeeze the lime juice over the jicama. Then sprinkle with the chili powder and cilantro.

Nutritional information is not available for this vegetable. Count as a low CHO vegetable serving.

LOW-FAT HUMMUS

Makes 1¾ cups

2 15-ounce cans garbanzo beans (chickpeas) with juice
1 teaspoon sesame oil
5 tablespoons lemon juice (bottled or fresh)
2 teaspoons minced fresh garlic
¼ teaspoon salt
½ teaspoon hot pepper sauce, such as Tabasco

Drain the beans and reserve the liquid. Blend the beans in a food processor. Gradually add the rest of the ingredients until smooth. Use the reserved liquid to thin the hummus, if needed. Consistency should be thick enough to spread on bread, but thin enough to eat as a dip.

Nutritional information per ½ cup: 128 calories, 6 gm protein, 21 gm CHO, 3 gm fat, 144 mg sodium, 300 mg potassium, 38 mg calcium, 4 gm dietary fiber. Each ½ cup counts as 1 plant protein *or* 1 high CHO vegetable

GRILLED TUNA

Makes 5 portions, 3.2 ounces each

This recipe was adapted from one by the National Fish and Seafood Council. I reduced the sodium content by using Worcestershire instead of soy sauce and omitting the salt.

1 pound fresh tuna, cut into 5 steaks

Marinade:
1 tablespoon lemon juice
2 tablespoons Worcestershire sauce
2 tablespoons orange juice
1 tablespoon tomato paste, no salt added
½ teaspoon minced garlic
½ teaspoon oregano
1 tablespoon chopped fresh parsley (or 1 teaspoon dried)
Pepper

Mix all ingredients for the marinade. Add the tuna, turning to coat well. Let the tuna stand at least 20 minutes in the marinade. Grill the fish for 5 minutes on each side, periodically basting with the marinade. Do not overcook, or the fish will be dry and tough. Note: Place the fish on a perforated pan on the grill to keep it from breaking apart when turning.

Nutritional information per serving: 179 calories, 27.5 gm protein, 3 gm carbohydrate, 6 gm fat (30 percent fat calories), 108 mg sodium, 396 mg potassium, 20 mg calcium, 0 gm dietary fiber. Count each serving as 3 ounces protein.

POACHED SALMON

Makes 4 servings, about 4 ounces each
This recipe is from a cookbook accompanying my Kenmore microwave.

1½ cups hot water
⅓ cup dry white wine
2 peppercorns
1 lemon, thinly sliced
1 bay leaf
1 teaspoon instant minced onion
1 teaspoon salt
2 large salmon steaks, about 8 ounces each

Pour the hot water and wine into a glass baking dish. Add the rest of the ingredients, except the salmon. Cook on high for 5 minutes, or until the water reaches a full boil. Carefully add the salmon steaks. Cover with plastic wrap or wax paper and cook on high for 2 to 3 minutes, until the fish becomes opaque. Let stand for 5 minutes to finish cooking. Discard the liquid. If desired, top with a small amount of plain yogurt mixed with dill weed or try Annie's No Fat Yogurt Dressing with Dill (found in natural foods section of grocery store).

Nutritional information for 4 ounces of salmon: 209 calories, 31 gm protein, 0 gm CHO, 8.5 gm fat, 60 mg sodium, 516 mg potassium, 52 mg calcium, 0 gm dietary fiber. Count ½ salmon steak as 4 protein.

PICO DE GALLO

Makes 16 servings, ¼ cup each
At my house, this dish goes quickly, so I always make a big batch. You may prefer to cut it in half. If the dish turns out too hot, dilute it with more tomato.

15 fresh jalapeño peppers
1 medium white onion
5 Roma tomatoes
4 tablespoons fresh cilantro (or to taste)
Pinch or two of salt

Wearing rubber gloves, carefully remove the stems and seeds from the peppers. (Depending on the peppers, this can be very hot and the seeds will only make it hotter. If you don't wear gloves, you will soon regret it!) Chop all the ingredients to a fine texture. An onion chopper or food processor is helpful, especially for the onions and peppers. However, the tomatoes can easily become too juicy, so chop them by hand. Gently mix all the ingredients. This dish should have very little juice; it isn't salsa. It is a wonderful condiment for eggs, fish, chicken, chili, and beans. You can use it in cooking or as a dip with fat-free tortilla chips.

Nutritional information per ¼ cup: 24 calories, 1 gm protein, 6 gm carbohydrate, <1 gm fat, 20 mg sodium, 216 mg potassium, 10 mg calcium, 1 gm dietary fiber. Count as 1 low-CHO vegetable serving.

SWEET POTATO FRIES

Makes 3 servings of about 6 fries each
This recipe is from the cookbook Meals Without Squeals *by Christine Berman and Jacki Fromer (Bull Publishing, 1991).*

1 small sweet potato (about 12 ounces)
1 teaspoon vegetable oil (canola or safflower)
Salt (optional)

Heat an oven to 375°. Peel the sweet potato and cut it into sticks or wedges. Toss them with the oil in a bowl. Spread the sticks on a baking sheet and bake for about 30 minutes, turning them halfway through the cooking period. If desired, sprinkle with a little salt before eating.

Nutritional information per serving: 84 calories, 1 gm protein, 17 gm CHO, 1.6 gm fat, 7 mg sodium, 240 mg potassium, 19 mg calcium, 2 gm dietary fiber. Count each serving, about 6 fries, as 1 high CHO vegetable.

STIR-FRY CHICKEN AND VEGGIES

Makes 2 large servings

This recipe was inspired, in part, by Jane Brody's "Simple Tofu Stir-Fry," in Jane Brody's Good Food Book, *published by W.W. Norton, 1985.*

Sauce:
¼ cup chicken or vegetable broth
1 tablespoon Worcestershire sauce
1 teaspoon lemon juice
1 tablespoon Mirin or dry sherry
6 ounces fettuccini noodles
Stir-Fry:
Pam or other nonstick cooking spray
1 teaspoon olive oil
1 teaspoon sesame oil (use chili oil if you like it really hot!)
1 tablespoon sesame seeds, preferably unhulled
1 tablespoon minced garlic
½ teaspoon crushed red pepper
6 ounces skinless chicken breast (or scallops)
2 carrots, sliced thin, on the diagonal
½ cup chopped onion
½ cup green peas, frozen
½ cup corn kernels, frozen
1 small zucchini, sliced thin

Mix together all sauce ingredients and set aside.

Cook the noodles in boiling water according to package directions. Meanwhile, coat a large nonstick skillet with cooking spray. Heat the olive and sesame oils over a medium flame. Add the sesame seeds, garlic, and red pepper. Sauté briefly and then add the chicken or scallops. Toss with the seeds and garlic to coat. Continue stirring while the chicken browns for about 2 minutes. Remove the chicken from the skillet and set aside.

Add the carrots and 2 tablespoons water to skillet. Reduce heat to low, cover, and cook until the carrots begin to soften, stirring occasionally. Remove the lid, add the onion, and cook, uncovered, 2 minutes more. Then add the peas, corn, and zucchini. Toss and cook for 1 minute. Then add the chicken and sauce. Toss all the ingredients well. Cover and cook

until heated thoroughly, about 3 minutes. Serve over fettuccini noodles.

Nutritional information per ½ serving: 646 calories, 43 gm protein, 91 gm CHO, 12 gm fat, 344 mg sodium, 140 mg calcium, 895 mg potassium, 10 gm dietary fiber. Count each serving as 3 grain, 2 low CHO vegetable, 1 high CHO vegetable, 3 protein, and 1 fat.

QUINOA SALAD WITH MINT

Makes 7 servings, 1 cup each

This recipe is adapted from one created by the chefs at Alfalfa's, a grocery store in Boulder, Colorado. It is light and easy to prepare. I especially like it served with seafood.

1 cup dry quinoa (a South American grain sold in natural foods stores)
1 quart water
½ tablespoon salt
1 cup cucumber, diced (peel if waxed)
¼ cup red onion, minced
1 cup celery, diced
2 tablespoons fresh mint, chopped
2 tablespoons fresh parsley, chopped
1 lime, juiced
2 tablespoons red vinegar
2 tablespoons extra virgin olive oil
Salt and pepper to taste

Rinse the quinoa according to the package directions. Bring the water and salt to a boil. Add the quinoa and cook for about 12 to 15 minutes. Drain the quinoa and let it cool. Prepare the other ingredients and mix them with the cooled quinoa. Serve chilled.

Nutritional information per cup: 142 calories, 6 gm fat, no cholesterol, 4 gm protein, 20 gm CHO, 2 gm dietary fiber. Count 1 cup as 2 grain.

ZUCCHINI HEALTH MUFFINS

Makes 8 large muffins

2¼ cups whole wheat flour
¼ cup sugar
¼ cup nonfat milk powder
1 teaspoon cinnamon
¼ teaspoon salt
1 teaspoon baking soda
½ teaspoon baking powder
½ teaspoon ginger
1½ medium zucchini, shredded
8 ounces plain nonfat yogurt
¼ cup pure maple syrup
¼ unsweetened applesauce
½ cup nonfat egg substitute (such as Egg Beaters)
1 cup seedless raisins
1 teaspoon vanilla extract
Extra applesauce for garnish

Preheat an oven to 350°. Spray 8 large muffin cups with nonstick cooking spray. In a medium bowl, combine the first 8 ingredients. Stir thoroughly. In a large bowl, combine remaining ingredients. Mix thoroughly with a wire whisk. Add the flour mixture to the zucchini mixture, mixing just until the flour is moistened. Spoon the batter into the cups. Bake for 30 minutes or until a toothpick inserted in the center of each muffin comes out clean. Cool the muffins thoroughly on a wire rack before removing them from the muffin pans. Eat plain *or* slice and heat under a broiler; serve with additional applesauce.

These muffins are flavorful, almost fat-free, and not as sweet as traditional zucchini muffins. To make them sweeter, use nonfat vanilla yogurt instead of plain or use additional sugar instead of the nonfat milk powder.

Nutritional information per muffin: 254 calories, 9 gm protein, 57 gm CHO, 0.8 gm fat (3 percent fat calories), 228 mg sodium, 502 mg potassium, 128 mg calcium, 5.7 gm dietary fiber. Count each large muffin as 1 grain and 1 sweet/sugar.

SPINACH OMELETTE

Makes 1 serving

Nonstick cooking spray
1 green onion, chopped (optional)
2 cups fresh spinach, torn into small pieces
½ cup Egg Beaters or other fat-free egg substitute (You can use 1 whole egg and 2 egg whites. This adds 5 grams of fat.)
Pinch of salt, pepper to taste
4 tablespoons fat-free or low-fat shredded cheese, any flavor

Coat a small, nonstick skillet with cooking spray. Over low-medium heat, cook the onion and spinach, covered, until the spinach is partially wilted, about 3 minutes. Pour the egg substitute over and around the spinach, covering the bottom of the skillet. Add pepper to taste and a pinch of salt. Cook on low until almost done. Sprinkle the cheese on top and continue to cook until the egg is set. To *finish* the omelette, either fold it in half and press it lightly to be sure all the egg is cooked *or* cook it under a broiler for a few minutes. Note: If you cook the egg with the lid on, it cooks fast and needs no *finish* step; however, the egg has a steamed flavor.

Nutritional information per recipe: 135 calories, 17 gm protein, 10 gm carbohydrate, 3.5 gm fat, 400 mg sodium, 747 mg potassium, 252 mg calcium, 2 gm dietary fiber. Count as 2 low CHO vegetable and 3 protein.

SHRIMP COWPOT

Makes 4 servings

Vegetable oil spray
1 tablespoon garlic, minced
1 small onion, chopped (about 1 cup)
1 tablespoon canola or olive oil
½ teaspoon lemon grass
½ teaspoon cumin
¼ teaspoon crushed red pepper
¼ teaspoon fennel seeds
¼ teaspoon salt
Pepper to taste
3 large carrots, sliced on the diagonal (about 2 cups)
1 bell pepper, chopped
1 small can (7 ounces) tiny shrimp, drained
2⅔ cups cooked brown rice (about 1 cup raw)
Soy sauce (optional)

Spray a large nonstick skillet with vegetable oil spray. Over medium heat, sauté the garlic and onion in the oil. When the onions are translucent, add the spices and carrots; reduce the heat. Cook, covered, until the carrots are just tender, about 5 minutes. Add the green pepper and cook until all the vegetables are tender. Add the shrimp and rice. Stir together and heat through. Season with soy sauce to taste, if desired.

Nutritional information per serving, without soy sauce: 300 calories, 12 gm protein, 52 gm CHO, 6 gm fat, 237 mg sodium, 509 mg potassium, 75 mg calcium, 6 gm dietary fiber. Count ¼ of recipe as 2 grain, 2 low CHO vegetable, 1 protein, 1 fat.

TANYA'S FROZEN YOGURT

Makes 1 large serving
My good friend Tanya Evtuhov shared this wonderful treat with me.

¾ cup frozen, unsweetened blueberries (or any other unsweetened, frozen fruit)
¾ cup nonfat, vanilla yogurt

Using a blender, thoroughly mix the fruit and yogurt. Eat right away or store in an airtight container in the refrigerator. Absolutely wonderful! Note: If you need to cut down on sweets, make this with artificially sweetened yogurt and save the CHO and calories found in the sugar.

Nutritional information per serving: 219 calories, 8.5 gm protein, 46 gm CHO, 0.7 gm fat, 106 mg sodium, 413 mg potassium, 259 mg calcium, 3 gm dietary fiber. Count as 1 fruit, 1 milk/yogurt and 1 sweet/sugar.

Power Nutrition Fitness Forms

Goals/Affirmation Sheet
Daily Record of Activity and Food Intake
Diet Worksheet

S A M P L E

G O A L S / A F F I R M A T I O N   S H E E T

Date: January 8 to February 18 (Use a 4- to 6-week time frame, the amount of time it takes to get a new habit started.)

Fitness Goals: (Set no more than 5 goals. Make them realistic and specific.)

1. Pack my lunch on Tuesdays and Thursdays.

2. Eat 5 servings of fruits and vegetables every day.

3. Drink a glass of water when I first wake up every morning.

4. Walk up and down 2 flights of stairs before lunch every day at work.

5. Do a 30-minute strength training routine twice a week.

Affirmation: (Make it a positive statement, using the present tense. The statement doesn't have to be completely true yet. The idea is to retrain yourself to think positively and to see yourself as successful.)

I Am Enjoying a Healthy Lifestyle.

G O A L S / A F F I R M A T I O N   S H E E T

Date: _____

Fitness Goals:

1. _____

2. _____

3. _____

4. _____

5. _____

Affirmation: _____

_____

_____

_____

D A I L Y   R E C O R D   O F   A C T I V I T Y   A N D   F O O D   I N T A K E

ACTIVITY	DURATION	DIFFICULTY

TOTAL TIME _____

FOOD INTAKE	AMOUNT	FOOD INTAKE	AMOUNT

DIET WORKSHEET

Use this form to determine your total calorie requirement and the grams of carbohydrate, protein, and fat to eat daily.

EXAMPLE

1. Multiply your weight by the appropriate factor to estimate baseline calorie needs.

   135-pound moderately active female

   Men: 11 _____ pounds × 11 = _____

   Women: 10 _____ pounds × 10 = _____

   135 pounds × 10 = 1350 baseline calories

2. Multiply your weight by the appropriate *activity factor** to estimate calories needed for activity.

	Sedentary	Light	Moderate	Heavy
Men:	3.2	6	7.2	10.5
Women:	3.0	5	6	9

   _____ pounds × _____(factor) = _____

   135 pounds × 6 = 810 activity calories

3. Add together the calories from 1 and 2 to estimate *total calorie needs* per day.**

   _____ + _____ = _____

   1350 + 810 = 2160 total calories

4. Multiply total calories by percent carbohydrate to get carb calories. Divide carb calories by 4 to get carbohydrate **grams.**

   _____ × _____ % = _____ carb calories

   2160 × 65% carbohydrate = 1404 carb calories

   _____ ÷ 4 = _____ carbohydrate grams

   1404 ÷ 4 = 351 carbohydrate grams

5. Multiply total calories by percent protein to determine protein calories. Divide protein calories by 4 to get protein **grams.**

   _____ × _____ % = _____ protein calories

   2160 × 15% protein = 324 protein calories

   _____ ÷ 4 = _____ protein grams

   324 ÷ 4 = 81 protein grams

6. Multiply total calories by percent fat to determine fat calories. Divide fat calories by 9 to get fat **grams.**

   _____ × _____ % = _____ fat calories

   2160 × 20% fat = 432 fat calories

   _____ ÷ 9 = _____ fat grams

   432 ÷ 9 = 48 fat grams

*Sedentary = little exercise and sit-down job; Light = some exercise or standing job; Moderate = exercise 3 to 5 times a week and/or moderately active job; Heavy = exercise 5 or more times a week or very active job, such as construction.
**If you need to lose weight, subtract 300 calories from your total calorie needs to determine calories for weight loss. Add 500 calories to total if you need to gain weight.

CHAPTER SIX

The Lower Back

BY BRYON HOLMES, M.S.

The Weak Link

The lower back is a key link in body wellness, and it plays an essential role in most weight-training movements. But people avoid training and using their lower backs, because of lower back problems, and/or fear of injury—when, in fact, these are the very reasons they should be exercising their lower backs. This chapter will dispel these misconceptions and fears, explaining how back pain starts and evolves, providing you with the knowledge and exercises to put you on the road to a healthy back.

The Interconnected System

All movement of the human body can be broken down to bones, ligaments, muscles, and tendons. Bones are connected to one another by ligaments to create the skeleton. Muscles are attached to the bones by tendons. It is contraction of the skeletal muscles that move the human frame. These systems are all intricately connected. The adage that a chain is only as strong as its weakest link can also be applied to the human body.

Structural strength in the human body is determined by the function of the work required by that body part. For example, the legs are stronger than the arms because they are required to do more work (carry the weight of the body). The racquet arm of a tennis player is stronger than his other arm. Not only are the muscles stronger, but the bone is denser and the ligaments and tendons are also stronger.

In many individuals, the lower back is the weak link. Lower back pain is a leading cause of lost work time, second only to the common cold. People will routinely exercise every muscle group but the lumbar extensors (low back). They have been instructed never to lift with their backs; and employers may require workers to use lumbar supports so they don't use their backs. No wonder the back is a weak link. If it is never exposed to workloads it never gets stronger; in fact, it gets weaker and becomes susceptible to injury.

The Unguarded Moment

An isolated human spine from a fresh cadaver can withstand only about five pounds of pressure before it buckles or collapses. This underscores the importance of soft tissue (muscles, ligaments, and tendons) that surround the spine and allow it to perform the normal physiological functions for which it is designed. All injuries occur when some external load or force exceeds an individual's structural capacity.

Ninety percent of all low-back pain may be attributed to soft-tissue damage. Most lower back injuries occur during an "unguarded moment." This usually occurs when an individual has to suddenly react to a change in his or her environment. It can occur when one turns, twists, stoops, or bends in an unusual manner. If the lower back is made stronger with regular exercise, it will be able to withstand greater external loads, and injury rates will decrease.

Acute and Chronic Pain

Back pain can be categorized into two phases: acute pain and chronic pain. Back pain is considered *acute* during the first six weeks. Most lower back pain (80 percent) will resolve itself within six weeks, regardless of any intervention. This explains why the most common medical advice during the acute phase is to take it easy and let the body heal itself. The use of passive modalities such as ice, heat, ultrasound, massage, acupuncture, acupressure, Rolfing, and chiropractic can make you feel better while your body recovers, but they provide no proven physiological benefit to accelerate the healing process.

When back pain continues beyond six weeks it is

considered *chronic.* An individual who is suffering from chronic lower back pain will subconsciously learn new muscle recruitment patterns that substitute for a weak and painful lower back. This is a primitive neuromotor survival strategy that allowed our ancestors to escape danger even in the event of injury. This phenomenon is obvious to anyone who has observed a wounded animal continue to be mobile despite its injuries. The natural reaction to back pain is to splint or guard any movements that require the back to work, temporarily preventing the back musculature from being exposed to external forces. This relieves short-term pain, but the long-term effects can be devastating. Pain leads to disuse; disuse leads to muscular atrophy; atrophy leads to weakness. Weakness predisposes an individual to recurrent injury because of the inability to withstand normal usage. This continuous cycle is referred to as the *chronic deconditioning syndrome.* Chronic disuse atrophy, or the deconditioning syndrome, can be compared to the case of an individual who has an arm in a cast for six to eight weeks. After removal of the cast, weakness in muscle strength is apparent. The human body physiologically adapts to the demands placed upon it. The muscle group in question has essentially adapted to no stimulation by allowing unused muscle to atrophy and weaken.

Rehabilitation

Strength of the trunk extensors is reduced in the patient with chronic back pain. Adequate strength of the trunk muscles is necessary for a return to full function. It is necessary to increase the functional and structural integrity of the lower back by increasing the competency of the soft tissues. In this manner, lower back pain is preventable and can be treated and managed successfully.

You can increase a muscle's contractile ability (strength) by exposing it to regular overload stimulation (strength training). In other words, by isolating and strengthening the muscles, you can treat and prevent back pain. Increasing your levels of strength increases your structural integrity and your ability to withstand the unguarded moment. Specific exercise is the only effective way to prevent lower back problems. It is also the only effective way to rehabilitate and control the recurrence of chronic low-back pain once it has developed.

In patients with chronic pain, the lumbar spine must be isolated during exercise to get stronger. During trunk extension, the hip flexors are the primary movers and the lumbar extensors are the secondary movers. If the lumbar extensors are to get strong, they must be isolated and exposed to greater workloads than usual. Then they become stronger and can withstand the unguarded moment. At the present time, there is only one device on the market that has a restraining mechanism that will isolate this area as the trunk extends—the MedX lower back machine.

Training Potential

In a study, a group of healthy subjects trained their lower backs one time a week for 10 weeks. This group had a 42 to 102 percent improvement in low-back strength doing just one set, one time per week. Most muscle groups will show a 20 to 30 percent improvement in strength with three sets of exercise, three times per week over a 12-week period. This suggests that the low-back muscles are chronically weak, compared to other muscle groups, even in the healthy populations. And it explains why 80 percent of the population suffers from low-back pain at some time during their lives.

Other Key Areas

It is important to know that other areas are important for a healthy lower back.

SHOULDERS AND ARMS

The shoulders and arms are an intricate part of the human kinetic chain. Most daily movements and routines require the use of the shoulders and arms. A balance of strength throughout the body is the key to leading a productive, injury-free life.

A main function of the low-back muscles is to stabilize the trunk as the shoulders and arms perform lifting and moving tasks in front of the body. If the shoulders and arms can function at levels significantly greater than the low back, then the low back will be injured as it attempts to stabilize greater forces than its structural capacity can maintain. On the other hand, if the shoulders and arms are weak, the natural reaction is to jerk the trunk in order to assist the shoulders and arms. This will lead to impact loads that result in injury to the shoulders or arms and also place the lower back at risk.

ABDOMINALS

Another vital area for a healthy lower back is the abdominals. Weak abdominal musculature allows the abdomen to sag, creating a greater load on the lower back, forcing it to hold up the mass in front of it. Strengthening the abdominals creates greater intraabdominal pressure, and increased pressure forces a more upright positioning of the spine, meaning better posture. The net result is a decreased load on the lumbar disks. Strong lower back muscles and strong abdominals work together in maintaining a pain-free healthy back.

UPPER BACK AND CHEST

As stated earlier, good posture is essential to lower back wellness. It is common for there to be an imbalance between the chest and back. Because we tend to do everything in front of us, the chest and shoulders tend to be stronger than the back, causing the upper torso to roll forward and shifting the torso into a forward posture. To alleviate this and to align the spine correctly, it is important to exercise the upper back as much as the chest. This will balance and center the torso, thereby improving posture.

HAMSTRING FLEXIBILITY

Flexibility in the hamstrings (backside of thigh) is important to the lower back because the hamstrings attach to the pelvis. The erector spinae in the lower back also attaches to the pelvis. A tight hamstring will prohibit the range of motion of the erector spine when one bends over (trunk flexion), thereby limiting its mobility and ability to gain strength through a full range of motion. One must maintain flexibility in the hamstrings in order to avoid this. A good exercise for this flexibility is the hamstring stretch on page 121.

Generally, range of motion is limited due to soft tissue: these can occur as intramuscular adhesions, as contractures in tendons, or as scar tissue. If you perform hamstring strengthening exercises through your full range of motion you will receive strengthening benefits about 15 degrees beyond where you stop. As your strength improves, you will now have the ability to overcome the resistance caused by the soft tissue and your range of motion will return to normal.

Lower back pain is usually caused by a combination of factors. If you have chronic lower back problems, it is important that you work with a qualified professional to treat the problem holistically.

The Exercises and Program

The following exercises will help strengthen the muscles of your lower back. They are listed in order of difficulty. Choose an exercise that fits your fitness level and incorporate it into your leg and buttocks routine. Do your lower back exercise at the end of your routine; this allows the back to remain strong and fresh while you perform your other exercises.

BASIC GUIDELINES FOR BACK STRENGTHENING

Always work within a range of motion in which you feel no pain. If it is painful to reach certain positions, then stop short of them during exercise. Exercises designed to increase strength will accomplish that increase 15 degrees beyond the end point of the movement. Therefore, stopping movement just prior to a position of discomfort will provide significant strengthening benefits beyond that range of motion. Never use a sudden movement when performing a strength exercise even though it is harder to do a slow, controlled movement. Sudden movements use momentum. By performing a slow, controlled movement, you will not be able to handle as much resistance, but muscular fatigue (overload) is still accomplished, and the risk of injury is greatly reduced.

LOWER BACK EXERCISES

Opposite Arm and Leg, on Knees: Start on all fours, resting on your hands and knees. You should look straight down; your head should be neither tucked nor looking up. From this position, simultaneously raise and straighten your right arm and left leg until they are parallel to the ground (or as close to parallel as you can without going past the parallel position). Hold for two seconds and come back slowly to the starting position. Repeat with left arm and right leg. Start with 10 repetitions on each side and build up to 20 repetitions. (Note: Never use momentum to complete your exercise; when you get tired, rest, then continue on.)

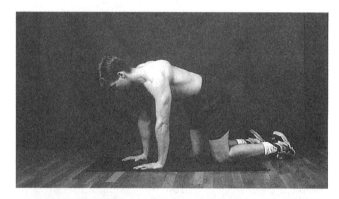

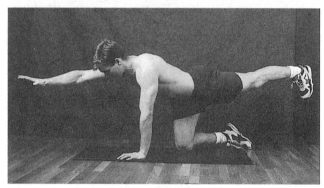

Opposite Arm and Leg, on Stomach: Lie facedown on the floor, arms extended overhead, palms on the floor. From this position, simultaneously raise your right arm and left leg to a comfortable height. Hold for two seconds and come back to the floor slowly. Repeat with left arm and right leg. Build up until you can complete 20 repetitions easily.

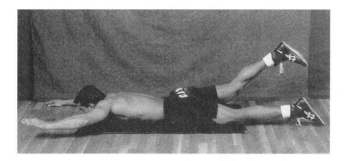

Basic Trunk Extension: Lie facedown, flat on the floor, arms at your sides. Place your heels under a support, such as a couch, or have a partner hold your ankles down; leave your arms at your sides. If you can do this exercise without raising your feet off the floor, you can do it without assistance. Slowly, raise your chest off the floor as high as you comfortably can. Hold for two seconds and come back to the floor slowly. Gradually increase until you can do 20 repetitions easily.

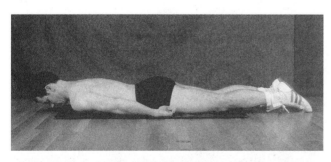

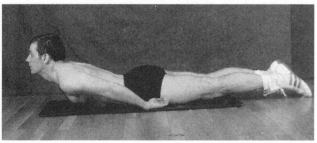

Intermediate Trunk Extension: Lie facedown with a firm pillow under your pelvis and arms at your sides. If necessary, place your heels under a support. Slowly, raise your chest off the floor to a comfortable height. Hold for two seconds and come back to the floor slowly. When you can do 20 repetitions easily, place another pillow or a rolled up towel under your pelvis. This will increase the difficulty and range of motion of the exercise.

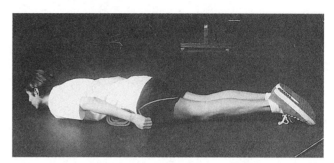

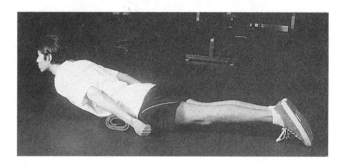

FOR THOSE WITH LOWER BACK PROBLEMS

If you have lower back problems, you face special challenges when working out. It is important for you to start slowly and build gradually. You may feel that you can do more during the early phases, but remember, it is quality, not quantity, that is important. If you skip to higher levels, you may not establish the necessary base of strength and you may injure yourself. So start with the first level and progress according to recommendations. Your lower back problems didn't develop overnight and restoration of function won't either.

When exercising, it is also important that you learn how to distinguish between good and bad pain, as discussed in Chapter 3. If you have a history of lower back pain, you should *not* exercise through spasm, lingering pain or shooting, peripheral pain. And remember, it is always imperative that you check with a doctor before beginning an exercise program.

Each exercise has a lower back rating. Check it before choosing exercises. *Low risk* does not mean the exercise is guaranteed to be safe for your back. It means you are at lower risk of injury. You should never jerk or perform sudden, extreme movements. Once you have developed a solid base of strength, you will be able to move to more advanced exercises. Just remember to go slowly and work with a doctor, physical therapist, or fitness trainer when in doubt.

The important thing to remember is, if you have a lower back problem, part of the problem is lower back weakness. You have to strengthen the weak area. Proper stretching and specific lower back exercises will help strengthen and prevent recurring back pain. If you take care of your back, it will last a lifetime, but strength and movement are the key. As we say in rehabilitation, "If it's not moving, it's probably dead."

Reference

Pollock, M., et al. "Effect of resistance training on lumbar extension strength." *The American Journal of Sports Medicine,* vol. 17, no. 5 (1989).

Putting It All Together

BY DEBORAH M. HOLMES, M.S.

MOTIVATION ⟶ **GOALS** ⟶ **ACTION** ⟶ **RESULTS**

Motivation and Body Image

Your wellness program begins with your own personal motivation. Without genuine motivation, it will surely fail. Do you believe that you are adequately motivated to achieve your fitness, health, and wellness goals? Because motivation is so important to your ultimate success, we've created this chapter to guide you in discovering your "motivation quotient."

We are all inundated by images in magazines, on television, and in films that imply a standard for what is healthy, what is fit, and what is acceptable. The impact that both the media and the fashion industry have had on the health and fitness industry—and the general public—has been profound. Just scan the magazine covers at your local supermarket. What is pre-sented as ideal is often an airbrushed fantasy image, a species of men and women who are all tall, slim, firm, tanned, and sparkling with health. But real human beings come in all shapes and sizes, and each of us has certain factors—genetic predisposition not the least—that contribute to our own, realistic "personal best." The emphasis should be on "personal." What the media has created is an unattainable, homogenized ideal that leaves all of us lacking and negatively impacts our self-esteem and body image. Because of this, health professionals are working overtime to try to counteract it.

The "body image" subject has become so important that most of the professional organizations in the fitness world now provide seminars and training in helping clients develop healthy body images. We know by working with clients of every body type and stature that overcoming this body image problem is a difficult and ongoing process.

What really motivates you? What "motivated" you to buy this book? Do you want to look like the cover of this book? Or do you want to look the best that *you* can possibly look? And are you merely looking for the next "quick fix" or are you interested in improving your knowledge of training essentials? These questions demonstrate some of the healthy and unhealthy motivations that might have led you to buy this book and embark on a new fitness program.

The first step is honestly and realistically evaluating your goals. Once you understand these motivations—both healthy and unhealthy—you can better direct your actions toward reaching your goal. From fitness, diet, and body image to financial, relationship, or even spiritual goals, a clear understanding of motivation makes all the difference.

Often family members, spouses, children, and the media itself can put undue pressure on you to lose weight, work out, change jobs, give up favorite foods, etc. But the fact is that these changes can occur—and can *last*—only when the motivation for them comes from you and your true desires. As you work your way through the following questionnaire, make sure that your motivations are strictly personal. Do not succumb to the opinions or preferences of others.

What Is Your Motivation?

Answer each question honestly and realistically.

1. List three reasons why you want to begin or change your exercise program.
   a.
   b.
   c.

   Are you being pressured into starting this program? _____
   If so, by whom or by what? _____

2. List three things that you dislike about your body.
   a.
   b.
   c.
3. What can you do to improve on these three body parts?
   a.
   b.
   c.
4. List three things that you like about your body.
   a.
   b.
   c.
5. What behaviors are you willing to give up in order to make the improvements that you want to accomplish?
   a.
   b.
   c.
6. What behaviors are you willing to add to your daily routine in order to achieve these improvements?
   a.
   b.
   c.
7. When will you begin to make these changes? _____
8. How many days a week will you perform these changes? _____
9. Who will be your biggest support during these changes? _____
10. What reward will you receive when you accomplish your goal?_____

Analyze your answers to these questions so that you can assure yourself that your motivations are healthy and self-directed.

Body Image Improvement Sheet

Take the following measurements when you begin your program. Use the last column to record what you would

BODY IMAGE IMPROVEMENT SHEET

	Date: _____	Date: _____	Date: _____	**GOAL** Date: _____
	Weight: _____	Weight: _____	Weight: _____	Weight: _____
	% body fat: _____	% body fat: _____	% body fat: _____	% body fat: _____

MEASUREMENTS

Shoulders	_____	_____	_____	_____
Chest	_____	_____	_____	_____
Waist	_____	_____	_____	_____
Hips	_____	_____	_____	_____
Right thigh	_____	_____	_____	_____
Left thigh	_____	_____	_____	_____
Right arm	_____	_____	_____	_____
Left arm	_____	_____	_____	_____
Right calf	_____	_____	_____	_____
Left calf	_____	_____	_____	_____

WHAT'S REALISTIC?

Weight loss: 1 to 2 pounds per week (this may vary by body size)

Inches lost: a combined total of 1 to 2 inches for every 5 pounds lost (this may vary by body size)

Percentage body fat decreased: 1 to 2 percent for every 5 pounds lost (for people 10 to 20 pounds overweight)

1 percent for every 5 to 10 pounds lost (for people less than 25 pounds overweight)

like to achieve (your target or goal measurements). If possible, have all your measurements taken by a fitness professional. In three months take follow-up measurements, and do it again every three months until and after your fitness goals are achieved. (Your results will be more accurate if the same fitness professional takes all of your measurements each time you have them taken.)

Make sure that your goals are both challenging and achievable. Setting goals that are unachievable will sabotage your success.

If you have a goal that is going to be very difficult to reach, be sure to break your end goal down into smaller subgoals. (See Chapter 4 for a full explanation of effective goal setting.) For example, if you are beginning a weight-loss program with a desired end goal of 30 pounds lost, begin with the more manageable goal of 15 pounds in three months, or even 8 pounds this month,

SEVEN KEYS TO WELLNESS

PHYSICAL DEVELOPMENT

Concerns your physical body. It includes your daily exercise and activity programs, your cardiovascular and strength fitness programs, your development of flexibility, and the maintenance of an active lifestyle in general. The physically well person is also concerned about good food and nutrition, not abusing tobacco, drugs, or alcohol, getting adequate sleep, wearing an auto seat belt, getting adequate medical care, etc.

EMOTIONAL DEVELOPMENT

Emphasizes awareness and acceptance of one's feelings. The emotionally well person maintains satisfying relationships with others while feeling positive and enthusiastic about his or her own life. He or she makes an effort to maintain minimal levels of stress and develop healthy feelings, using emotional outlets in a constructive way.

INTELLECTUAL DEVELOPMENT

Encourages creative, stimulating mental activities. An intellectually well person uses all resources and knowledge available to improve personal skills and creative thought processes. Intellectual stimulation is vital for a healthy human being.

SOCIAL DEVELOPMENT

Relates to your community and physical environment. A socially well person emphasizes interdependence and pursues harmony with family, friends, and associates. This person has developed healthy ways to interact, react, and live with all people involved within his or her life as well as with nature.

VOCATIONAL DEVELOPMENT

Encourages the pursuit and growth of one's attitude toward his or her work. A vocationally well person seeks jobs that bring personal satisfaction and enrichment into life. The desire for financial security is another motivating factor in vocational development.

SPIRITUAL DEVELOPMENT

Involves seeking meaning and purpose in human existence. A spiritually well person forms a strong appreciation for the experience of being alive and acknowledges an interdependence with the natural forces that exist in the universe. The spiritually developed person asks the big questions about the meaning of existence and explores his or her own relationship with the universe.

ENVIRONMENTAL DEVELOPMENT

Recognizes the impact that the environment has on our individual lives. An environmentally healthy person takes personal and social responsibility for the earth.

then 8 pounds next month, until the goal has been reached. Give yourself a reward when a subgoal has been reached. If you fall off the wagon, don't punish yourself for it. The damage from one small lapse is nothing compared to the damage of a lifetime of overeating and underexercising; when you have a lapse, remember that you are just a single moment away from getting back on track, if you choose to support yourself by keeping your commitment.

Remember, you're in this game for the long haul. Over the course of your life, your goals and motivations will change. What you do consistently over this span of time will determine the quality of your life.

What Is Wellness?

What is wellness? For the most part, wellness is a lifestyle. Enhancing wellness depends upon your ability to be responsible for how you live and the choices you make about your health. It means taking responsibility for yourself and taking an active role in improving every aspect of your daily life in order to achieve and remain in a healthy state of living.

Each of us is different. These differences are what make up our personal profiles, and each of our profiles are as different as we are as individuals. Our genetics, our upbringing, our physical structure, our needs, our wants and everything in between make us who we are.

In spite of these differences, we're all human beings and we have much in common. The biggest similarity is our dependence on good health and overall wellness. Each of us must make continual choices in our lives in order to maintain good health. These include eating properly, taking medications, trying to reduce stress in our lives, getting enough sleep, and exercising. Happily, as important as good health is, simple adjustments in lifestyle can make a big difference. The more balanced these seven elements become in your life, the higher your personal wellness profile will become.

We are all affected by these seven dimensions in our daily lives to some degree. If we look at the whole picture as a pie chart divided into seven sections, each piece represents a dimension of wellness. If there is a problem within one piece of the pie then the rest of the pie will be affected somehow. The hub of "wellness"

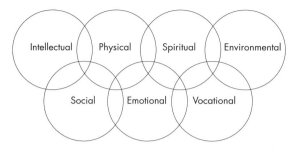

will be disturbed until that piece of the pie is healed.

One dimension of your life can directly affect many of the other wellness dimensions. For example, if you recently fell and broke your ankle, we would say that your physical wellness has been taxed. Because of this, vocational wellness might suffer if your job requires you to be active and/or you missed days from work due to your injury. It's also likely that you would be stressed emotionally, not to mention the social impact of an injury vis-à-vis family and friends. Everything is intermingled to create that web of wellness that makes up our different wellness profiles.

It's important to understand that every pie chart will be different. For instance, a professor at a university may have a larger piece of pie for intellectual stimulation than a mother, whose social and family interactions are most important. An athlete would have a larger piece of "physical well-being" than a minister of a church whose religious beliefs are a higher priority. Each one of our pie charts will reflect our individuality.

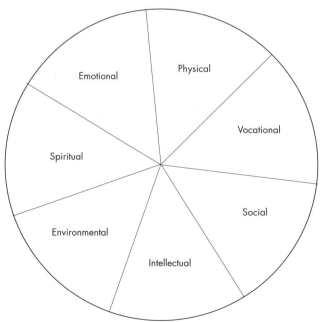

When you are reading this book and studying the benefits of strength training, pay attention to your wellness profile. Your entire wellness profile will be affected by the addition of or changes to your exercise program. You need to assure yourself that when you begin this new exercise program, all dimensions within your wellness profile will support it. For example, will you be able to fit this exercise program into your work schedule? Will you be able to afford this exercise program financially? Will you have a social support system?

Creating stronger muscles is extremely important and affects the physical dimension of your profile. However, having strong muscles will not, by itself, put you in a state of optimal health; it is only one small step toward improving your entire wellness profile. Living in the world today involves strengthening all the dimensions of your wellness profile. After all, wellness *is* the lifestyle you have chosen to live.

Developing Your Exercise Routine

As we have seen, factors affecting physical wellness include medical care, nutrition, and exercise. Exercise has a tremendous impact on overall physical wellness; let's look at what is involved with exercising for health.

The many benefits of exercise include stress reduction, weight loss, cardiovascular benefits, increased muscular strength and endurance, and increased flexibility. Other lifestyle benefits include increasing overall life span, increased quality of life, decreased risk of developing lifestyle diseases such as diabetes, hypercholesterolemia, hypertension, and coronary artery disease.

The three components of physical exercise are cardiovascular exercise, muscular strengthening and endurance, and flexibility. To have a well-rounded physical wellness profile you need to include each of these three components in your exercise program.

CARDIOVASCULAR FITNESS

Cardiovascular fitness is achieved by performing activities that tax the heart, lung, and circulatory systems. When cardiovascular exercise is performed, the body puts a demand on the oxygen exchange systems of our bodies. Oxygen is taken in from the lungs into the circulatory system, then distributed to the muscles that are being used during exercise. The oxygen then helps break down the stored fats into energy for use by the working muscle. This entire exchange system forces the lungs and heart to become extremely efficient, so that the working muscles can continue their activities.

The American College of Sports Medicine states that 30 minutes of cardiovascular exercise at least three times a week is sufficient to receive health benefits. A cardiovascular program consists of activities that allow you to reach 65 to 85 percent of your maximum heart rate for a duration of no less than 20 minutes. The kinds of exercises that we are discussing are walking, jogging, swimming, bicycling, and aerobic dancing. Maintaining these kinds of exercises longer than 20 minutes may provide additional benefits if performed correctly.

The following formula is a simple, effective, and accurate way of calculating your target heart rate.

Finding your target pace:

220 − your age = (_____) number of beats per minute
(_____) × .65 = *lower end of target*
(_____) × .85 = *upper end of target*

How to figure out your 10-second pulse check: Divide both the upper and lower target numbers by 6. (This will give you the number of beats you should count when checking your pulse for 10 seconds during exercise.)

When you are in the middle of your exercise session, take a 10-second heart rate count, by checking your pulse at your wrist or on your neck. You need to be somewhere within the upper and lower ends of your target pace.

STRENGTH TRAINING

Strength training provides increased strength gains and increased endurance to the muscles, joints, bones, and ligaments of the body. The kind of benefits we can achieve with strength training include developing a stronger posture and structural features, stronger bones, increased strength for daily activities, increased muscle tone and flexibility, and improved strength in the joints.

Strength training should include exercises designed for all major muscle groups of the body, and should be performed at least two to three times per week. Strength training can be done in a variety of ways: free weights, strength machines, or body weight. There are a variety of strength-training programs that will help you to achieve the benefits you seek.

Your strength-training program needs to include exercises for all parts of your body. You should train the larger muscle groups first, followed by your smaller muscles near the end of your workout.

Do not begin any strength program without proper instruction from someone educated in the field of strength training. Learning proper form and concepts from the beginning will allow for a safe and effective exercise program.

When beginning your program, be sure to choose an exercise weight that will allow you to reach a point of

EXERCISES TO CHOOSE FROM

BACK
Pullovers
Upright rows
Bent-over rows
Single-arm rows
Lat pull-down (behind the neck)
Lat pull-down (to the chest)
Rear flys
Low back extensions

LEGS
Leg extensions (quadriceps)
Leg curls (hamstrings)
Squats
Lunges
Abduction exercises
Adduction exercises
Calf raises

CHEST
Bench press
Flat bench flys
Incline bench press
Incline flys
Pullovers
Wide arm push-ups

TRICEPS
Dumbbell supine extensions
Dumbbell upright extensions
Triceps kickbacks
Close grip bench press
Close grip push-ups
Dips

SHOULDERS
Lateral raises
Military press
Front raises
Delt raises
Rear flys

BICEPS
Barbell curls
Dumbbell curls
Concentration curls
Hammer curls

EXTRAS TO ADD
Side bends
Neck exercises
Forearm strengthening
Abdominals

fatigue within a reasonable number of repetitions. Reaching fatigue means performing the maximum number of lifts after which you cannot lift the weight another time during the set. It's important that you not get hung up on numbers; don't get stuck on always doing sets of 10, or 16, or 20. You need to determine the set number each time you exercise; write down the number of repetitions that you have done after each exercise; then on the next day that you exercise, attempt to do more repetitions. When you are comfortably lifting between 12 and 16 repetitions, you need to increase the training weight in your next exercise session.

FLEXIBILITY

Flexibility is usually the most neglected element of a training program. Flexibility training works the muscles, ligaments, and joints, which is important for the maintenance of posture, joint mobility, range of motion, and helps keep the ligaments and tendons from tightening. Flexibility training needs to be done at least three times a week, and should provide stretches for all major muscle groups and joints.

Don't Overdo It: Its important that you begin your comprehensive exercise program slowly and increase your exercise levels as you feel comfortable. A safe way to begin your stretching program is to start with one stretch for all major body parts, and to learn to perform the stretch properly. While performing the stretch, maintain the stretch for 10 to 15 seconds, then perform it a second time.

As you feel more confident with your stretching program, you can increase the intensity by adding more specific stretches; by increasing the duration, to hold the stretches for 15 to 30 seconds; or by increasing the number of times that you perform each stretch. It's important to begin and end your exercise program with stretching.

Neck Stretch: Each movement should be done once; then move on to the next movement without resting. From a standing position, drop head forward, chin to chest. Hold for 10 seconds. Looking straight ahead, lower your right ear to your right shoulder. Hold for 10 seconds. Lower your left ear to your left shoulder. Hold for 10 seconds. Gently raise your head up to center. Use your hands for support as shown.

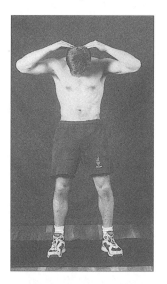 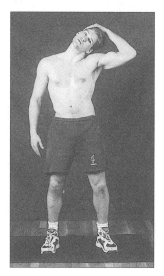

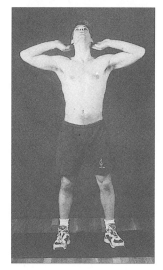

Shoulder Roll: Standing, raise your shoulders high on your neck and roll them backward. Perform five reps. Then repeat the movement, but roll your shoulders forward. Perform five reps. Then bring your shoulders up toward your ears and hold for a count of five and release.

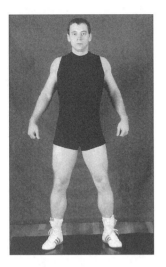

Shoulder Stretch: On your knees, grasp hands in front of your body and turn palms forward while fingers remain interlocked; stretch shoulders forward, as you reach out as far as possible, rounding your back. Hold for 15 seconds and perform two reps. Maintain hand position, stretch up, straight overhead. Hold for 15 seconds and perform two reps.

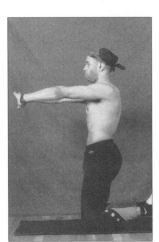
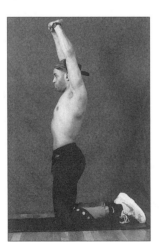

Side Bend: Stand with your feet together, arms fully extended over your head, hands touching. Bend at your waist over your right side. Hold position for 10 seconds. Then bend at your waist over left side. Hold this position for 10 seconds.

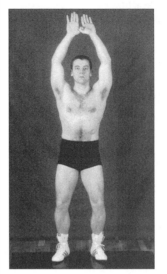
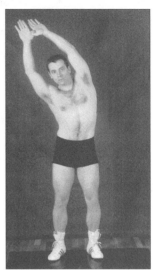

Side Bend Two: Spread legs wide. Bend at your waist, letting one hand slide down the leg while the over hand goes easily over your head. Slowly come up and perform the movement on the other side.

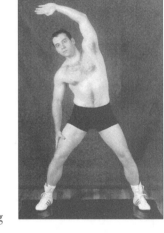

Knees-to-Chest Hug: Lie flat on your back; bring both knees to your chest. From this position, wrap your arms around your legs and hug your knees to chest, as you bring your chin to your chest. Hold for 15 seconds.

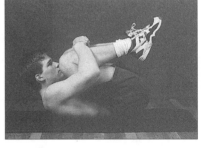

Knees to Side: Lie flat on your back, knees bent, feet flat on floor. Let both legs fall to one side. Hold for 10 seconds. Then let the legs fall to the other side. Hold for 10 seconds.

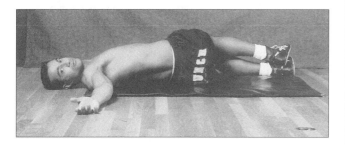

Elongation Stretch: Lie flat on your back, arms fully extended over your head, legs fully extended on the floor. Extended from your fingertips to your toes, lengthen your body in both directions. Hold for 15 seconds.

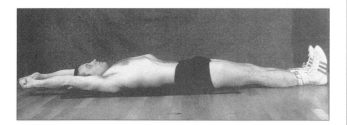

Hamstring Stretch: Lie on your back, legs extended. Grab one leg behind the knee and gently pull it toward your head. Hold for 15 seconds. Repeat with the other leg.

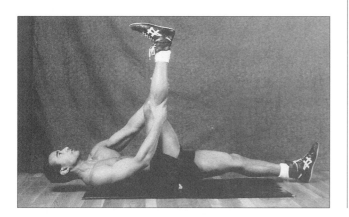

Quadriceps Stretch: Turn on one side and lie comfortably with shoulder under ear. Reach back for your top ankle and gently pull back. Then switch sides. Hold on each side for 15 seconds.

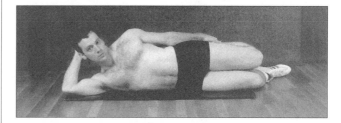

Back and Stomach Stretch: Lie on your stomach, hands under your chest (palms down). Slowly pressing up with your arms, straighten elbows as much as you can and arch your back. Relax lower body. Look up, attempting to get your chin as high as possible. Hold for 15 seconds.

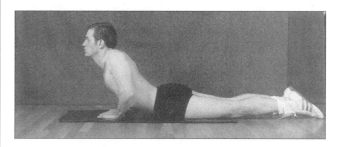

Back Arch: Come up on your hands and knees (on all fours). Place hands under your shoulders and hunch your back up like a cat and lower your head. Hold for 15 seconds and perform two reps. Then arch your back in the opposite direction. Hold for 15 seconds and perform two reps.

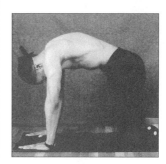 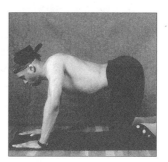

Chest Stretch:
Kneeling erect,
clasp your hands
behind your lower
back and slowly try
to extend your hands
up and back. Hold
for 15 seconds.

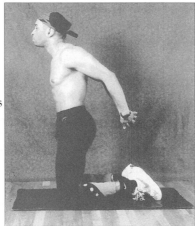

Rag Doll: Standing
with your knees
slightly bent, let your
torso hang down like
a rag doll. Give in to
gravity and let any
excess tension roll
out your fingertips.
Then slowly, vertebra
by vertebra, build
your spine back up to
standing, your head being the last thing up.

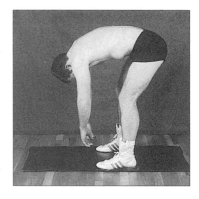

ADVANCED STRETCHING

As you continue to get stronger with your exercise program it would be beneficial to increase your stretching program to include more specific stretching techniques. Stretching at the end of a hard workout is a very good way to alleviate tightness, cool down the muscles, and help avoid unnecessary soreness the following day.

When beginning your stretching program, please consult an exercise instructor so that you will know proper form and procedures for stretching.

Groin Stretch: Sitting
upright on the floor,
bring the soles of your
feet together, as close to
the body as possible.
Gently add pressure to
the inner thighs with
elbows pushing down for
greater stretch. Hold for
15 seconds.

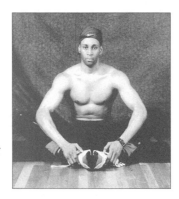

Back Stretch: Sit on
floor with both legs extended. Lean your torso forward
and lightly grasp your knees, elbows pointed out. As
you become more flexible, you can grasp farther down
your legs. Hold for 15 seconds and repeat.

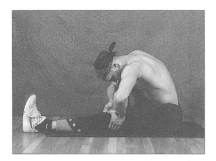

Getting Started

We hope that with this information you will be able to "put it all together." Discover your motivations, set your goals, and begin your program.

OUTLINE FOR CARDIOVASCULAR EXERCISE

WEEKS 1 AND 2:

	5 minutes easy pace
	5 minutes target pace
	5 minutes easy pace
Total time:	15 minutes

WEEKS 3 AND 4:

	5 minutes easy pace
	5 minutes target pace
	2 minutes easy pace
	5 minutes target pace
	5 minutes easy pace
Total time:	22 minutes

WEEKS 5 AND 6:

	5 minutes easy pace
	10 minutes target pace
	2 minutes easy pace
	10 minutes target pace
	5 minutes easy pace
Total time:	32 minutes

WEEKS 7 AND 8:

	5 minutes easy pace
	15 minutes target pace
	2 minutes easy pace
	15 minutes target pace
	5 minutes easy pace
Total time:	42 minutes

MAINTENANCE: (AFTER 8 WEEKS):

	5 minutes easy pace
	10 to 30 minutes target pace
	5 minutes easy pace
Total time:	20 to 40 minutes

OUTLINE FOR STRENGTH TRAINING

WEEKS 1 AND 2: PERFORM 1 SET OF EACH

1 exercise for your back
1 exercise for your chest
1 exercise for your shoulders
1 exercise for your biceps
1 exercise for your triceps
1 exercise for your quadriceps
1 exercise for your hamstrings
Beginning abdominals exercise

WEEKS 3 AND 4: PERFORM 1 SET OF EACH

2 exercises for your back
2 exercises for your chest
1 exercise for your shoulders
1 exercise for your biceps
1 exercise for your triceps
1 exercise for your quadriceps
1 exercise for your hamstrings
1 exercise for your calves
Abdominals exercise

WEEKS 5 AND 6: PERFORM 1 SET OF EACH

3 exercises for your back
2 exercises for your chest
2 exercises for your shoulders
1 exercise for your biceps
1 exercise for your triceps
1 exercise for your quadriceps
1 exercise for your hamstrings
1 exercise for your total legs/gluteals
1 exercise for your calves
Abdominals exercise

WEEKS 7 AND 8:

Begin two sets of each exercise.
Continue adding variety into your program.

MAINTENANCE:

Continue at two to three sets of each exercise.
Mix up your workout, allowing for variety.
Continue to increase weight when needed.

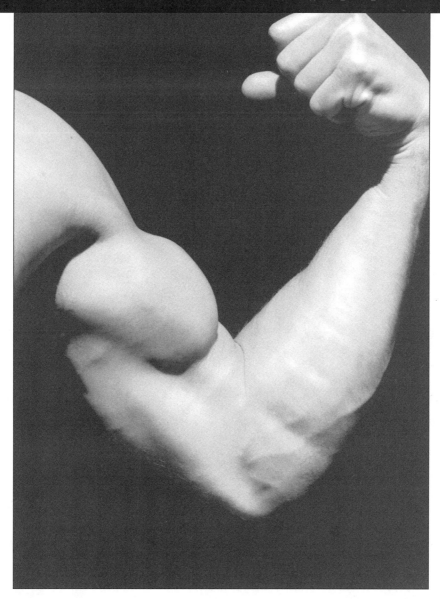

PART THREE

The Exercises

Introduction to the Exercises

There is a huge variety of exercises that work your shoulders and arms. Most exercise books or videos give you between 10 and 20 from which to choose. In this book you will receive more than 100 different exercise variations. You are given such an extensive selection and variety of exercises so that you can find exactly the program that works for you, and reduce the boredom factor. This will keep you motivated for the long haul, which is what you will need to achieve the shoulders, arms, and traps of your dreams.

When reading through the exercises in the following chapters, use this chapter as a reference to answer any question that may arise.

A Key to the Exercises

Each exercise is presented in a uniform format. Take the time now to familiarize yourself with this format; it will help you to make informed choices. Here is an explanation of the format and its categories:

DIFFICULTY LEVELS

The exercises are ranked from 1 to 3: 1 is the easiest, 2 is intermediate, and 3 is advanced. Choose exercises that correspond to your fitness level and exercise experience. These are, of course, general categories. Depending on your individual strengths and weaknesses, you will find particular exercises more or less difficult than the next person does. Remember, increasing difficulty is a way to increase intensity, which causes desired muscle adaptation. So, as a general guideline, start with the easier exercises, build strength, and advance to more difficult movements.

LOWER BACK

Because everybody's lower back is different, we rank each exercise according to "risk" factor. The ranking system is a warning: Proceed carefully. If you have a history of lower back problems, you need to exercise with extra care. You should also consult a doctor to discuss exercise in relation to your specific problem and help identify which exercises you may want to avoid. Again, these rankings are general guidelines to help you find the appropriate exercises that fit your needs and experience.

The three lower-back rankings are: Low Risk, Moderate Risk, and High Risk. These rankings are based on a combination of the following criteria:

1. *The direction of motion involved in the movement.* Movements that involve raising a weight above your head involve more risk than movements that do not.
2. *Posture and type of movement.* If you are performing an exercise that requires you to lift the weights up, there is a greater risk when the torso is upright in a standing or seated position, or when the torso is bent in a standing or seated position. If, however, you are performing an exercise that requires you to push the weight down, the risk is diminished.
3. *External support.* The more external support the lower back has, the safer the movement will be. Therefore, any movement where you keep your lower back pressed against the floor, wall, or a seat back is generally safer than movement without such support.

   It is important to discuss the use of weight belts to support the lower back at this time. Weight belts are a useful tool to support the lower back while exercising. However, they are often overused. When performing exercises for the shoulders and arms, you will stabilize the exercise with your lower back. This helps to further strengthen the lower back. When you utilize a weight belt, you eliminate most of this opportunity to strengthen the lower back. You need to develop a logical strategy of when to utilize a weight belt. Generally speaking, the best strategy is not to use a belt when performing high volume (low poundage) exercises, and to use a belt when performing low volume (high poundage) exercises, especially those movements that involve pressing a weight over your head. This, of course, is an individual decision and should be based on your needs and level of fitness.

4. *Motor skill rating of the exercise.* An exercise that is more difficult to coordinate is also potentially more difficult to stabilize. Consequently it has more potential to put the lower back at risk.
5. *Speed of movement.* Explosive or hard-to-control movements such as a Push Press or upper body plyometrics (the designing of exercises to link speed and strength) for the shoulders and arms have the potential to be stressful to the lower back.

It is also important to note that an increase in the intensity (weight) of any exercise can create stress on the lower back. Improper technique also can always create stress on the lower back. Knowing the general principles that are involved with lower back strain gives you the tools to modify your exercise selection to fit your lower back needs.

AREA

The exercises are grouped according to the muscles they work: shoulders, trapezius, triceps, biceps, and forearms. The shoulder exercises are further grouped into the area of the shoulder they work: front, side, back, rotator cuff. Being able to visualize and feel the muscles you are working is essential to understanding the exercise and getting the most out of your workouts.

INSTRUCTION

This is the exercise itself: the starting position, movement, and finish.

TRAINER'S TIPS

This section acts as your personal trainer. Some of the tips will be specific to the exercise. Others will be constant reminders, tips that are true for every exercise. You need to hear these tips over and over until they become second nature. The following tips are essential for working the shoulders and arms:

- Keep motion controlled (especially on the eccentric phase) so you can feel constant tension.
- Feel your muscles work (focus on the correct area) and try to maintain tension through both ranges of the motion.
- Use caution if you have lower back problems. Bouncing the weight at the bottom of a movement or jerky motions can make the exercise potentially dangerous.
- Maintain correct upper torso posture. Keep knees bent slightly in all standing positions.
- When performing an exercise where the elbow is going to lock out, decelerate as you near the lockout.
- Always use proper breathing technique (see page 24).
- Always keep neck and back in alignment. Don't look up, down, or to the side. Look straight ahead.

Speed of Movement

It is important to follow certain guidelines in regard to the speed at which you do the exercises. There are two basic types or classifications:

1. *Concentric, or Positive, Phase*—Move with authority or explosiveness (one to two seconds).
2. *Eccentric, or Negative, Phase*—Move under control (three to four seconds).

How explosive you are on the concentric phase depends on several factors: (1) how long you've been working out (a minimum of four weeks); (2) why you are training (sports, general condition, rehabilitation); (3) variety in training. This means you also have to cycle explosive movements when planning your program.

Controlling the eccentric phase (e.g., lowering the weight from a bent arm to a straight arm on a Dumbbell Curl) is very important to get the maximum training effect in a workout and also to prevent injury. If you force the muscle to work on the eccentric phase rather than relying on gravity or momentum, you will receive the maximum benefit throughout the full range of motion. Also it is common to hurt yourself on the eccentric phase by letting gravity take the weight down; using gravity puts the joint and muscle under undue stress because of the potential bouncing at the end of the motion and because when the muscle relaxes (loses control), it has to suddenly regain control again.

Following these guidelines on speed is very important in getting the most out of your workout, and guaranteeing that you will have a safe workout.

Eccentric Emphasis Training

At some point you may wish to perform eccentric emphasis training. Generally, it is best to emphasize the eccentric (negative) phase after you have reached concentric failure, meaning that you have reached your maximum output during the concentric (positive) phase of the exercise, and cannot continue. For example, you're doing Barbell Curls and you cannot curl the bar up for another rep. You have reached muscular failure in the concentric (positive) phase. Now you require assistance in curling the weight up in the concentric phase. At this point, a partner can "spot" you, helping you to curl the weight up for at least one more rep. Now you can lower the bar in a controlled and slow motion for another eccentric rep. This allows you to reach maximum potential for both phases of the exercise. In such cases, you may take as long as five to 10 seconds on the eccentric phase. Or you may add weight, so you need help curling the weight up in the concentric phase. Then lower the weight in a slow, controlled motion. In either case you are attempting to overload the eccentric phase by increasing the intensity through its range of motion.

Pulsing

Pulsing is holding a movement at the top of its range of motion, then moving back and forth, about one to two inches, keeping constant tension on the muscle being exercised. This tiny movement pumps the muscle. An example would be performing Triceps Push-Downs taking the elbow to a lockout and then bending and straightening within a range of one to two inches.

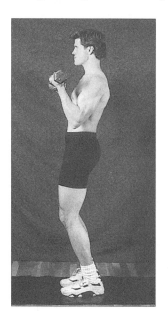
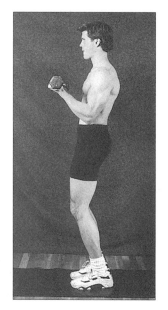

Bars, Grips, Hand Positions, and Attachments

There are numerous ways you can create variety: (1) different types of bars; (2) different types of grips; (3) different types of hand positions; or (4) different types of cable attachments. These allow you to create variety for the same exercise (e.g., Lateral Raise with the hands pronated, supinated, or neutral) or change the muscle focus (e.g., Close Grip Bench Press allows you to focus more on the triceps, as opposed to a Medium Grip Bench Press, which would focus more on the chest).

BARS

Using different bars can change the angle at which the muscle is working.

Straight Bar: Commonly used in shoulder, trap, triceps, biceps, and forearm work.

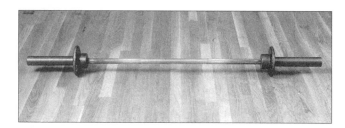

Curl Bar: Used primarily in triceps, biceps, and forearm work, but can also be used in shoulder and trapezius exercises. You can create different angles using this bar by gripping on the different angles of the bar.

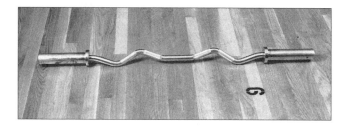

French Curl Bar: Adds variety to your arm workout and allows you to safely use a neutral grip, taking pressure off wrists.

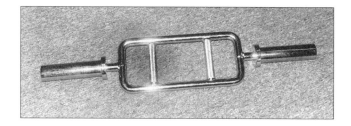

GRIPS

When visiting your local gym you will see fitness enthusiasts performing the exercises shown in this book with a wide variety of grips. Different grips can also change the angle of the exercise (e.g., performing a Straight Bar Curl with a close grip or a wide grip) or they can create an entirely different exercise (e.g., using an underhand grip to perform a Straight Bar Curl as opposed to using an overhand grip to perform a Reverse Curl). Varying the grip you use can alleviate two major problems—training plateaus and mental boredom—thus allowing you to train with more enthusiasm and intensity. Grip variation also helps in specificity, or training for specific adaptations. If an activity requires you to push overhead with a narrow grip, then you would want to narrow the grip on your military press.

With these principles in mind, let us look how changing hand position affects the specifics of and adds variety to your workout.

There are five variations of grip:

Underhand Grip:
Grab the bar or dumbbell with palms facing up and thumbs facing out. This grip is most commonly used in biceps and forearm work, but can also be used to change the angle in some triceps, shoulder, and trapezius exercises.

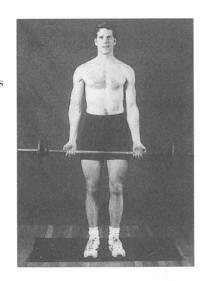

Overhand Grip:
Grab the bar or dumbbell with your palms facing down and your thumbs facing in. This grip is most commonly used in triceps, shoulder, and trapezius work, but can also be used to change the angle in some biceps and forearm exercises.

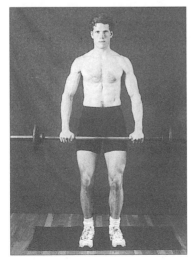

Close Grip: With an overhand or underhand grip, grab the bar in the center. The distance between both hands on the bar can vary from both hands next to each other and touching, to about six inches apart—how far apart depends on what is comfortable for you. This grip is used primarily in triceps and biceps work, but can also be used in some trapezius and forearm exercises.

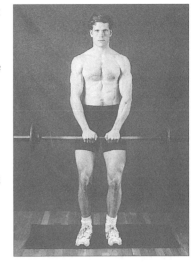

Medium Grip:
Using an overhand or underhand grip (whichever the exercise requires), grab the bar with your hands, shoulder width or slightly wider. This grip is used primarily for shoulder, trapezius, biceps, and forearm work, but can also be used in some triceps exercises.

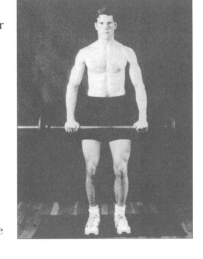

Wide Grip: Using an overhand or underhand grip (whichever the exercise requires), grab the bar about six to 18 inches outside shoulder width—how wide depends on what is comfortable for you. This grip can be used to change

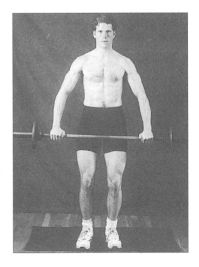

the angle for the muscle in shoulder, trapezius, triceps, biceps, and forearm exercises.

Shoulders: The main function of the deltoid muscles is to move the upper arm. Assisting the deltoids in moving the upper arm are the muscles of the shoulder girdle (see Chapter 2: "Body Basics"). Movement of the lower arm is generally initiated by either the biceps or the triceps.

MILITARY PRESS (PAGE 153)

Wide Grip: In this position, your grip is wider than the elbows. Lifting the bar vertically would involve the use of the deltoids (mostly medial and anterior). Since the elbows are nearly fully extended there is little use of the triceps to reach full extension. Thus this movement emphasizes mostly the deltoids but through a limited range of motion (motion of the bar). The posterior deltoids are activated by bringing the elbows back when moving the bar behind the neck. Keeping the bar behind the head will also take emphasis off the chest muscles.

Medium Grip: With this grip the arms are bent at a right angle. The bar can be placed behind or in front of the neck (if performing in the front keep your head forward, not up, as this promotes back arch and more use of the pectoralis muscles). With the movement of the upper arm, the deltoid muscles are recruited in the same manner as with the wide grip. With the elbows bent more at the start of the movement, the involvement of the triceps will be greater through a full range of motion.

Close Grip: With the bar in front of your neck, you grip the bar with your hands shoulder width apart. From this position the anterior (front) head of the deltoid is emphasized along with more emphasis on the triceps muscles.

UPRIGHT ROW (PAGE 158)

Wide Grip: With a wide grip (hands at least a foot wider than the hips), the bar is elevated vertically by bringing the elbows and hands up. The medial head of the del-

toid (shoulder abduction) is the prime mover, with the biceps assisting as you raise the bar.

Medium Grip: The hands grasp the bar where they naturally hang down (just outside the hips). This grip will involve all three heads of the deltoid (medial, anterior, and posterior), with the medial very active. With increased arm flexion there is more activity from the biceps.

Close Grip: Grasp the bar with hands thumb width apart. This grip emphasizes the shoulders as in the previous grip, with more biceps involvement than the previous two grips. With all grips the shoulder girdle is utilized.

Triceps: The triceps extend the arm (opposite of flexion, increasing the angle of the joint).

TRICEPS PUSH-DOWN (PAGE 186)

Close Grip: Hands are placed thumb width apart, with an overhand grip. Stabilizing upper arm and extending hands down isolates the triceps.

Medium Grip: Place hands shoulder width apart and push down as technique description states. With a medium grip and upper arm stationary, the emphasis is again on the triceps. If elbows flair out, shoulders and chest become more actively involved.

Wide Grip: As with the medium grip, the key for the wide grip (wider than shoulder width) is to keep the elbows in tight. If the grip becomes too wide and forces the elbows out, the shoulders and chest become actively involved and the isolation of the triceps is diminished.

Biceps: The biceps flex the arm (the opposite of extension, decreasing the angle of the joint). The effect of hand variation with the biceps is much more subjective in that it doesn't bring about recruitment of other muscle groups. All grips with biceps exercises isolate the biceps. The following is based upon empirical evidence by bodybuilders.

BARBELL CURL (PAGE 211)

Wide grip: Placing the hands wider than the elbows constitutes a wide grip. In theory this grip will widen the biceps (from inside to outside).

Medium Grip: Grasp the bar with the hands even with the elbows. This grip will enlarge the biceps from front to back.

Close Grip: Grip the bar with hands inside the elbows. The narrow grip will increase the size of the biceps peak.

Let us emphasize here that the component that most positively or negatively affects the ultimate outcome of the exercise is the intensity of the exercise. That's right, the same old philosophy that we hammer into your brains through this series of books. If you used a big rock, with the appropriate intensity you would make gains. You must reach momentary muscular exhaustion (MME) for the prescribed number of repetitions.

Let's face another fact: At one time or another we all have stopped short because of MME. MME is uncomfortable if not downright painful, and reaching it is an acquired skill.

Remember that by changing your hand positions you can affect the muscle groups being exercised. Be very careful about this: Sometimes too much variation is not good. Proper adaptations take place with consistency. Don't change for the sake of changing. See Chapter 19, "Creating Your Own Routine." Exercises in this book are described for specific reasons, in almost all instances you will be better off if you adhere to the specific descriptions for these exercises.

HAND POSITIONS

Changing the hand position can influence the angle of the exercise on the muscle. It also may allow you to perform certain exercises (with a new hand position) that will feel less stressful on the shoulder or elbow in your particular case. The three hand positions are:

Pronation: When the hand is pronated it is rotated so that the thumb is turned toward the body. To perform an exercise with a pronation, you would maintain this hand position throughout the exercise.

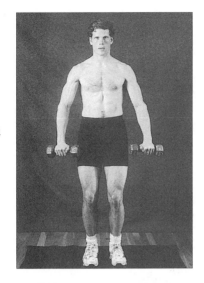

Supination: When the hand is supinated it is rotated so that the thumb is turned away from the body. To perform an exercise with a supination, you would maintain this hand position throughout the exercise.

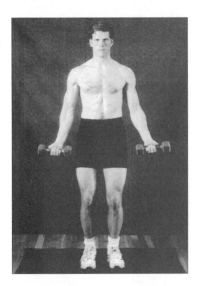

Neutral: When the hand is neutral it is turned so that the thumb is facing forward. To perform an exercise with a neutral hand, you would maintain this hand position throughout the exercise.

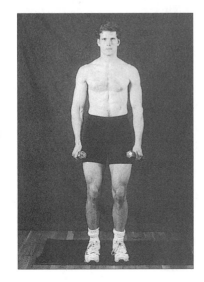

CABLE ATTACHMENTS

There are numerous attachments you can use on a cable pulley system to create new angles and allow you to perform a variety of exercises. In fact there are so many that it would be impossible to cover all the various and unique devices you may run across. The following are the most common attachments you will find at various clubs:

V-Bar: The name describes it. Shaped like a V, it is most commonly used to work triceps (e.g., Triceps Push-Down)

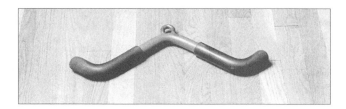

Cable Straight Bar: As the name implies, this is a straight bar that can be used for traps, triceps, biceps, and forearm work.

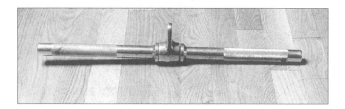

Cable Curl Bar: Shaped like a regular curl bar, this can be used for trapezius, triceps, biceps, and forearm work.

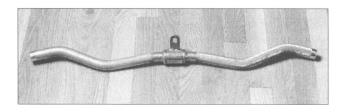

Rope: This is a rope that has a hook in the middle so that it can be attached to a cable system. It is used primarily for triceps work but can be adapted (use your imagination) to exercises for other muscle groups. One benefit it provides for triceps work is the ability to flair your hands out when the arms are extended so that the triceps can be taken through a greater range of motion.

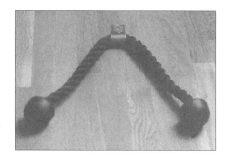

Single Handle: This is a handle you can perform with one arm. It can be used in shoulder, triceps, biceps, and forearm work.

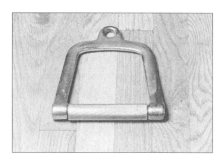

POSITION FOR
CABLE CROSS OR PULLEY WORK

When performing cable work it is important to observe two things: distance and posture. You must position yourself far enough away from the weight stack so you will be safe during the raising and lowering of the stack. You must also be far enough away so you can perform the exercise and not let the weights rest on the stack before you have completed your full range of motion. Posture is also important. It will vary according to the demands of the exercise.

As you try out these exercises, remember: Train hard, train smart.

DESCRIPTION OF ATHLETIC POSITION
FOR LIFTING

Checklist: Here is what your position should be: knees bent, feet shoulder width apart, chest out, shoulders back, lower back straight (not hunched, but maintaining its natural curvature). Your weight should be evenly distributed on both feet, and head, shoulders and hips should be aligned with the spine, your eyes focused straight ahead.

ABDOMINAL SUPPORT

In the exercise tips you will often be told to support your movements with your abdomen. This means your abdominal muscles should be activated, helping to stabilize and balance your body. It is a place of readiness and strength.

CHAPTER NINE

The Shoulders

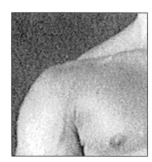

Exercise:
Front Raise

DIFFICULTY: 2
LOWER BACK: MODERATE RISK
AREA: ANTERIOR DELTOID

STARTING POSITION: Sit on edge of bench or stand with feet shoulder width apart and knees slightly bent. Hold both dumbbells so that they hang down at your sides with the back of your hands facing forward.

MOVEMENT: Raise both dumbbells directly in front, to shoulder level. Then lower to starting position under control.

   Variation: This movement can be done one arm at a time and leaning on a bench for support. Or the movement can be performed with a barbell weight plate.

TRAINER'S TIPS:
• Maintain good posture throughout the exercise.
• Focus your mind on the front of your shoulder throughout the exercise.
• Avoid arching your lower back as you lift.
• Try to keep your trapezius disengaged or down throughout the exercise.
• Do not raise outside the body. Instead, angle toward the center of the body.

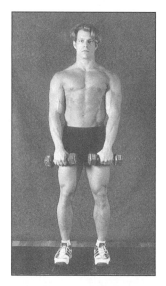
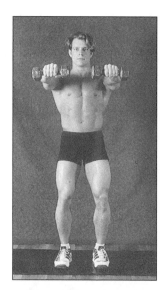
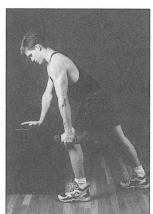
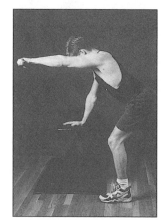

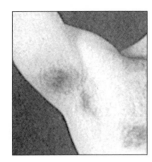

Exercise:
One-Arm Overhead Front Raise

DIFFICULTY: 2
LOWER BACK: MODERATE RISK
AREA: FRONT

STARTING POSITION: Sit on edge of bench or stand with feet shoulder width apart and knees slightly bent. Your upper torso should be vertical with your back straight and chest up. Hold the dumbbell so that it hangs down at your side with your thumb facing in (or pronated). Your arm should be straight, or slightly bent at the elbow. Position other arm on hip.

MOVEMENT: Maintaining arm position, raise dumbbell forward and up over your head. Lower to starting position under control. Perform required repetitions and repeat with other arm.

Variations: You can change the angle of the exercise by performing it with neutral hands (thumbs facing forward). This exercise can also be performed with both shoulders at the same time or by alternating repetitions with each shoulder. Another alternative would be to use a low cable or a rubber band.

TRAINER'S TIPS:
• Maintain good posture throughout the exercise.
• Focus your mind on the front of your shoulder throughout the exercise.
• Avoid arching your lower back as you lift. Support your midsection throughout the exercise.
• Try to keep your trapezius disengaged or down throughout the exercise.
• Do not raise your arms outside the body. Swing the dumbbell in a straight forward motion and up over your head.

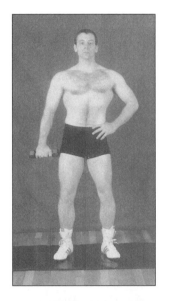

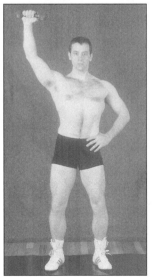

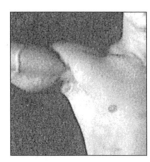

Exercise:
45-Degree Raise

DIFFICULTY: 2
LOWER BACK: MODERATE RISK
AREA: MEDIAL DELTOID, ANTERIOR DELTOID

STARTING POSITION: Sit on edge of bench or stand with feet shoulder width apart and knees slightly bent. Hold both dumbbells hanging down at your sides. Hands can be neutral (thumbs facing forward), pronated (thumbs facing in), or supinated (thumbs facing out).

MOVEMENT: Raise both dumbbells so that they are halfway between the side of your body and the front of your body. Elevate to shoulder level. Lower to starting position under control.

TRAINER'S TIPS:
• Maintain good posture throughout the exercise.
• Avoid arching your lower back as you lift.
• Focus your mind from the middle to the front of your shoulder throughout the exercise.

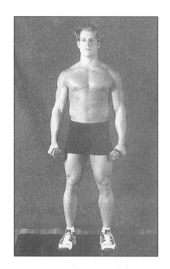

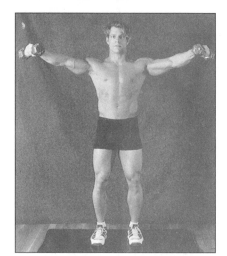

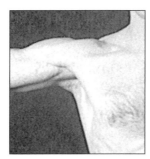

Exercise:
Lateral Raise

DIFFICULTY: 2
LOWER BACK: MODERATE RISK
AREA: MEDIAL DELTOID

STARTING POSITION: Sit on edge of bench or stand with feet shoulder width apart and knees slightly bent. Let the dumbbells hang down in front of your body. Hands can be neutral (thumbs facing forward), pronated (thumbs facing in), or supinated (thumbs facing out).

MOVEMENT: Raise both dumbbells laterally (to the side) from your sides until they reach shoulder level. Lower under control to starting position.

   Variation: This exercise can be done on the cable machine with a cross grip, with one or two arms. Another variation is to extend the cable from behind your body.

TRAINER'S TIPS:
• Maintain good posture throughout the exercise.
• Avoid arching your lower back as you lift. Support midsection with your abdomen throughout exercise.
• Try to keep your trapezius disengaged or down throughout the exercise.
• Focus your mind on the sides of your shoulders.
• Keep elbows slightly bent throughout the movement.

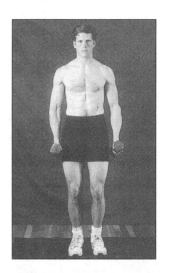

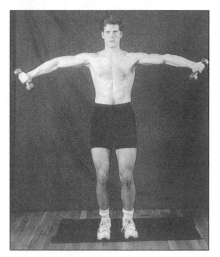

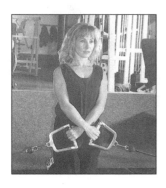

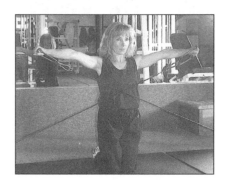

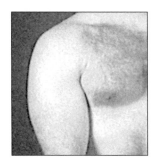

Exercise:
One-Arm Overhead Cross-Lateral Raise

DIFFICULTY: 2
LOWER BACK: MODERATE RISK
AREA: SIDE AND BACK

STARTING POSITION: Stand with feet shoulder width apart and knees slightly bent. Your back should be straight and your chest up. Hold a dumbbell with your right hand, crossing your right arm toward your left hip. Your arm should be straight, or slightly bent at the elbow, and the back of your hand should be facing forward (pronated). Position other hand on hip.

MOVEMENT: Maintaining this arm position (keeping arm straight), raise the dumbbell forward and diagonally until it is fully extended above your head. Lower to starting position under control. Perform the required repetitions and repeat with your other shoulder.

   Variations: This exercise may also be performed with a low cable or rubber bands.

TRAINER'S TIPS:
• Maintain good posture throughout the exercise.
• Focus your mind on your shoulder throughout the exercise.
• Avoid arching your lower back as you lift. Support your midsection throughout the exercise.
• Try to keep your trapezius disengaged or down throughout the exercise.

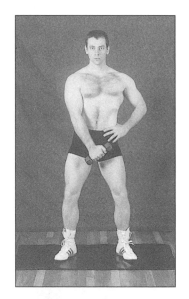

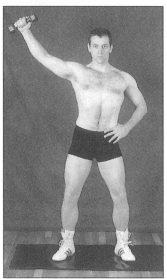

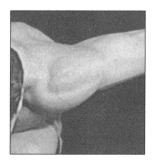

Exercise:
Rear Delt Raise

DIFFICULTY: 2
LOWER BACK: MODERATE RISK
AREA: POSTERIOR DELTOID

STARTING POSITION: Sit on edge of bench. Bend forward at the waist so that your chest is a couple of inches above your knees. Your back should be flat and your head should be aligned with your back. Hold both dumbbells so that they hang at your sides, behind your lower legs, hands neutral (thumbs facing forward), and arms slightly bent.

MOVEMENT: Keeping your chest down and back flat, raise both dumbbells up (not back) until they are parallel to the ground or close to parallel. Lower to starting position in a controlled manner.

   Variation: Leaning on a bench for support, do single arm raises.

TRAINER'S TIPS:
• Maintain your body position throughout the lift.
• Avoid arching or rounding your lower back as you lift.
• Think of bringing your elbows toward your ears as you raise the dumbbells.
• As you raise the dumbbells you can pronate or maintain neutral position.

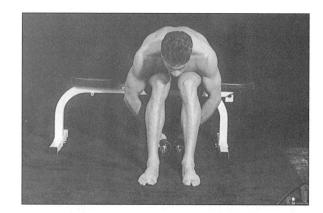

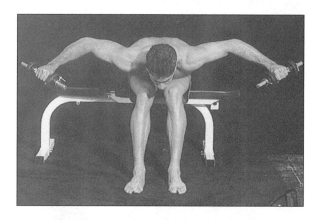

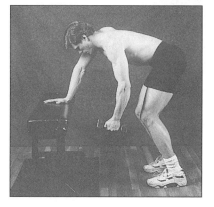

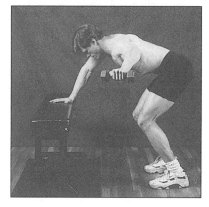

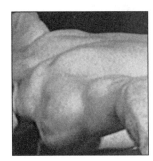

Exercise:
Prone Rear Delt Raise

DIFFICULTY: 2
LOWER BACK: MODERATE RISK
AREA: POSTERIOR DELTOID

STARTING POSITION: Assume the prone position on a bench. Your torso should be resting on the bench with your head hanging over the edge. Hold dumbbells so that they hang down at your sides (perpendicular to your body), shoulders protracted, hands neutral (thumbs facing forward), and arms slightly bent.

MOVEMENT: Raise both dumbbells until they are parallel to the ground. Concentrate on lifting the elbows; the arms can remain slightly bent. Lower to starting position under control.

   Variation: This can also be done on an incline bench.

TRAINER'S TIPS:
• Maintain your body position throughout the lift.
• Think of bringing your elbows toward the ceiling as you raise the dumbbells.
• Concentrate on pinching your shoulder blades together as you raise the dumbbells.
• Focus your mind on the back of your shoulders during the exercise.

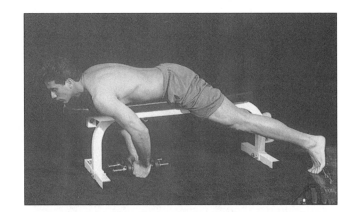

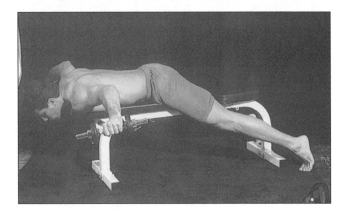

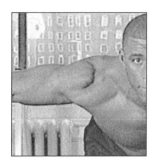

Exercise:
Rear Delt Cable Raise

DIFFICULTY: 2
LOWER BACK: MODERATE RISK
AREA: POSTERIOR DELTOID

STARTING POSITION: Attach handles to lower pulley and center yourself between cable cross machine. Grasp cable handles with a cross-hand grip (left hand, right cable; right hand, left cable). Keep your hands neutral (thumbs facing forward) and arms slightly bent. Your back should be flat and your head should be aligned with your back.

MOVEMENT: Keeping your chest down and back flat, raise both handles up (not back) until arms are parallel to the ground or close to parallel. Lower to starting position in a controlled manner.

   Variation: This movement can also be done with dumbbells.

TRAINER'S TIPS:
• Maintain your body position throughout the lift.
• Avoid arching or rounding your lower back as you lift.
• Think of bringing your elbows toward your ears as you raise the cable handles.
• Concentrate on pinching your shoulder blades together as you raise the cable handles.
• Focus your mind on the back of your shoulders during the exercise.

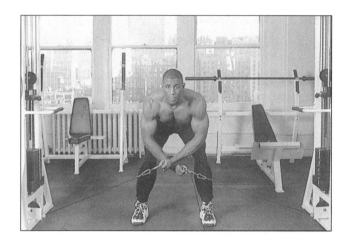

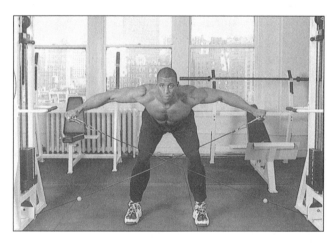

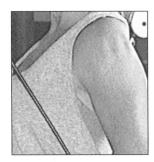

Exercise:
Cable Straight-Arm Pullback

DIFFICULTY: 1
LOWER BACK: LOW RISK
AREA: POSTERIOR DELTOID

STARTING POSITION: Stand facing the cable and weight stack. Position yourself away from the stack so the plates are raised (not resting on the stack). Your working hand should hang at your side, elbow slightly bent, holding the cable handle, attached to the upper or lower pulley, with the palm facing forward or back. Feet should be placed shoulder width apart; pinch your shoulder blades together and back.

MOVEMENT: Keeping your arm extended and your shoulder blades pinched together and back, pull the cable back. Return under control to original starting position. After completing desired number of repetitions, repeat with other arm.

TRAINER'S TIPS:
• Maintain good posture throughout the exercise.
• Keep shoulder blades pinched together and back throughout the exercise.
• Avoid twisting the upper torso when you pull.
• Concentrate on pinching your shoulder blades together as you move the cable handles.
• Focus your mind on the back of your shoulders during the exercise.

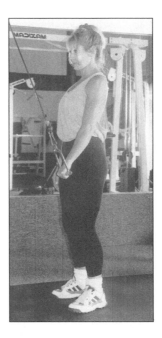

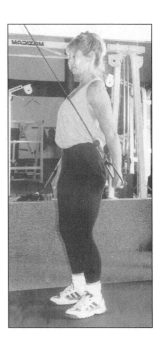

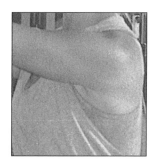

Exercise:
Rear Delt Rope Pull

DIFFICULTY: 2
LOWER BACK: LOW RISK
AREA: POSTERIOR DELTOID

STARTING POSITION: Facing the cable weight stack with the rope attachment secured to the upper pulley, grasp the rope and kneel, positioning yourself away from the weight stack so that the weight plates you are going to use are raised (not resting on the plates that aren't being used). Keeping your torso stable and in correct lifting position, extend your arms so that your hands are together and at forehead level.

MOVEMENT: Keeping your arms extended (with a slight bend at the elbow), your back properly aligned, and your torso still, pull the rope by moving out and back with your hands. As the resistance is raised keep the elbows at shoulder level and pinch your shoulder blades together. Return under control to the starting position.

TRAINER'S TIPS:
• Maintain proper lifting position throughout the exercise.
• Avoid initiating movement with torso.
• Focus your mind on the back of your shoulders throughout the exercise.
• Squeeze shoulder blades together.

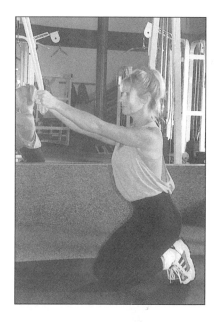

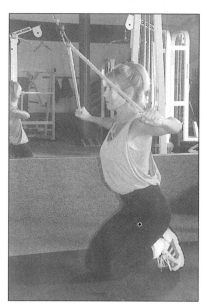

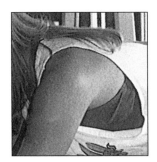

Exercise:
Rear Delt Rope Raise

DIFFICULTY: 2
LOWER BACK: HIGH RISK
AREA: POSTERIOR DELTOID

STARTING POSITION: Stand facing the cable weight stack with the rope attachment secured to the lower pulley. Grasping the rope, position yourself away from the weight stack so that the weight plates you are going to use are raised (not resting on the plates that aren't being used), while your arms hang at your side. Keeping your knees slightly bent and feet shoulder width apart, bend at the waist until your torso is parallel to the ground. Your arms should be extended (in the direction of the low pulley), hands together.

MOVEMENT: Keeping your arms extended (with a slight bend at the elbow), your back flat, and your torso still, raise the rope by pulling out and up with your hands. As the resistance is raised take the elbows up, not back, and pinch your shoulder blades together. Return under control to the starting position.

TRAINER'S TIPS:
• Keep back flat and neck aligned throughout the exercise.
• Avoid initiating movement with torso.
• Focus your mind on the back of your shoulders throughout the exercise.

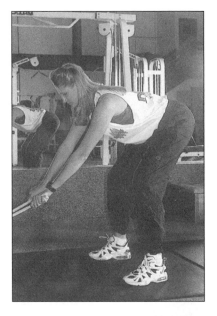

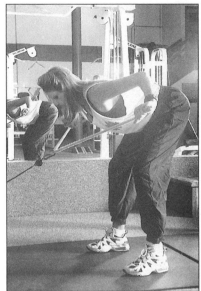

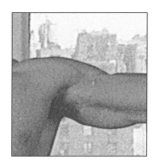

Exercise:
Horizontal Extension/Flexion

DIFFICULTY: 2
LOWER BACK: MODERATE RISK
AREA: ROTATOR CUFF

STARTING POSITION: Sit on edge of bench or stand with feet comfortably apart and knees slightly bent. Hold both dumbbells so that they hang down at your sides with the back of your hands facing forward. Hands can be neutral (thumbs facing forward) or supinated (thumbs facing out). Raise both dumbbells directly in front to shoulder level and slightly toward the center.

MOVEMENT: Move both dumbbells laterally (out), or away from the midline, keeping them at shoulder level and parallel to the ground. From the extended position, return the dumbbells to the center along the same plane. This constitutes one repetition.

Variation: This exercise can be performed with a cable machine or on a bench in a supine or prone position.

TRAINER'S TIPS:
• Maintain good posture throughout the exercise.
• Move at a controlled speed.
• Focus your mind on the front of your shoulders throughout the exercise.

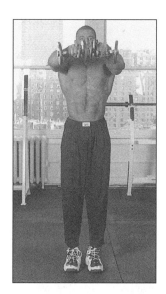

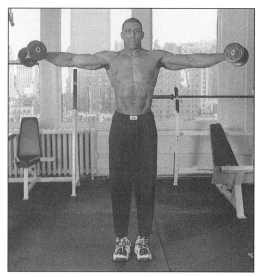

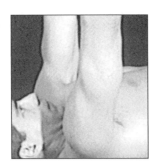

Exercise: Protraction

DIFFICULTY: 2
LOWER BACK: MODERATE RISK
AREA: ANTERIOR DELTOID

STARTING POSITION: Assume the supine position on a bench, your torso resting on the bench and your chin tucked. Extend arms and hold dumbbells so they are directly overhead (perpendicular to your body), shoulders relaxed and retracted (back). Hands should be pronated (thumbs facing inward).

MOVEMENT: Keeping your arms straight, raise both dumbbells by pushing both shoulders forward (protraction). Lower to starting position under control.
    Variation: This exercise can be performed one arm at a time.

TRAINER'S TIPS:
• Concentrate on pushing your shoulders up as you raise the dumbbells.
• This movement has a naturally small range of motion.

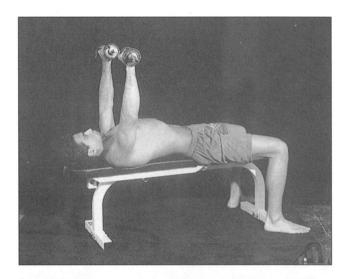

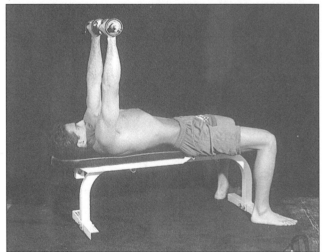

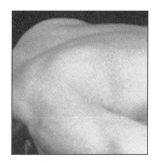

Exercise:
Retraction/Horizontal Shrug

DIFFICULTY: 2
LOWER BACK: LOW RISK
AREA: POSTERIOR DELTOID

STARTING POSITION: Assume the prone position on a bench, with your head hanging over the edge. Hold both dumbbells so that they hang down perpendicular to the sides of your body, shoulders relaxed and protracted forward and hands should be neutral (thumbs facing forward). Your arms should be slightly bent.

MOVEMENT: Raise both dumbbells by pulling both shoulders back (retraction); do not bend elbows. Lower to starting position under control.

   Variation: This exercise can also be performed one arm at a time.

TRAINER'S TIPS:
• Concentrate on pinching your shoulder blades together as you raise the dumbbells.
• This exercise has a naturally small range of motion.
• Focus your mind on the back of your shoulders during the exercise.

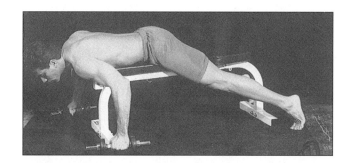

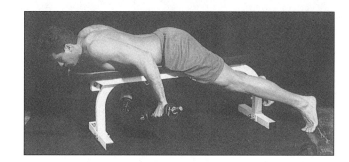

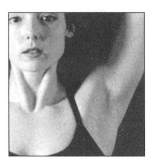

Exercise:
Dumbbell Shoulder Press

DIFFICULTY: 2
LOWER BACK: MODERATE RISK
AREA: DELTOIDS, TRICEPS

STARTING POSITION: Sit on edge of bench or stand with feet shoulder width apart and knees slightly bent. Hold both dumbbells at shoulder level with the palms facing forward. Your chest should be up with both shoulders pulled slightly back and your eyes looking straight ahead.

MOVEMENT: Raise both dumbbells directly over your head by straightening both arms. Return to starting position under control.

   Variation: Start from a neutral position (palms facing in) and rotate palms forward as you extend your arms over your head.

TRAINER'S TIPS:
• Maintain good posture throughout the exercise.
• Avoid arching your lower back as you lift. Support midsection with your abdomen throughout the exercise.
• Focus your mind on your shoulders throughout the exercise
• Another option is to bring the dumbbells together at the top of the movement.

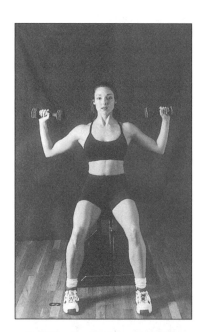

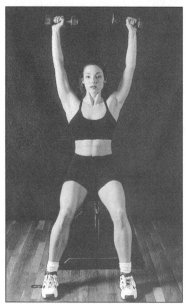

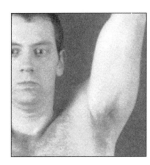

Exercise:
Military Press

DIFFICULTY: 2
LOWER BACK: MODERATE RISK
AREA: ANTERIOR DELTOID, MEDIAL DELTOID, TRICEPS

STARTING POSITION: Sit on bench (flat or shoulder press) facing the rack. Position hands slightly wider than shoulder width. Remove bar from rack and position it in front of you at shoulder level. Keep back straight and chest up with your head level and looking straight ahead. Feet should be at least shoulder width apart to provide a good base.

MOVEMENT: Raise the bar by pushing it directly over your head. Lower under control to starting position.

TRAINER'S TIPS:
• Maintain good posture throughout the exercise.
• Avoid arching or hunching your lower back as you lift. Support midsection with your abdomen throughout the exercise.
• A wider grip will isolate the shoulder muscles even more. But avoid an extreme angle, which will put extra stress on the shoulder joint.
• Focus your mind on the shoulders throughout the exercise.
• Don't lock out at the top of the movement. Keep constant tension on shoulder muscles.

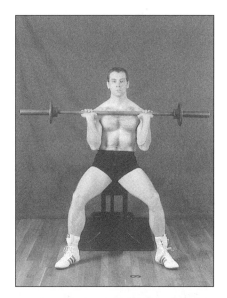

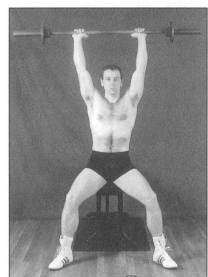

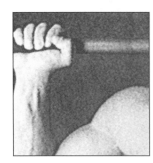

Exercise:
Behind-the-Neck Press

DIFFICULTY: 2
LOWER BACK: MODERATE RISK
AREA: DELTOIDS, TRICEPS

STARTING POSITION: Stand, or sit on a flat or shoulder press bench, facing the rack. Positioning hands slightly wider than shoulder width, remove bar from rack and hold behind your head with bar slightly touching traps. Keep back straight and chest up, with your head looking straight ahead. Feet should be shoulder width apart to provide a good base.

MOVEMENT: Raise the bar by pushing it directly over your head. Lower to starting position under control.

TRAINER'S TIPS:
- Maintain good posture throughout the exercise.
- Avoid arching your lower back as you lift. Support midsection with your abdomen throughout the exercise.
- Try to avoid tilting your head forward when lowering the bar.
- Focus your mind on the shoulders throughout the movement.
- Avoid arching your lower back as you lift.
- Do not lock out at top of the movement; keep constant tension on the shoulders.
- Complete through a full range of motion.
- If standing, avoid using your legs to assist the lift.

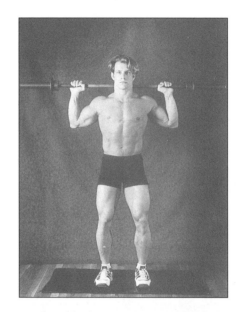

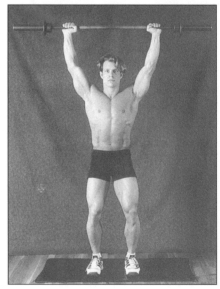

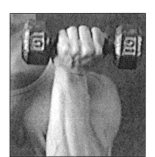

Exercise:
Rotation Press (Arnold Press)

DIFFICULTY: 2
LOWER BACK: MODERATE RISK
AREA: DELTOIDS, TRICEPS

STARTING POSITION: Sit on edge of bench or stand with feet shoulder width apart and knees slightly bent. Hold both dumbbells underneath your chin with your hands rotated so that the back of your hands face forward. Your chest should be up with shoulders pulled slightly back and your eyes looking straight ahead.

MOVEMENT: Raise both dumbbells directly over your head as you rotate the weight so the palms of your hands face out when your arms reach full extension (just short of lock out). Bring both dumbbells together at the top of the movement. Return to starting position. This constitutes one repetition.

   Variation: You may also perform this exercise by raising both dumbbells over your head but in an angle away from the head so that when you have rotated the palms out and arms have reached full extension, the dumbbells are now outside the plane of the body.

TRAINER'S TIPS:
• Maintain good posture throughout the exercise.
• Avoid arching your lower back as you lift.
• Focus your mind on your shoulders throughout the exercise.
• Do not lock out at top of the movement; keep constant tension on the shoulders.

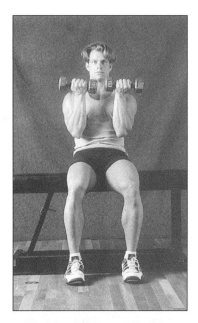

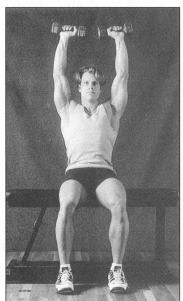

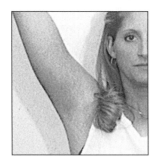

Exercise:
Compound Press

DIFFICULTY: 2
LOWER BACK: MODERATE RISK
AREA: DELTOIDS, TRICEPS

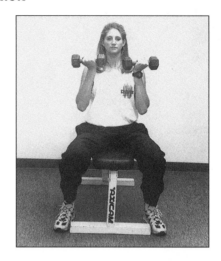

STARTING POSITION: Sit on a bench or stand with feet shoulder width apart and knees slightly bent. Hold both dumbbells underneath your chin with your hands rotated so that the back of your hands face forward. The dumbbells should be touching each other under your chin. Your chest should be up with both shoulders pulled slightly back. Look straight ahead.

MOVEMENT: Move the dumbbells to the outside (laterally) as you rotate your palms forward. Arms should form a right angle. From this position lower the dumbbells slightly so that they touch the outsides of your shoulders. Raise both dumbbells directly over your head. Bring dumbbells together at the top as you straighten your arms. Lower the dumbbells to the outside of the shoulders under control. Return to starting position by bringing your hands together (medially) and rotating your hands so that the palms face you. This constitutes one repetition.

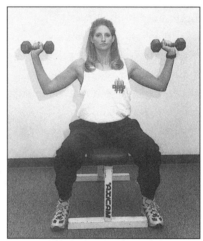

TRAINER'S TIPS:
• Maintain good posture throughout the exercise.
• Focus your mind on your shoulders throughout the exercise.

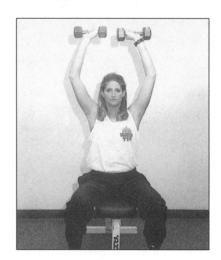

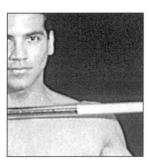

Exercise:
Push Press

DIFFICULTY: 3
LOWER BACK: HIGH RISK
AREA: DELTOIDS, TRICEPS

STARTING POSITION: Position bar on power rack at mid-chest level. Place both hands a little wider than shoulder width apart. Squat underneath bar and remove from the power rack with the help of your legs. Position feet about shoulder width apart. Legs should be bent to about a quarter squat with your butt slightly back and your back straight, your head positioned so that you are looking straight ahead.

MOVEMENT: Begin the exercise by slightly bending your legs. This should be done fairly quickly. Immediately explode back up using your legs and arms to help push the bar up directly over your head. Return to starting position under control.

TRAINER'S TIPS:
• When exploding up, think of jumping.
• Avoid arching your lower back as you lift.
• Focus on being as quick and explosive as you can on each repetition.

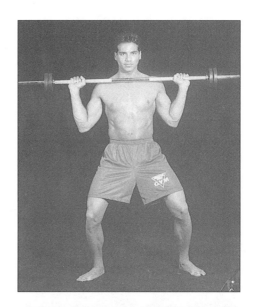

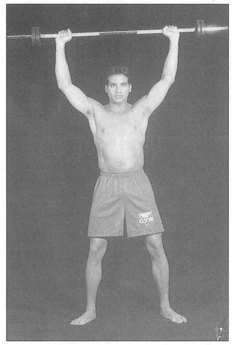

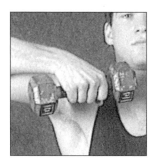

Exercise:
Upright Row

DIFFICULTY: 2
LOWER BACK: MODERATE RISK
AREA: SHOULDERS, BICEPS, FOREARMS

STARTING POSITION: Standing in proper lifting posture (knees slightly bent, feet shoulder width apart), center yourself in front of a barbell and grasp the bar with a double overhand grip two to six inches apart.

MOVEMENT: Keeping proper back alignment (back straight, chest out, eyes straight ahead), extend arms fully. Then elevate bar by pulling up with the elbows to just under the chin. During upward movement, keep hands close to the body and point elbows up and out. Return to starting position in a controlled manner. Repeat for the prescribed number of repetitions.

   Variations: Can be performed with dumbbells or machine.

TRAINER'S TIPS:
• This is an upright row. Keep torso still, do not extend hips.
• Concentrate on the front of your shoulders.
• Keep good postural alignment.
• Don't come up on toes.
• Focus your mind on your front deltoids.

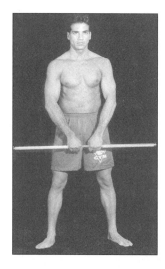
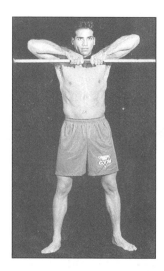
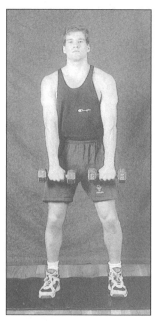
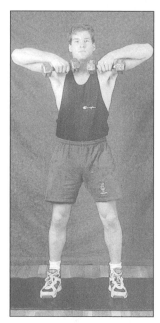

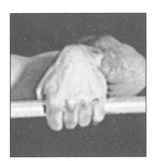

Exercise:
Stationary Clean

DIFFICULTY: 3
LOWER BACK: HIGH RISK
AREA: DELTOIDS, BICEPS,
FOREARMS

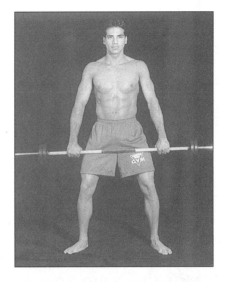

STARTING POSITION: Place barbell on power rack at mid-thigh level. Standing in proper lifting posture, center yourself in front of the bar and grasp it with a double overhand grip, allowing your hands to hang down naturally.

MOVEMENT: Keeping proper back alignment (back straight, chest out, eyes straight ahead), extend arms fully. Elevate bar by pulling up with the elbows to a point just under the chin. During upward movement, keep hands close to the body and pull elbows up and out. Once the bar has reached chin level, quickly rotate the elbows down and in, and catch the bar at shoulder level. Return to starting position in a controlled manner. Repeat for the prescribed number of repetitions.

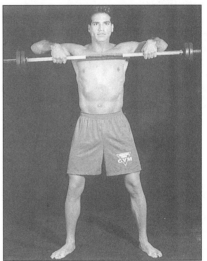

TRAINER'S TIPS:
• This is a stationary clean. Keep torso still, do not extend hips.
• Keep hands close to the body throughout the movement.
• Do not come up on toes.
• Do not reverse curl the bar. Pull the bar high on your body, then catch it in the underneath position. This movement is closer to an upright row than a reverse curl.
• Focus your mind on the shoulder muscles.

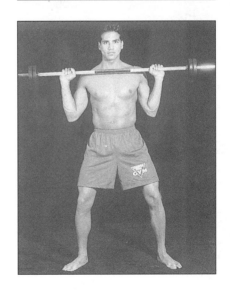

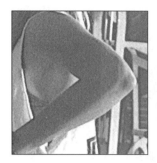

Exercise:
High Cable Internal Rotation

DIFFICULTY: 2
LOWER BACK: LOW RISK
AREA: ROTATOR CUFF

STARTING POSITION: Stand facing the weight stack. Grasp a long bar in an overhand grip, with hands evenly spaced and elbows bent at 90 degrees. Your elbows should be pointed out with your forearms perpendicular to your upper arm.

MOVEMENT: Keeping your arms bent, move your hands forward and down by rotating the shoulder. Rotate until your hands are down and your elbows are pointing up. Return to the starting position in a controlled manner.

TRAINER'S TIPS:
• Maintain arm bend and elbow position throughout the lift.
• Use very light weights to start. Even as you progress you should probably stick with fairly light weights and high reps as the muscles around the rotator cuff are small and can easily be injured if too much stress is placed on them.
• Control the motion both ways. Avoid jerky motions.
• Avoid moving the upper body.
• Avoid raising the trapezius muscles.

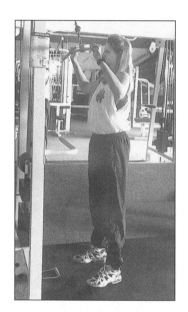

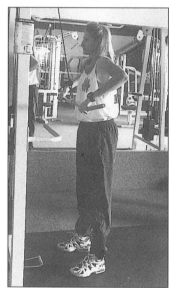

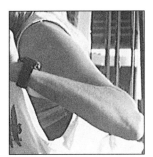

Exercise:
Low Cable External Rotation

DIFFICULTY: 2
LOWER BACK: LOW RISK
AREA: ROTATOR CUFF

STARTING POSITION: Stand with knees bent or kneel facing the weight stack. Grasp a long bar, positioned on the low pulley, with an overhand grip, hands evenly spaced and elbows bent at 90 degrees. Your elbows should be pointed out and up with your forearms perpendicular to your upper arm.

MOVEMENT: Keeping your arms bent, move your hands up and back by rotating the shoulder. Rotate until your hands are up and your elbows are pointing down. Return to the starting position in a controlled manner.

   Variation: This exercise can be performed one hand at a time (unilaterally).

TRAINER'S TIPS:
- Maintain arm bend and elbow position throughout the lift.
- Focus your mind from the middle to the back of your shoulder.
- Use very light weights to start with. Even as you progress you should probably stick with fairly light weights and high reps as the muscles around the rotator cuff are small and can easily be injured if too much stress is placed on them.
- Control the motion both ways. Avoid jerky motions.
- Keep torso still.
- Avoid raising the trapezius muscles.

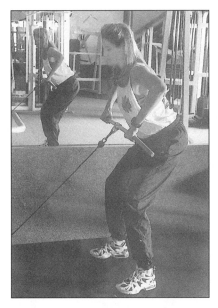

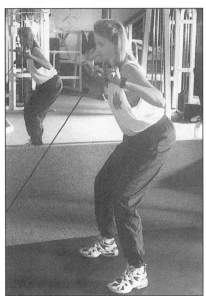

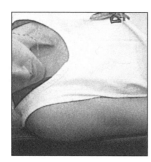

Exercise:
Internal Rotation

DIFFICULTY: 2
LOWER BACK: LOW RISK
AREA: ROTATOR CUFF

STARTING POSITION: Lie on your side. Your bottom arm should be positioned with the inside of your upper arm and elbow pressed against your side. Your forearm and hand holding the dumbbell should be bent at the elbow at 90 degrees so that the dumbbell touches your opposite side. Your hand should hold the dumbbell so that the thumb is toward your head.

MOVEMENT: Keeping your arm bent and elbow pressed to the side, lower your forearm away from your body by rotating the shoulder. Rotate until you feel a stretch in the shoulder. Move back to the starting position while keeping the arm bent and elbow pressed to the side. The rotation in both directions constitutes one repetition.

TRAINER'S TIPS:
• Maintain arm bend and elbow position throughout the lift.
• Focus your mind on the inside front of your shoulder.
• Use very light weights to start with. Even as you progress you should probably stick with fairly light weights and high reps as the muscles around the rotator cuff are small and can easily be injured if too much stress is placed on them.

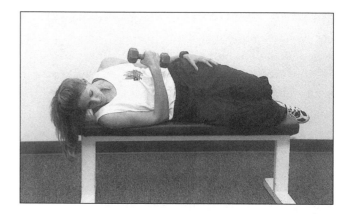

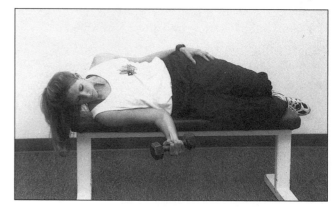

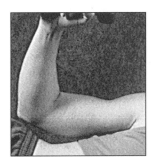

Exercise:
External Rotation

DIFFICULTY: 2
LOWER BACK: LOW RISK
AREA: ROTATOR CUFF

STARTING POSITION: Lie on your side. Your bottom arm can be used as a pillow on which to rest your head or may be positioned where it is comfortable as long as you remain on your side. Your top arm should be positioned so that the inside of the upper arm and elbow is pressed against your side. Your top arm should be bent at 90 degrees so that the dumbbell hangs down and almost touches your opposite side. Your hand should hold the dumbbell so that your thumb is toward your head.

MOVEMENT: Keeping your arm bent and elbow pressed to the side, raise the dumbbell vertically by rotating the shoulder. Rotate as far as you can keeping the arm bent and elbow pressed to your side. Rotate back the other way keeping the arm bent and elbow pressed to the side until you return to starting position. The rotation in both directions constitutes one repetition.

TRAINER'S TIPS:
• Maintain arm bend and elbow position throughout the lift.
• Focus your mind from the middle to the back of your shoulder.
• Use very light weights to start with. Even as you progress you should probably stick with fairly light weights and high reps as the muscles around the rotator cuff are small and can easily be injured if too much stress is placed on them.
• Control the motion both ways. Avoid jerky motions.

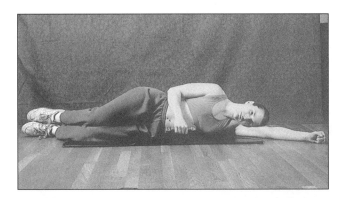

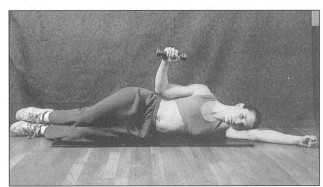

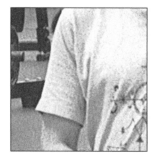

Exercise:
Internal Cable Rotation

DIFFICULTY: 2
LOWER BACK: LOW RISK
AREA: ROTATOR CUFF

STARTING POSITION: Standing in proper lifting posture, or kneeling with your right side facing the weight stack, grasp the handle with your right hand. Keep upper arm and elbow pressed against your side and bent at a 90-degree angle at the elbow. Your palm is facing forward, thumb is toward your head and little finger toward your feet.

MOVEMENT: Maintaining proper lifting posture and keeping elbow pressed into your side, use the shoulder to rotate the handle toward your stomach. Slowly return to starting position by rotating back in opposite direction, still keeping the arm and elbow bent. The rotation in both directions constitutes one repetition. Perform the same number of repetitions with opposite arm.

TRAINER'S TIPS:
• Maintain arm bend and elbow position throughout the lift.
• Use very light weights to start. Even as you progress you should probably stick with fairly light weights and high reps as the muscles around the rotator cuff are small and can easily be injured if too much stress is placed on them.
• Control the motion in both directions. Avoid jerky motions.

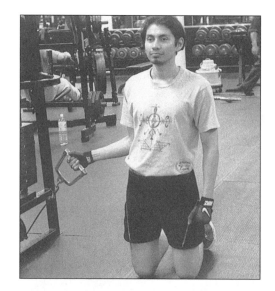

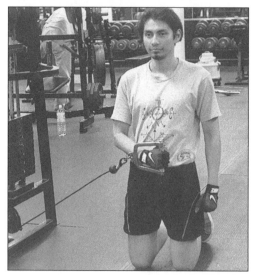

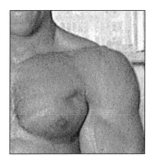

Exercise:
External Cable Rotation

DIFFICULTY: 2
LOWER BACK: LOW RISK
AREA: ROTATOR CUFF

STARTING POSITION: Standing or kneeling in proper lifting position with your right side facing the weight stack, grasp the handle with your left hand. Keep upper arm and elbow pressed against your side and bent at a 90-degree angle so that your hand touches your belly button. Hold the handle so that the thumb is toward your head.

MOVEMENT: Maintaining proper lifting posture and keeping elbow pressed into your side, use your shoulder to rotate the handle away from your stomach. Rotate as far as you can, keeping your elbow pressed to your side. Slowly return back to the starting position keeping the elbow bent and pressed to your side. The rotation in both directions constitutes one repetition. Perform the same number of repetitions with opposite arm.

TRAINER'S TIPS:
• Maintain arm bend and elbow position throughout the lift.
• Focus your mind from the middle to the back of your shoulder.
• Use very light weights to start with. Even as you progress you should probably stick with fairly light weights and high reps as the muscles around the rotator cuff are small and can easily be injured if too much stress is placed on them.
• Control the motion both ways. Avoid jerky motions.

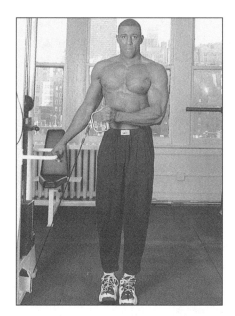

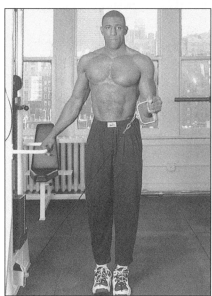

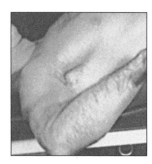

Exercise:
Overhead Rotation

DIFFICULTY: 2
LOWER BACK: LOW RISK
AREA: ROTATOR CUFF

STARTING POSITION: Lying on a bench, grasp a dumbbell in one hand and extend your upper arm, keeping it level with your shoulder. Then bend your arm at a 90-degree angle, bringing it back toward your ear.

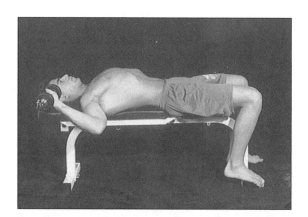

MOVEMENT: Keeping your arm bent, rotate your shoulder so that the dumbbell travels toward the outside of your hips. Rotate back the other way, keeping the arm bent and elbow and upper arm aligned with your body, until you reach your starting position. A rotation in both directions constitutes one repetition.

Variation: This exercise can also be done lying on the floor.

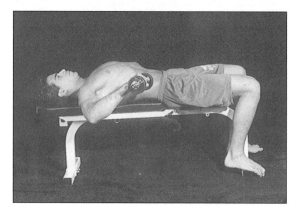

TRAINER'S TIPS:
- Maintain arm bend and elbow position throughout the lift.
- Use very light weights to start with. Even as you progress you should probably stick with fairly light weights and high reps as the muscles around the rotator cuff are small and can easily be injured if too much stress is placed on them.
- Control the motion both ways. Avoid jerky motions.
- Focus your mind on the inside front of your shoulder.

CHAPTER TEN

The Traps

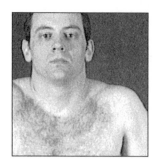

Exercise: Shrug

DIFFICULTY: 1
LOWER BACK:
    MODERATE RISK
AREA: TRAPEZIUS

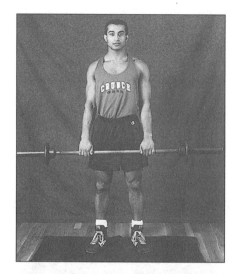

STARTING POSITION: Standing with knees slightly bent, evenly grasp bar with a double overhand grip slightly wider than shoulder width apart.

MOVEMENT: Keeping proper back alignment (back straight, chest out, eyes straight ahead), elevate bar by raising your shoulders toward your ears and hold for a count. Return to starting position in a controlled manner. Repeat for the prescribed number of repetitions.

Variations: Can be performed with dumbbells or machine. Once shoulders are completely elevated you can protract (move toward the front) or retract (move toward the back) the shoulders before performing the eccentric contraction.

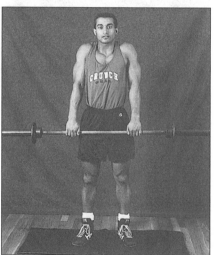

TRAINER'S TIPS:
- Make sure to squeeze at top of the contraction.
- Keep good posture alignment.
- Don't lean back.
- Don't come up on toes.
- Once the shoulders are elevated completely, drop chin (should increase shoulder lift).
- Keep elbows straight—lift with the shoulders, not the biceps.
- Focus your mind on the working muscles.

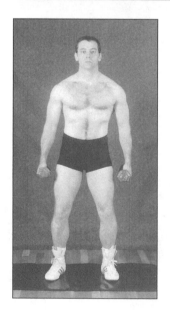
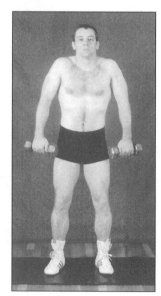

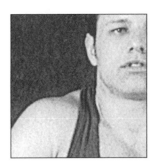

Exercise:
Wide Shrug

DIFFICULTY: 1
LOWER BACK: MODERATE RISK
AREA: TRAPEZIUS

STARTING POSITION: Standing with knees slightly bent, evenly grasp bar with a wide double overhand grip.

MOVEMENT: Keeping proper back alignment (back straight, chest out, eyes straight ahead), elevate bar by raising your shoulders toward your ears and hold for a count. Return to starting position in a controlled manner. Repeat for the prescribed number of repetitions.

Variations: Can be performed with dumbbells and machine. Once shoulders are completely elevated you can protract (move toward the front) or retract (move toward the back) the shoulders before performing the eccentric contraction.

TRAINER'S TIPS:
- Make sure to squeeze at top of the contraction.
- Keep good postural alignment.
- Don't lean back.
- Don't come up on toes.
- Once the shoulders are elevated completely, drop chin (should increase shoulder lift).
- Keep elbows straight—lift with the shoulders, not the biceps.
- Focus your mind on the working muscles.

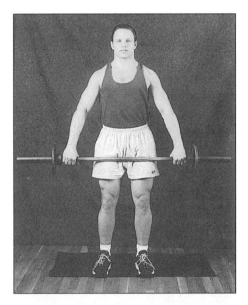

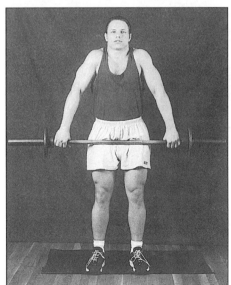

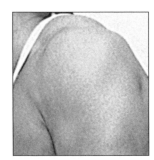

Exercise:
Angled Shrug

DIFFICULTY: 1
LOWER BACK: MODERATE RISK
AREA: TRAPEZIUS

STARTING POSITION: Standing with knees slightly bent and centered, grasp a barbell with a double overhand grip, hands naturally hanging down. Keeping proper back alignment (back straight, chest out, eyes straight ahead), lean forward with the torso, so that the chest is slightly ahead of the knees.

MOVEMENT: Elevate bar by raising your shoulders straight up. This means vertically, not toward the ears. Return to starting position in a controlled manner. Repeat for the prescribed number of repetitions.

   Variations: Can be performed with dumbbells or machine. You can also change the angle of the exercise by varying the degree of forward lean.

TRAINER'S TIPS:
• Make sure to squeeze at top of the contraction.
• Keep good postural alignment.
• Don't lean back.
• Don't come up on toes.
• Keep elbows straight—lift with the shoulders, not the biceps.
• Once the shoulders are elevated completely, drop chin (this should further raise shoulders) and hold for a count.
• Focus your mind on your traps.
• Tighten abs to support your lower back.

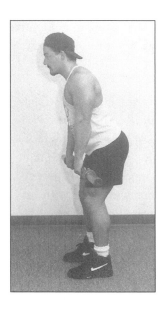
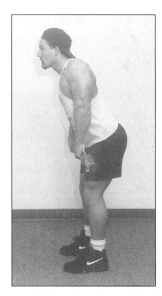

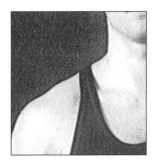

Exercise:
Seated Shrug

DIFFICULTY: 1
LOWER BACK: MODERATE RISK
AREA: TRAPEZIUS

STARTING POSITION: Seated at the end of the bench, grasp two dumbbells, thumbs forward, arms hanging down naturally.

MOVEMENT: Keeping proper back alignment (back straight, chest out, eyes straight ahead), elevate dumbbells by raising your shoulders toward your ears and hold for a count. Return to starting position in a controlled manner. Repeat for the prescribed number of repetitions.

Variations: Once shoulders are completely elevated, you may protract (move toward the front) or retract (move toward the back) shoulders before performing the eccentric contraction. You may also vary the exercise angle by the torso lean.

TRAINER'S TIPS:
• Make sure to squeeze at top of the contraction.
• Keep good postural alignment.
• Don't lean back.
• Once the shoulders are elevated completely, drop chin (should increase shoulder lift).
• Concentrate on letting the movement of the shoulders do the work, not the arms.
• Focus your mind on traps.

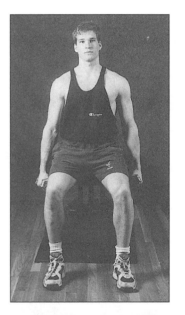

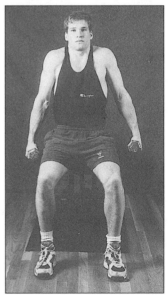

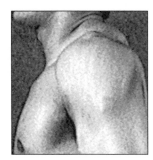

Exercise:
Behind-the-Back Shrug

DIFFICULTY: 1
LOWER BACK: MODERATE RISK
AREA: TRAPEZIUS

STARTING POSITION: Standing centered with back toward the bar, knees slightly bent, grasp barbell with a double overhand grip that allows hands to hang down naturally.

MOVEMENT: Keeping proper back alignment (back straight, chest out, eyes straight ahead), elevate bar by raising your shoulders toward your ears. Once the shoulders are elevated completely, drop chin (should raise shoulders higher) and hold for a count. Return to starting position in a controlled manner. Repeat for the prescribed number of repetitions.

    Variations: Can be performed with machine. Once shoulders are completely elevated you can protract (move toward the front) or retract (move toward the back) the shoulders before performing the eccentric contraction.

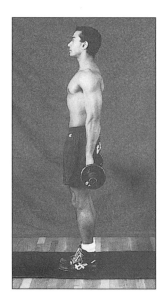
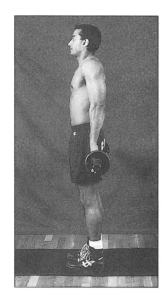

TRAINER'S TIPS:
- Make sure to squeeze at top of the contraction.
- Keep good postural alignment.
- Don't lean back.
- Don't come up on toes.
- Try to "hide" your neck with your shoulders.

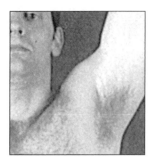

Exercise:
Overhead Shrug

DIFFICULTY: 2
LOW BACK: HIGH RISK
AREA: TRAPEZIUS

STARTING POSITION: Grasp dumbbells with a double overhand grip. Press dumbbells directly overhead.

MOVEMENT: Keeping proper back alignment (back straight, chest out, eyes straight ahead), move dumbbells vertically by raising your shoulders toward your ears and hold for a count. Lower shoulders to starting position in a controlled manner. Repeat for the prescribed number of repetitions.

Variations: Can be performed with a barbell or machine. Once shoulders are completely elevated, you can protract (move toward the front) or retract (move toward the back) them before performing the eccentric contraction.

TRAINER'S TIPS:
- Make sure to squeeze at top of the contraction.
- Keep good postural alignment.
- Don't lean back.
- Don't come up on toes.
- Keep arms straight.
- Once the shoulders are elevated completely, drop chin (should raise shoulders higher).
- Focus your mind on complete movement with the traps.

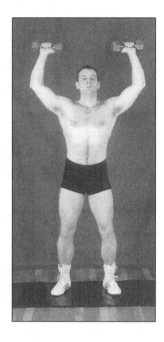
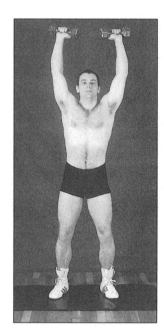

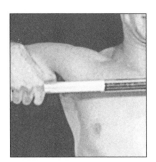

Exercise:
Modified Snatch Pull

DIFFICULTY: 3
LOW BACK: HIGH RISK
AREA: SHOULDER GIRDLE, TRAPEZIUS

STARTING POSITION: Stand centered in front of a barbell with knees slightly bent and feet shoulder width apart. Grasp the bar with a double overhand grip, hands placed as far apart as is safely possible.

MOVEMENT: Keeping proper back alignment (back straight, chest out, eyes straight ahead), elevate bar by first shrugging with your shoulders. Once the shoulders are elevated, pull up with arms until the bar reaches chin level. Return to starting position in a controlled manner. Repeat for the prescribed number of repetitions.

   Variations: Can be performed with dumbbells or machine.

TRAINER'S TIPS:
• This is a modified snatch pull. Keep torso still; do not extend hips.
• Initiate movement with the trap muscles.
• Keep good postural alignment.
• Don't come up on toes.
• Focus your mind on your traps, shoulders, and arms.

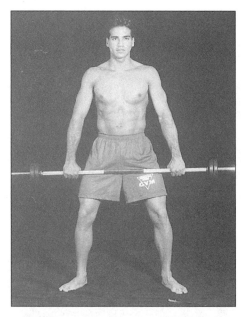

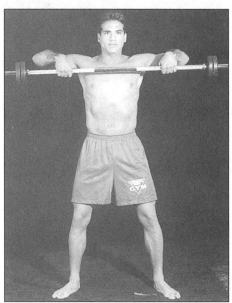

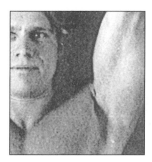

Exercise:
Front Trap Raise

DIFFICULTY: 2
LOWER BACK: MODERATE RISK
AREA: TRAPEZIUS, SHOULDERS

STARTING POSITION: Sit on edge of bench or stand with feet shoulder width apart and knees slightly bent. Raise both dumbbells so that arms extend straight out in front at shoulder level. Hands can be neutral (thumbs facing forward), pronated (thumbs facing in), or supinated (thumbs facing out).

MOVEMENT: Raise both dumbbells until they come together overhead. Hold for a count, then lower to starting position in a controlled manner.

   Variations: This exercise can be performed unilaterally, with a barbell, plate, or machine.

TRAINER'S TIPS:
• Maintain good lifting posture throughout the exercise.
• Avoid arching your lower back as you lift.
• Support midsection with abdominal muscles throughout the exercise.
• Keep torso still throughout the movement.
• Focus your mind on the trapezius muscle.
• Elevate shoulders (shrug) at top of the movement.

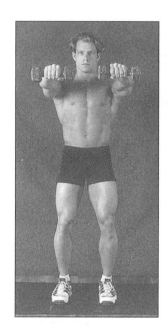
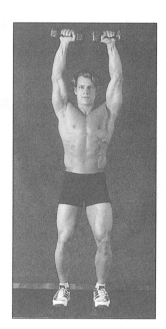

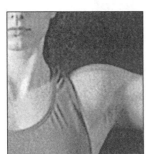

Exercise:
Lateral Trap Raise

DIFFICULTY: 2
LOWER BACK: MODERATE RISK
AREA: TRAPEZIUS, SHOULDERS

STARTING POSITION: Sit on edge of bench or stand with feet shoulder width apart and knees slightly bent. Raise both dumbbells so that arms extend straight to the side at shoulder level. Palms should face either up or forward.

MOVEMENT: Raise both dumbbells in a circular motion until they come together overhead. Hold for a count, then lower to starting position under control.

TRAINER'S TIPS:
• The movement is similar to drawing a halo around your head.
• Maintain good posture throughout the exercise.
• Avoid arching your lower back as you lift. Support midsection with your abdomen throughout the exercise.
• Keep the torso still throughout the movement.
• Focus your mind on the trapezius muscle.
• Elevate shoulders (shrug) at top of the movement.

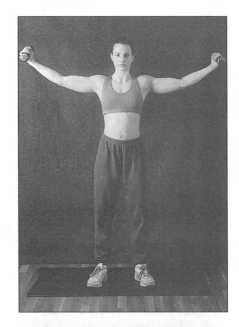

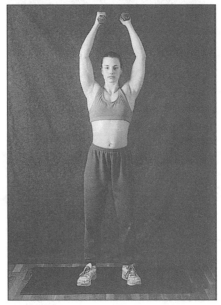

CHAPTER ELEVEN

The Triceps

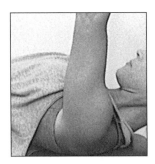

Exercise:
Supine Dumbbell Extension

DIFFICULTY: 1
LOWER BACK: LOW RISK
AREA: TRICEPS

STARTING POSITION: Lie on your back on a flat bench (or incline if you wish to change the angle). Weight should be displaced on your shoulder blades with chin tucked toward chest. Your working arm is extended perpendicular to the floor.

MOVEMENT: Lower the dumbbell by bending the elbow so that the dumbbell hangs down beside your ear. Keeping your elbow static, push the dumbbell up until your arm is fully extended, and you have returned to starting position.

    Variations: You may perform this exercise with both arms in unison or in an alternating fashion. This exercise may be performed by flaring the elbow out and taking the dumbbell across the chest.

TRAINER'S TIPS:
- Maintain good posture throughout the exercise.
- Keep the elbows static throughout the exercise.
- Focus your mind on your triceps.
- Move the dumbbell in a vertical path.

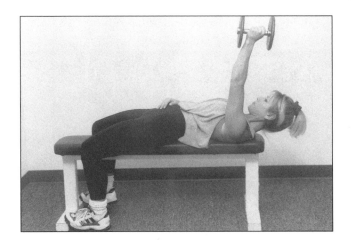

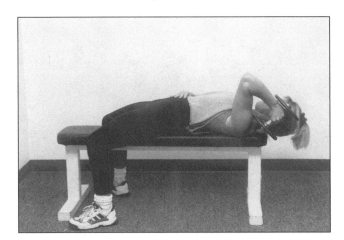

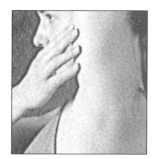

Exercise:
Dumbbell Upright Extension

DIFFICULTY: 1
LOWER BACK: MODERATE RISK
AREA: TRICEPS

STARTING POSITION: Stand or sit with feet shoulder width apart. Back should be straight with chest up. The working arm is extended straight up.

MOVEMENT: Keeping your upper arm vertical, bend your elbow and lower the dumbbell so that it hangs down behind and just to the side of your head, creating a 90-degree angle. Maintaining elbow position, push the dumbbell up until your arm is fully extended.

Variation: You may also perform this exercise with both arms at the same time or in an alternating fashion.

TRAINER'S TIPS:
• Maintain good posture throughout the exercise.
• Keep the elbows static throughout the exercise.
• Focus your mind on the back of the arm (above the elbow and below the shoulder) throughout the exercise.
• You can use your free arm to support your working arm.

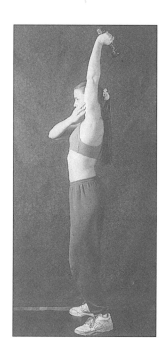
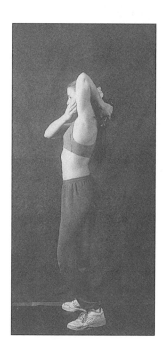

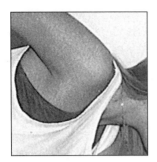

Exercise:
Dumbbell Kickback

DIFFICULTY: 1
LOWER BACK: MODERATE RISK
AREA: TRICEPS

STARTING POSITION: Rest your left knee on a bench. Bend forward, placing your left hand on the bench for support. Holding a dumbbell, bend your arm and elevate your elbow as high as possible. Avoid dipping your shoulder and keep the forearm perpendicular to the ground.

MOVEMENT: Keeping your upper arm pressed to your side with the elbow elevated, push the dumbbell up until your arm is fully extended. Return under control to original starting position. Execute for prescribed number of repetitions, then repeat with the opposite arm.

Variations: Facing palms toward the front and toward the rear will add variety. This exercise can also be performed on a cable machine, with a rubber band, or with tubing. You may also perform this exercise with both arms by placing your head against a preacher curl to balance you when you bend forward.

TRAINER'S TIPS:
• Maintain good position throughout the exercise.
• Keep the elbow elevated throughout the exercise.
• Focus your mind on your triceps.

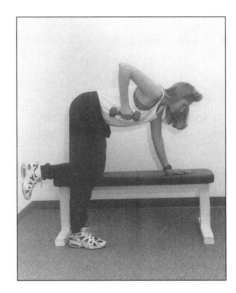

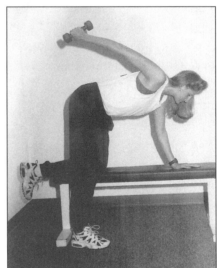

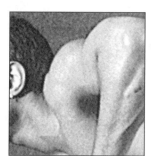

Exercise:
Lateral Kickout

DIFFICULTY: 1
LOWER BACK: MODERATE RISK
AREA: TRICEPS

STARTING POSITION: Stand with feet shoulder width apart facing a bench, holding a dumbbell in either your right or left hand. Bend at the waist, creating a 45-degree angle, and place your free hand on the bench to support and balance you. Raise your working arm out to the side and bend at the elbow. Elevate the elbow as high as possible without dipping your shoulder.

MOVEMENT: Keeping your elbow pointed to the side and elevated, push the dumbbell up until your arm is fully extended. Return under control to original starting position, keeping your elbow elevated.

Variation: You may perform this exercise with both arms by placing your head against a preacher curl to balance you when you bend forward.

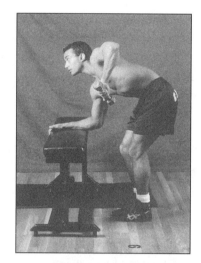

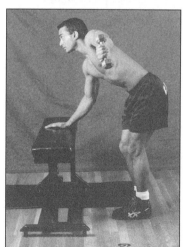

TRAINER'S TIPS:
• Maintain good position throughout the exercise.
• Keep the elbow elevated throughout the exercise.
• Do not raise dumbbell higher than shoulder level.
• Focus your mind on the back of the arm (above the elbow and below the shoulder) throughout the exercise.

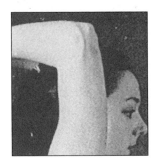

Exercise:
French Press

DIFFICULTY: 2
LOWER BACK: MODERATE RISK
AREA: TRICEPS

STARTING POSITION: Stand (knees slightly bent) or sit with feet shoulder width apart, back straight, and chest up. Hold dumbbell behind your head with both hands. The dumbbell should be held by the plate not the handle and should be extended overhead.

MOVEMENT: Keeping upper arms static, lower the dumbbell by bending the elbows so that the dumbbell is behind your head. Return to the starting position.

TRAINER'S TIPS:
• Maintain good posture throughout the exercise.
• Keep the elbows static throughout the exercise.
• Control both up and down phases of movement.
• Focus your mind on your triceps.

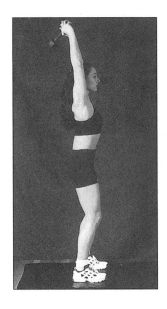
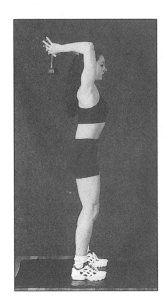

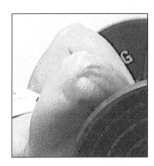

Exercise:
Supine Bar Extension

DIFFICULTY: 1
LOWER BACK: LOW RISK
AREA: TRICEPS

STARTING POSITION: Lie on your back on a flat bench (or incline if you wish to change the angle). Weight should be displaced on your shoulder blades with chin tucked toward chest. Extend arms straight up, positioning parallel on each side of your head, with the bar aligned slightly behind the top of your head.

MOVEMENT: Lower the bar by bending the elbows so that the bar hangs down behind your head. Keeping your elbows static, push the bar up until your arms are fully extended and you have returned to starting position.

TRAINER'S TIPS:
• Maintain good posture throughout the exercise.
• Keep the elbows static throughout the exercise.
• Focus your mind on your triceps.
• Move the bar straight up and down.

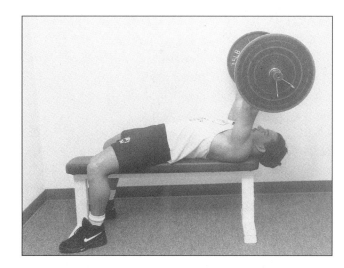

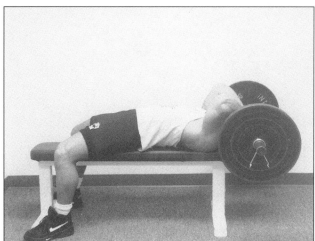

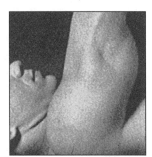

Exercise:
Close-Grip Bench Press

DIFFICULTY: 1
LOWER BACK: LOW RISK
AREA: TRICEPS

STARTING POSITION: Lie on your back on a flat bench, feet flat on the bench or on the floor. Grip the bar in the center with both hands so that both thumbs, if extended, are touching or almost touching. Remove the bar from the rack and hold it above your chest, both arms extended.

MOVEMENT: Lower the bar in a controlled manner until it touches the bottom of your chest, then push it back up to the starting position.

TRAINER'S TIPS:
- Lower the bar under control, taking care not to bounce it off your chest.
- Keep your body stable and balanced on the bench throughout the exercise.
- Focus your mind on your triceps.

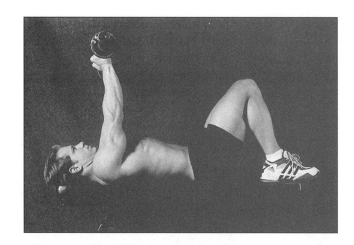

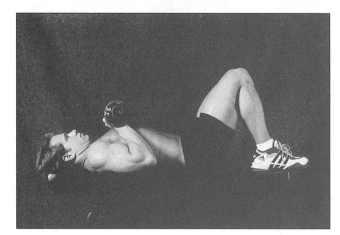

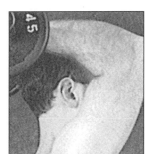

Exercise:
Barbell Upright Extension

DIFFICULTY: 1
LOWER BACK: MODERATE RISK
AREA: TRICEPS

STARTING POSITION: Stand or sit with feet shoulder width apart, back straight, and chest up. Arms extended straight up and positioned parallel on each side of the head. Grip the bar (straight bar or easy curl bar) with an overhand grip.

MOVEMENT: Keeping upper arms static, bend your elbows so that the bar hangs down behind your head and you create a 90-degree angle between upper and lower arm. Push the bar up until your arms are fully extended.

   Variation: Exercise may be performed with elbows pointed to the side.

TRAINER'S TIPS:
• Maintain good posture throughout the exercise.
• Keep the elbows static throughout the exercise.

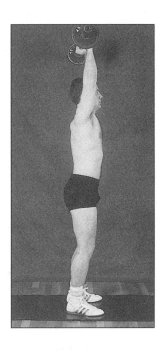
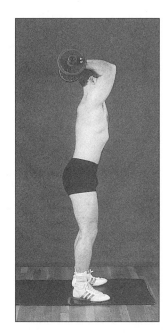

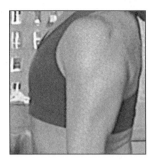

Exercise:
Triceps Push-Down

DIFFICULTY: 1
LOWER BACK: LOW RISK
AREA: TRICEPS

STARTING POSITION: Attach a V-bar, straight bar, E-Z curl bar, or rope attachment to the upper pulley. Stand facing the cable weight stack with your feet shoulder width apart. Grab the bar with an overhand grip, keeping your upper arms tight against your sides. Your elbows should be bent just past a 90-degree angle.

MOVEMENT: Keeping your upper arms against your sides, push the bar down until your arms are fully extended. Return under control to original starting position.

TRAINER'S TIPS:
• Maintain good posture throughout the exercise.
• Keep the elbows locked into the sides throughout the exercise.
• Avoid raising the shoulders and elbows during the exercise.
• Focus your mind on your triceps.

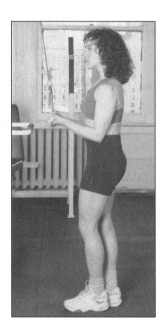 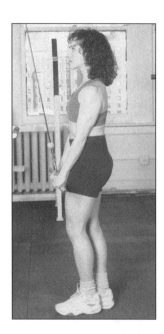

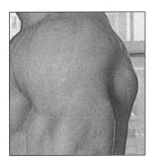

Exercise:
Triceps Pull-Down

DIFFICULTY: 1
LOWER BACK: LOW RISK
AREA: TRICEPS

STARTING POSITION: Attach an E-Z curl bar or straight bar to the upper pulley. Stand facing the cable and weight stack with your feet shoulder width apart. Grab the bar with an underhand grip. Position both elbows so that they are tight against your sides and are bent up past a 90-degree angle.

MOVEMENT: Keeping your upper arms locked into your sides, pull the bar down until your arms are fully extended. Return under control to original starting position.

TRAINER'S TIPS:
• Maintain good posture throughout the exercise.
• Keep the elbows locked into the sides throughout the exercise.
• Avoid raising the shoulders and elbows during the exercise.
• Focus your mind on your triceps.

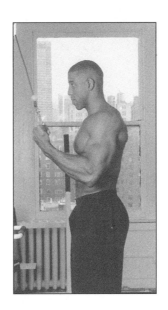
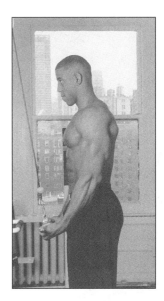

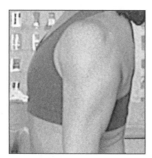

Exercise:
One-Arm Triceps Push-Down

DIFFICULTY: 1
LOWER BACK: LOW RISK
AREA: TRICEPS

STARTING POSITION: Attach a cable handle to the upper pulley. Stand facing the cable and weight stack with your feet shoulder width apart. Grab the handle with an overhand grip. Position elbow of working arm so that it is locked into your side. Your elbow should be bent up past a 90-degree angle.

MOVEMENT: Keeping your elbow locked into your side, push the handle down until your arm is fully extended. Return under control to starting position. Perform exercise with opposite arm.

TRAINER'S TIPS:
• Maintain good posture throughout the exercise.
• Keep the elbows locked into the sides throughout the exercise.
• Avoid raising the shoulders and elbows during the exercise.
• Focus your mind on your triceps.

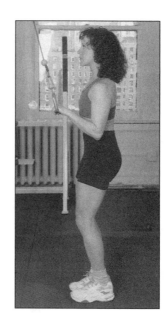
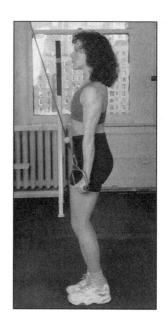

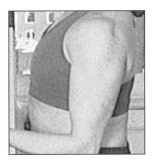

Exercise:
One-Arm Triceps Pull-Down

DIFFICULTY: 1
LOWER BACK: LOW RISK
AREA: TRICEPS

STARTING POSITION: Attach a cable handle to the upper pulley. Stand facing the cable and weight stack with your feet shoulder width apart. Grab the handle with an underhand grip. Position elbow of working arm so that it is locked into your side. Your elbow should be bent up past a 90-degree angle.

MOVEMENT: Keeping your elbow locked into your side, pull the handle down until your arm is fully extended. Perform exercise with opposite arm.

TRAINER'S TIPS:
• Maintain good posture throughout the exercise.
• Keep the elbows locked into the sides throughout the exercise.
• Avoid raising the shoulders and elbows during the exercise.
• Focus your mind on your triceps.

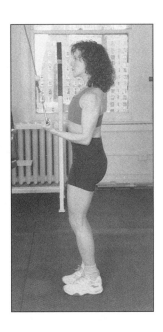
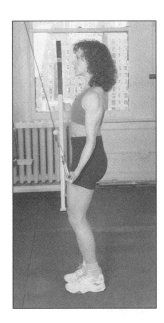

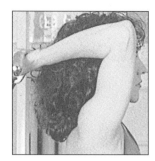

Exercise:
Upright Cable Extension

DIFFICULTY: 1
LOWER BACK: LOW RISK
AREA: TRICEPS

STARTING POSITION: Attach a V-bar, straight bar, rope, or curl bar to the low pulley. Kneeling, position yourself with your back toward the weight stack. Grip the handle with an overhand grip. Maintain an upright position with your back straight and chest up. Position your elbows so they are pointing up and parallel to each other. Elbows should be bent so that your hands are behind the head at about ear level.

MOVEMENT: Keeping your elbows static, push your hands up until your arms are fully extended and return under control to original starting position.

Variation: May be performed with a reverse grip using a straight or E-Z curl bar attachment.

TRAINER'S TIPS:
• Maintain your body position throughout the exercise.
• Keep the elbows pointed up throughout the exercise.
• Focus your mind on the back of the arm (above the elbow and below the shoulder) throughout the exercise.

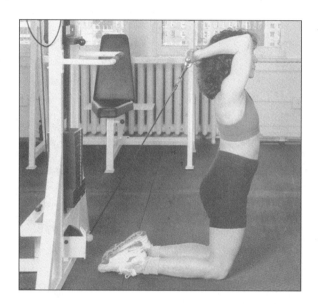

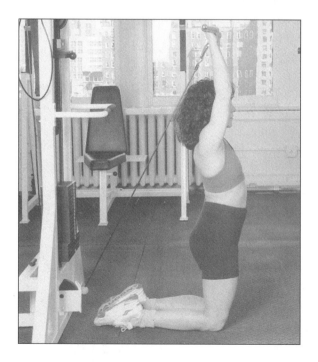

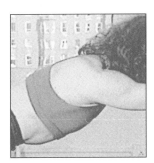

Exercise:
High Cable Extension

DIFFICULTY: 1
LOWER BACK: LOW RISK
AREA: TRICEPS

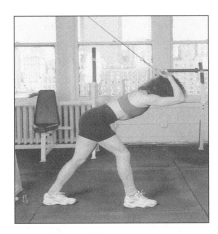

STARTING POSITION: Attach a V-bar, straight bar, rope, or curl bar to the high pulley. Position yourself with your back toward the cable weight stack, knees slightly bent, and feet shoulder width apart. (You can also position yourself on your knees.) Using either an underhand or overhand grip, step forward, then bend at the waist to create about a 45-degree angle. Position your elbows so they are pointing forward at about eye level. Elbows should be bent so that your hands are behind the head at about ear level.

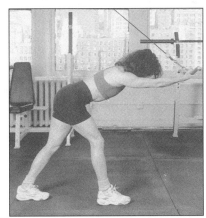

MOVEMENT: Keeping your elbows static, move your hands forward until your arms are fully extended. If using the rope attachment, spread apart hands and hold for a count. Return under control to original starting position, keeping your elbows static.

TRAINER'S TIPS:
• Maintain your body position throughout the exercise.
• Keep the elbows static throughout the exercise. You can assist in this by placing them on a preacher curl in front of you.
• Avoid raising your elbows when returning to starting position.
• Focus your mind on the back of the arm (above the elbow and below the shoulder) throughout the exercise.

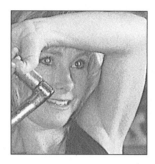

Exercise:
Overhead Cable Push

DIFFICULTY: 2
LOWER BACK: MODERATE RISK
AREA: TRICEPS

STARTING POSITION: Attach handle to the low pulley. Kneeling, position yourself with your right shoulder toward the cable weight stack. Grip the handle with your left hand using an overhand grip. Maintain an upright position with your back straight and chest up. Elevate weight so that your elbow is pointing up and out with the arm bent at a right angle, palm facing up.

MOVEMENT: Keeping your upper arm static, raise your left hand up until your arm is fully extended. Return under control to original starting position, keeping your upper arm static. Complete for prescribed number of repetitions, then repeat with opposite arm.

TRAINER'S TIPS:
• Maintain your body position throughout the exercise.
• Keep the elbow pointed up throughout the exercise.
• Focus your mind on the back of the arm (above the elbow and below the shoulder) throughout the exercise.

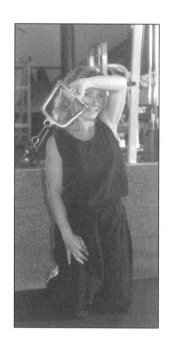
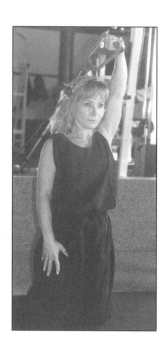

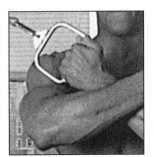

Exercise:
Cable Cross Pull-Down

DIFFICULTY: 1
LOWER BACK: LOW RISK
AREA: TRICEPS

STARTING POSITION: Attach a single-hand cable handle to the upper pulley of each side of cable cross machine. Stand centered between the two weight stacks with your feet shoulder width apart, keeping your back straight, chest up, and knees slightly bent. Your right hand should be holding the handle from the left cable and your left hand should be holding the handle from the right cable. Your arms should be bent at the elbow and crossed in front of your chest with the back of your hands facing forward (away from your chest). Your elbows should be pointed straight down and your hands should be just under both sides of your chin.

MOVEMENT: Keeping your elbows static, pull the handles down and out until your arms are fully extended. Return under control to starting position.

TRAINER'S TIPS:
• Maintain good posture throughout the exercise.
• Keep the elbows static throughout the exercise.
• Avoid raising the shoulders and elbows during the exercise.
• Focus your mind on your triceps.

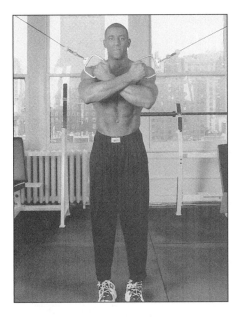

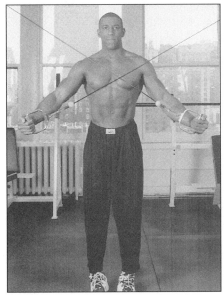

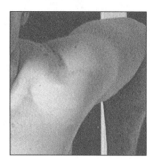

Exercise:
Dip

DIFFICULTY: 1
LOWER BACK: LOW RISK
AREA: TRICEPS

STARTING POSITION: Placing both hands on the handles of the dip apparatus, raise yourself up until your arms are fully extended and all of your weight is supported by your arms. Your back should be flat and your chest up. Your legs may be straight or bent.

MOVEMENT: Lower yourself in a controlled movement until you reach a 90-degree bend in the elbows, then raise yourself up to the starting position.

   Variations: You may add additional weight by wearing a dip belt or holding a dumbbell between the knees while performing this exercise.

TRAINER'S TIPS:
• Maintain a flat back with your chest up throughout the exercise.
• Don't bounce at the bottom.
• Try to move up and down in a strict vertical motion.
• Focus your mind on your triceps.
• Don't initiate upward movement with legs.
• For best triceps isolation, keep elbows in tight to body.

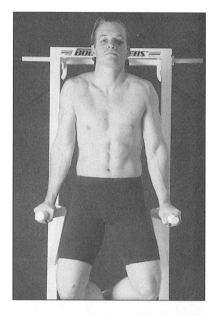

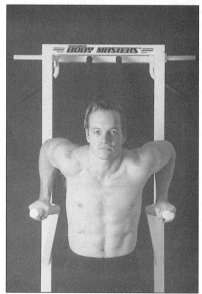

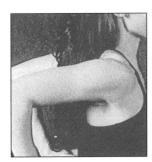

Exercise:
Bench Dip

DIFFICULTY: 1
LOWER BACK: LOW RISK
AREA: TRICEPS

STARTING POSITION: Sit on the side of a bench. Place your palms (fingers forward) on the bench beside your hips. Your legs should be bent at the knees. Push up with both arms until they are fully extended and move your torso forward so that your butt and back are just in front of the bench.

MOVEMENT: Bend your arms to a 90-degree angle, lowering your butt toward the floor. Then raise yourself up to the starting position.

Variations: You may make this exercise more difficult in a variety of ways: (1) Extend your legs forward until they are straight. (2) Place both legs on a second bench in front of you. (3) Place weight plates on your lap. (4) Have a partner press down on your shoulders as you press upward.

TRAINER'S TIPS:
• Maintain flat back and raised chest throughout the exercise.
• Move in a strict vertical line. Don't let your hips slide forward.
• Keep the forearms vertical throughout the exercise.
• Don't bounce at the bottom of the movement.
• Focus your mind on your triceps.

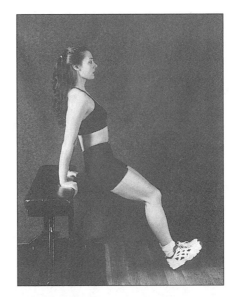

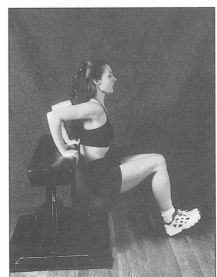

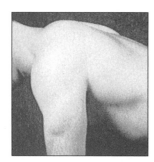

Exercise:
Triangle Push-Up

DIFFICULTY: 1
LOWER BACK: MODERATE RISK
AREA: TRICEPS

STARTING POSITION: Lie on your stomach with your hands under your chest, elbows pointing out. Your palms should be flat on the floor with the tips of your thumbs and index fingers touching in a triangle formation. Push yourself up until both arms are fully extended. Your torso and legs are extended, with your back flat.

MOVEMENT: Lower your torso down until your chest almost touches the floor, then push yourself up to the starting position.

   Variations: An easier version, using less body weight, is to start with your arms extended and torso raised but with knees bent, supporting your lower body on the floor. You can add additional resistance in three ways: (1) Have a partner push against your shoulder blades as you push up. (2) Have a partner place weight plates on your upper back. (3) Jackknife the torso with arms fully extended. Instead of lowering your chest to the triangle, lower your head.

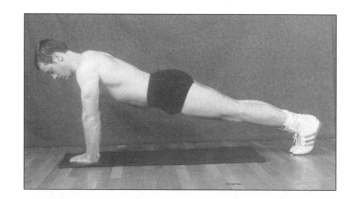

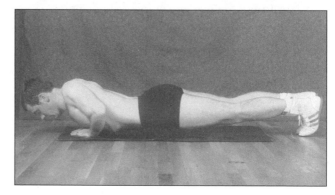

TRAINER'S TIPS:
• Maintain an extended torso throughout the exercise. Avoid arching or rounding the back.
• Focus your mind on your triceps.

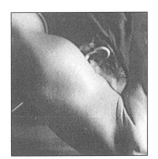

Exercise:
Body Weight Push-Back

DIFFICULTY: 2
LOWER BACK: LOW RISK
AREA: TRICEPS

STARTING POSITION: Stand facing a bar that is secured in a power rack. The bar should be at waist level or below. Place both hands on the center of the bar, two to four inches apart. Extend both arms, creating a horizontal lean against the bar.

MOVEMENT: Keeping your upper arms stationary, lean into the bar, bending your elbows until you create a 90-degree angle. Keep head below the bar for full range of motion. Push yourself up and back until your arms are fully extended. Repeat.

Variations: The farther you step back from the bar, the more difficult the exercise will be. The most difficult position would be when your body is fully extended back from the bar. You may also add more resistance to the exercise by having a partner provide manual resistance to you by pushing against your butt. This exercise can be performed unilaterally (one arm). It can also be performed up against a wall.

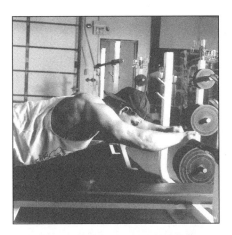

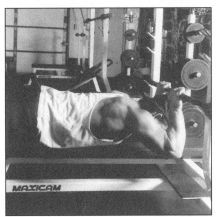

TRAINER'S TIPS:
- Keep elbows tight to the torso throughout the exercise.
- To increase resistance, use legs to push against the extension of your arms.
- Focus your mind on your triceps.

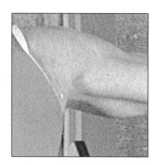

Exercise:
One-Arm Wall Extension

DIFFICULTY: 1
LOWER BACK: LOW RISK
AREA: TRICEPS

STARTING POSITION: Lean against wall, supporting your body with your forearm and fist. Your upper arm should be placed at shoulder level, and your elbow bent at a 90-degree angle.

MOVEMENT: Press your fist against the wall and use your triceps to extend your arm and push your body away from the wall. Return to starting position.

   Variations: This exercise can be done with your forearm placed vertically (six o'clock or twelve o'clock).

TRAINER'S TIPS:
• The greater the angle of body lean into the wall the more difficult the exercise becomes.
• Apply firm pressure with your fist to push body from wall.
• Focus your mind on your triceps.

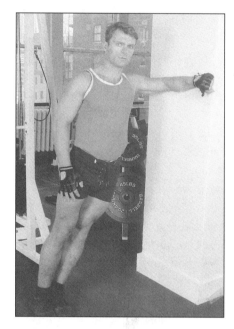

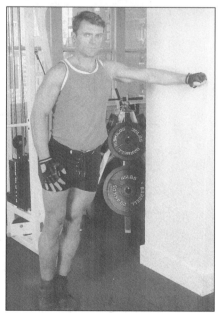

CHAPTER TWELVE

The Biceps

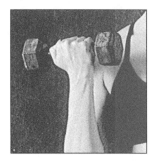

Exercise:
Seated Dumbbell Curl

DIFFICULTY: 1
LOW BACK: LOW RISK
AREA: BICEPS

STARTING POSITION: Grasp two dumbbells and sit on the edge of a flat bench in good lifting posture, feet on the floor and back straight. Extend arms down at your sides, with palms facing in toward your thighs.

MOVEMENT: As you begin the curl movement with both dumbbells, supinate your forearms (rotate palms to the outside) and continue to curl in a smooth arc to the shoulder. At shoulder level, rotate palms to the outside. Then lower and rotate dumbbell back to the starting position, facing the side of your upper thigh.

Variations: Seated dumbbell curls may also be performed with one arm at a time. You may choose a synchronized movement, raising one dumbbell as the other is descending, or concentrate on each arm separately.

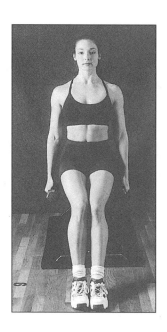
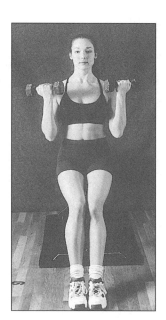

TRAINER'S TIPS:
• Keep upper arm motionless and pressed against upper torso throughout the range of movement.
• Aim for a smooth, flowing movement.
• Do not allow a sudden drop or drag on shoulder socket at bottom of movement.
• Contract biceps at the top of the movement.
• Focus your mind on working muscles.

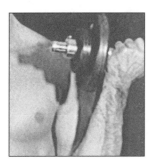

Exercise:
Standing Dumbbell Curls

DIFFICULTY: 1
LOWER BACK: LOW RISK
AREA: BICEPS, FOREARMS

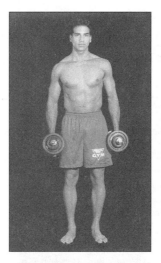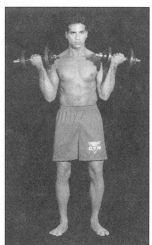

STARTING POSITION: Stand with feet shoulder width apart, grasping two dumbbells with arms hanging straight at your sides, palms facing in.

MOVEMENT: As you begin the curl movement with both dumbbells simultaneously, supinate your forearms and continue to curl in a smooth arc to the shoulder. At shoulder level, your wrists should have rotated (supinated) as far as they can to the outside. Then slowly lower the weights back to the starting position.

Variations: Standing dumbbell curls may also be performed with one arm at a time. You may choose a synchronized movement, raising one dumbbell as the other is descending, or concentrate on each arm separately. Another variation of this exercise is the Kneeling Barbell Curl (page 213).

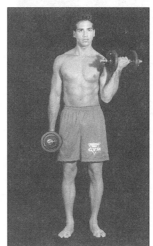

TRAINER'S TIPS:
• Keep upper arm motionless and pressed against upper torso throughout the range of movement.
• Aim for a smooth, flowing movement.
• Do not allow a sudden drop or drag on shoulder socket at bottom of movement.
• You may stand with back flat against the wall for added back support.
• Focus your mind on working muscles.
• Slight elevation or lifting of the elbows when the arm is fully flexed will increase the intensity of the contraction.

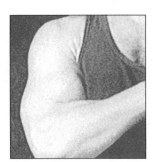

Exercise:
Cross Curl

DIFFICULTY: 2
LOWER BACK: HIGH RISK
AREA: BICEPS

STARTING POSITION: Stand with feet shoulder width apart, grasping two dumbbells, arms hanging at your sides, palms facing in.

MOVEMENT: Curl the right dumbbell in a smooth arc across the chest to the opposite shoulder. Then lower the dumbbell back across the body to starting position. Keep palm facing the body at all times. Repeat with left-hand dumbbell to complete one repetition. Continue to alternate until set is completed.

TRAINER'S TIPS:
• Keep upper arm motionless and pressed against upper torso throughout the range of movement.
• Aim for a smooth movement throughout the range of motion.
• Do not allow a sudden drop or drag on shoulder socket at bottom of the movement.
• Focus your mind on working muscles.
• You may stand with back flat against the wall for added back support.

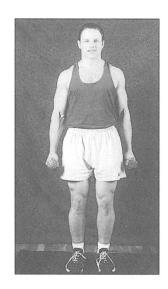

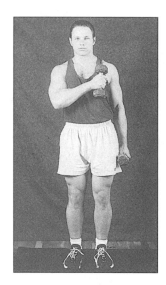

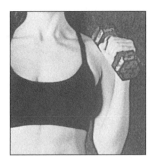

Exercise:
Hammer Curl

DIFFICULTY: 2
LOWER BACK: MODERATE RISK
AREA: BICEPS, FOREARMS

STARTING POSITION: Grasp two dumbbells and place feet shoulder width apart with arms hanging straight at your sides, palms facing in toward legs. Keep upper arms motionless and pressed tight to torso throughout movement.

MOVEMENT: Curl both dumbbells in an upward arc at the same time, keeping palms facing each other throughout entire movement. The motion is similar to hammering or pounding a nail. At the top of the movement, when both dumbbells have completed their arc to shoulder level, contract muscles strongly, then begin to lower both dumbbells back to starting position.

    Variations: Hammer Curls can be performed while sitting on a flat bench, especially if you have a tendency to move your torso excessively during the exercise. This movement can also be done one dumbbell at a time, alternating.

TRAINER'S TIPS:
• Maintain a smooth movement, with both dumbbells rising and lowering even and parallel to each other.
• Control the downward movement; do not allow a sudden drop at the end of your arc.
• Focus your mind on working muscles.
• You may stand with back flat against the wall for added back support.

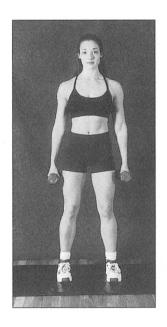
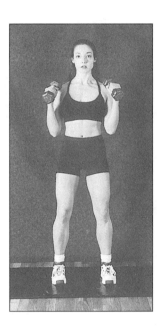

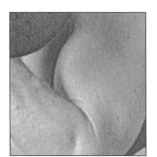

Exercise:
Incline Dumbbell Curl

DIFFICULTY: 2
LOWER BACK: LOW RISK
AREA: BICEPS

STARTING POSITION: Sit with back firmly pressed against the support of an incline bench at approximately 45 to 70 degrees of angle, feet on the floor and back straight. Grasp two dumbbells and let your arms hang at your sides, palms facing in toward your thighs. Keep upper arms motionless and allow arms to hang straight down.

MOVEMENT: As you begin the curl movement with both dumbbells, fully supinate forearms and continue to curl in a smooth arc to the shoulder. At shoulder level, slightly elevate elbows and fully contract biceps. Then slowly return to the starting position.

Variations: Incline dumbbell curls may also be performed with one arm at a time. You may choose a synchronized movement, raising one dumbbell as the other is descending, or concentrate on each arm separately.

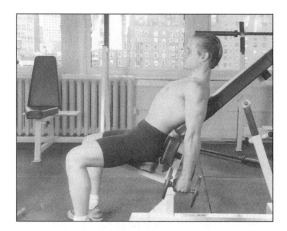

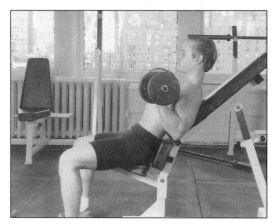

TRAINER'S TIPS:
• Keep upper arm motionless and pressed against upper torso throughout the range of movement.
• Aim for a smooth, flowing movement.
• Do not allow a sudden drop or drag on shoulder socket at bottom of movement.
• Contract biceps at the top of the movement.
• Focus your mind on working muscles.

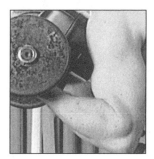

Exercise:
Prone Incline Dumbbell Curl

DIFFICULTY: 2
LOWER BACK: LOW RISK
AREA: BICEPS

STARTING POSITION: Lie facedown with your chest firmly pressed against the surface of an incline bench at approximately 30 to 45 degrees of angle. Grasp two dumbbells, arms hanging straight down, dumbbells facing your body.

MOVEMENT: As you begin the curl movement with both dumbbells, supinate your forearms and continue to curl in a smooth arc to the shoulder. At shoulder level, rotate wrists at the outside. Then slowly rotate and lower weights back to the starting position.

Variations: Prone incline dumbbell curls may also be performed with one arm at a time. You may choose a synchronized movement, raising one dumbbell as the other is descending, or concentrate on each arm separately. This exercise may also be performed with weights in the Hammer Curl position.

TRAINER'S TIPS:
- Keep upper arm motionless and pressed against upper torso throughout the range of movement.
- Aim for a smooth, flowing movement throughout range of motion.
- Do not allow a sudden drop or drag on shoulder socket at bottom of the movement.
- Focus your mind on working muscles.

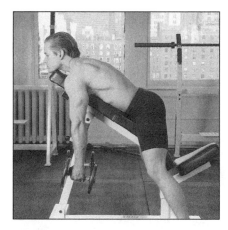

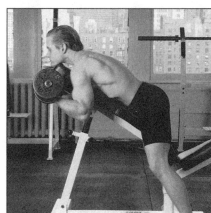

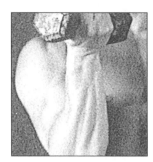

Exercise:
Kung Fu Curl

DIFFICULTY: 3
LOWER BACK: HIGH RISK
AREA: BICEPS, FOREARMS

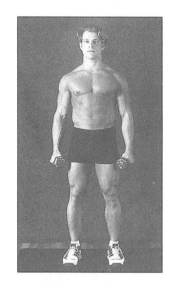

STARTING POSITION: Stand with feet shoulder width apart, grasping two dumbbells, with arms hanging straight at your sides, palms facing in. Keep inside of upper arms pressed tight to the torso throughout movement.

MOVEMENT: This exercise involves two separate movements. First bring the dumbbell with your right hand across the front of your body to your belly button. Then raise the dumbbell up and back toward your right shoulder. Lower the dumbbell in a reverse motion, keeping the dumbbell and palm close to the body, then in a smooth, synchronized movement begin to lift the opposite dumbbell in the same manner as the right, returning to starting position. Continue to alternate until set is completed.

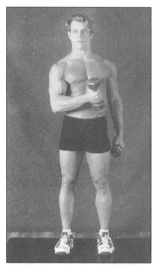

TRAINER'S TIPS:
- Keep upper arm motionless and pressed against upper torso throughout the range of movement.
- Aim for a smooth, flowing movement at all times.
- Focus your mind on the working muscle.
- The movement is similar to a Kung Fu block, hence the name.

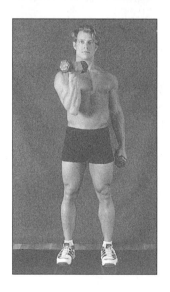

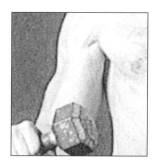

Exercise:
Zottman Curl

DIFFICULTY: 3
LOWER BACK: MODERATE RISK
AREA: BICEPS, FOREARMS

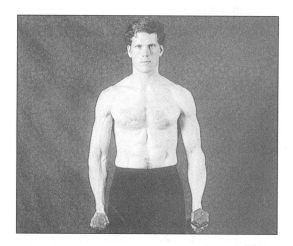

STARTING POSITION: Stand with feet shoulder width apart, grasping two dumbbells with arms hanging straight at your sides, palms facing in.

MOVEMENT: As you begin the curl movement, supinate your forearm. Curl in a smooth arc to the shoulder. Then lower the dumbbells back to starting position. As you lower the weight, begin to turn your wrist so that your palm is facing down (pronate) by the time your elbow makes a 90-degree angle. Return to neutral starting position and repeat.

Variations: Zottman Curls can also be performed while sitting on a flat bench. You may also choose a synchronized movement, raising one dumbbell as the other is descending, or perform the prescribed number of repetitions with one arm and then move to the other.

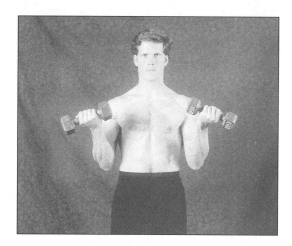

TRAINER'S TIPS:

• The key to Zottman Curls is the extreme rotation on both the upward and the downward movements, so that the palm faces fully up on upswing and fully down toward the ground on the downward phase.

• Keep upper arm motionless and pressed against upper torso throughout the range of movement.

• Aim for a smooth, flowing movement in which one hand is going up as the other is coming down.

• Focus your mind on working muscles.

• You may stand with back flat against the wall for added back support.

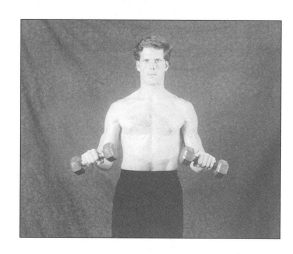

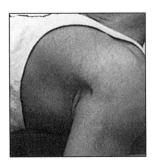

Exercise:
Supine Dumbbell Curl

DIFFICULTY: 2
LOWER BACK: LOW RISK
AREA: BICEPS

STARTING POSITION: Holding dumbbells at chest level, assume the supine position on a flat work bench. Place feet on the floor and distribute weight on the shoulder blades.

MOVEMENT: Lower the dumbbells in a controlled manner until arms hang down to your sides with your palms facing inward. Return to starting position by curling arms up and turning palms out. Keep upper arms static during this motion. Squeeze biceps at the end of the movement.

Variations: Can be performed with one arm, alternating, or with an overhand or hammer grip.

TRAINER'S TIPS:
• Keep body weight distributed on your shoulder blades.
• Keep the upper arm static throughout the exercise.
• Focus your mind on the biceps throughout the exercise.
• Keep head up.

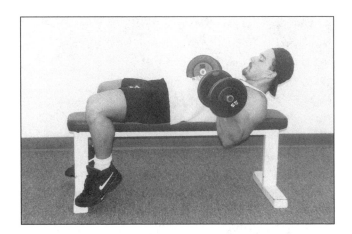

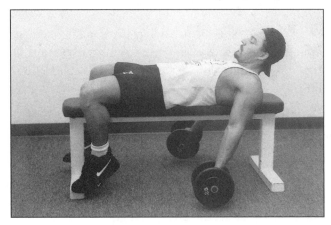

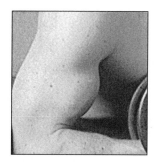

Exercise:
Concentration Curl

DIFFICULTY: 2
LOWER BACK: MODERATE RISK
AREA: BICEPS

STARTING POSITION: Sitting on the end of a bench or stool, grasp a dumbbell with the right hand and place the upper right arm on the inside of the right leg. Angle your body forward to a comfortable position and rest your left arm on your left leg.

MOVEMENT: Keeping your right upper arm and right leg static, raise the dumbbell with your right hand to your left shoulder. While curling, supinate your forearm and squeeze your biceps at the top of the movement. Lower in a controlled motion to starting position. Perform for the prescribed number of repetitions, then repeat with opposite arm.

   Variations: Can be performed with an overhand grip or hammer grip.

TRAINER'S TIPS:
• Maintain your body position throughout the exercise.
• Keep the elbows static throughout the exercise.
• Focus your mind on the biceps throughout the exercise.
• Don't initiate the movement with the leg.

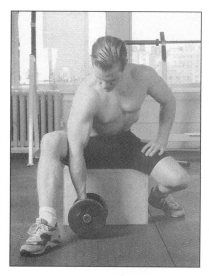

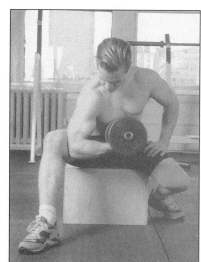

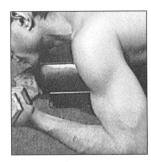

Exercise:
Prone Dumbbell Curl

DIFFICULTY: 3
LOWER BACK: MODERATE RISK
AREA: BICEPS, FOREARMS (FLEXOR MUSCLES),
            SHOULDERS (BRACHIALIS)

STARTING POSITION: Lie facedown with your chest firmly pressed against the surface of a flat bench. Grasp two dumbbells and let your arms hang down at your sides, dumbbells facing in toward your body.

MOVEMENT: Curl both dumbbells in a smooth arc toward your shoulders as you simultaneously supinate your forearms. At shoulder level, begin to lower the weights toward the ground, slowly turning wrists so that your palms return to the starting position, facing in toward your body.

    Variations: Prone dumbbell curls may also be performed with one arm at a time. You may choose a synchronized movement, raising one dumbbell as the other is descending, or concentrate on each arm separately. This exercise may also be performed with weights in the Hammer Curl position.

TRAINER'S TIPS:
• Keep upper arm motionless and pressed against upper torso throughout the range of movement.
• Aim for a smooth, flowing movement.
• Focus your mind on working muscles.

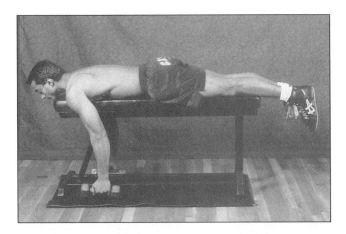

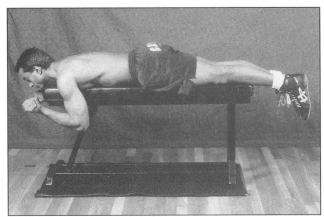

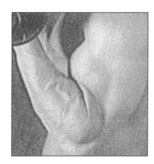

Exercise:
Standing Barbell Curl

DIFFICULTY: 2
LOWER BACK: HIGH RISK
AREA: BICEPS, FOREARMS

STARTING POSITION: Stand with feet shoulder width apart or wider, holding a barbell with an underhand grip. Hands should be slightly farther apart than your elbows. Arms should be fully extended. Keep upper arms motionless and pressed against torso throughout movement.

MOVEMENT: Curl the bar in an arc toward your chin. As your forearms reach perpendicular, elevate your elbows slightly and contract your biceps at the top of the movement. Slowly lower the bar handle back to starting position.

   Variation: Can also be performed with a wide or close grip.

TRAINER'S TIPS:
• Upper body should remain motionless throughout the exercise.
• Maintain a smooth movement throughout; avoid jerky motions.
• Avoid cheating movements such as bouncing or "throwing" weight upward.
• Keep elbows tight to the body.
• Keep knees slightly bent.
• Focus your mind on working the muscles.

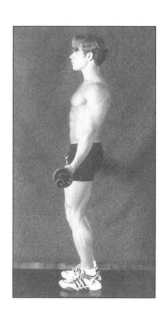
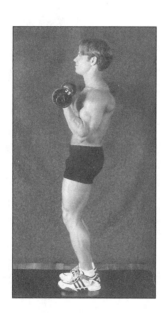

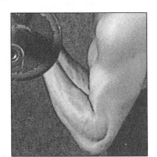

Exercise:
Barbell Concentration Curl

DIFFICULTY: 2
LOWER BACK: HIGH RISK
AREA: BICEPS

STARTING POSITION: Grasp a barbell in a narrow underhand grip, hands no more than four to six inches apart. Sit with feet slightly less than shoulder width apart, knees bent, and lean forward until your upper body is parallel to the floor. Your elbows will just touch your knees but *not* rest on them; allow arms to hang straight down from shoulders to floor.

MOVEMENT: Keeping the upper arm stationary, curl the barbell slowly in an upward arc toward your chin. Contract your biceps at the top of the movement.

TRAINER'S TIPS:
• Keep back of elbows in contact with knees.
• Keep head in line with the body; eyes looking down.
• Keep torso steady; don't arch or sway.
• Focus your mind on the biceps.
• Tighten abs to support your lower back.

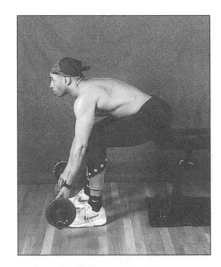

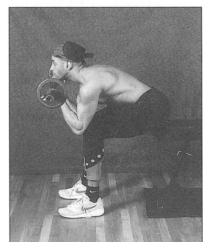

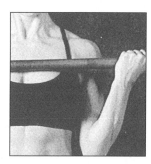

Exercise:
Kneeling Barbell Curl

DIFFICULTY: 2
LOWER BACK: MODERATE RISK
AREA: BICEPS

STARTING POSITION: Kneel on the floor with knees together, and grasp the barbell in a shoulder width underhand grip, with your arms fully extended at your sides.

MOVEMENT: Curl the barbell in an upward arc toward your neck, aiming for the spot just below your chin. Contract your biceps at the top of the movement while slightly elevating your elbows, then slowly lower the barbell back to starting position.

   Variations: This movement can also be done with dumbbells.

TRAINER'S TIPS:
• Keep upper arm pressed close to upper torso throughout the range of motion.
• Upper body should remain motionless throughout the exercise.
• Maintain a smooth movement throughout the entire range of motion.
• Focus your mind on working muscles.
• When elevating elbows, allow wrists to drop slightly.

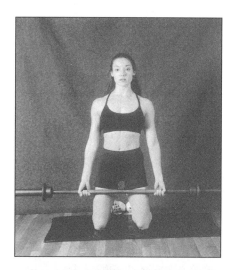

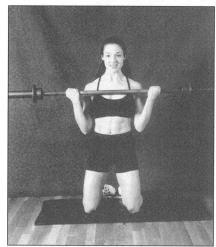

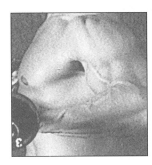

Exercise:
Barbell Drag Curl

DIFFICULTY: 3
LOWER BACK: MODERATE RISK
AREA: BICEPS, FOREARMS (FLEXOR)

STARTING POSITION: Stand with feet shoulder width apart or slightly wider and grasp the barbell with an underhand grip. Slightly bend your knees and let your arms extend fully.

MOVEMENT: Curl the barbell up your torso, letting it slide up your abs as high as you can (*allowing elbows to move behind body*). This will usually be no higher than your lower pectorals. Slowly slide the barbell back down to starting position, still tight to torso. This completes one repetition.

TRAINER'S TIPS:
• Keep upper arm pressed close to upper torso even as elbows move out in back.
• Upper body should remain motionless throughout the exercise.
• It is important to keep wrists straight in this exercise.
• Maintain a smooth movement from bottom to top of range of motion; avoid jerky movements.
• Keep knees slightly bent.
• Focus your mind on working muscles.

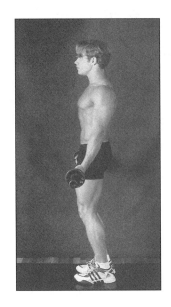
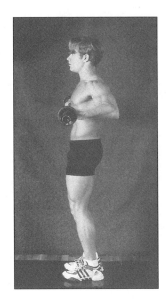

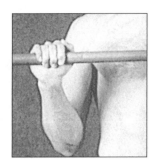

Exercise:
Barbell Reverse Curl

DIFFICULTY: 3
LOWER BACK: HIGH RISK
AREA: BICEPS, FOREARMS

STARTING POSITION: Grasp a barbell in a shoulder width, overhand grip. Stand with feet shoulder width apart, with knees slightly bent and arms fully extended.

MOVEMENT: Curl the barbell in an upward arc toward your chin. Contract your biceps muscle at the top of the movement. Then slowly lower the barbell back to starting position.

   Variations: Movement can also be done with an E-Z curl bar or with a cable attachment, using the lower pulley.

TRAINER'S TIPS:
• Keep upper arm motionless and pressed close to upper torso throughout the range of movement.
• Upper body should remain motionless throughout the exercise.
• It is important to keep wrists straight in this exercise.
• Maintain a smooth movement from bottom to top of range of motion; avoid jerky motions.
• Do not lock out body; keep knees slightly bent.
• Avoid cheating movements such as bouncing or "throwing" weight upward.
• Focus your mind on working muscles.
• For safety, wrap thumbs around the bar.

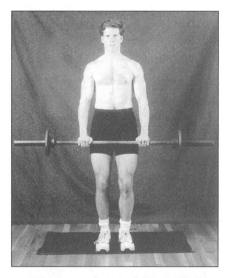

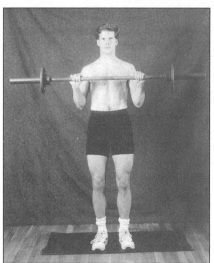

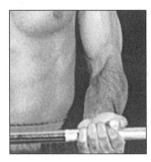

Exercise:
21s (Barbells)

DIFFICULTY: 3
LOWER BACK: MODERATE RISK
AREA: BICEPS

STARTING POSITION: Grasp barbell with an underhand grip, hands shoulder width apart, arms hanging down in front of your body.

MOVEMENT: Using any curl movement (traditionally this is done with standing barbell curls), divide the movement into three equal parts. In part one, you raise the barbell three quarters of the way up for seven reps. On the seventh rep, raise the barbell all the way up (under your chin). For part two, you then lower the barbell three quarters of the way down for seven reps. On the seventh rep, lower the barbell all the way. Then complete the exercise by doing seven reps with a full range of motion.

    Variations: Can be performed with any curl exercise.

TRAINER'S TIPS:
- Concentrate on the small movements.
- Control both upward and downward phases of movement.
- Focus your mind on the biceps throughout the exercise.

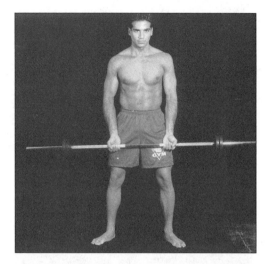

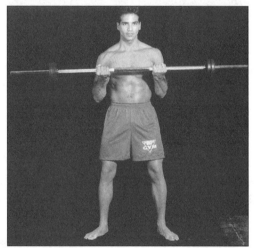

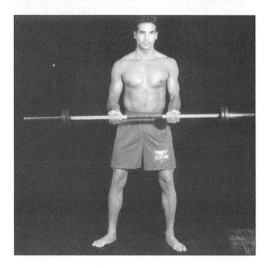

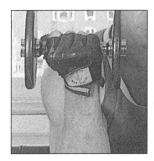

Exercise:
Dumbbell Preacher Curl

DIFFICULTY: 2
LOWER BACK: LOW RISK
AREA: BICEPS

STARTING POSITION: Place your chest firmly against a preacher stand. Grasping two dumbbells, let arms hang down and across preacher stand, palms facing up.

MOVEMENT: Curl both dumbbells in a smooth arc to the shoulder. Then lower the weights back to starting position.

   Variations: Preacher dumbbell curls may also be performed with one arm at a time. You may choose a synchronized movement, raising one dumbbell as the other is descending, or concentrate on each arm separately. This exercise may also be performed with weights in the Hammer Curl position.

TRAINER'S TIPS:
• Be very careful not to allow weights to bounce or drop at the end of the movement or when approaching failure. Your biceps are especially vulnerable when the forearm is fully extended.
• Keep upper arm motionless and in contact with bench throughout the range of movement.
• Aim for a smooth, flowing movement.
• Focus your mind on working muscles.
• Do not allow torso to move up and down (stay seated).

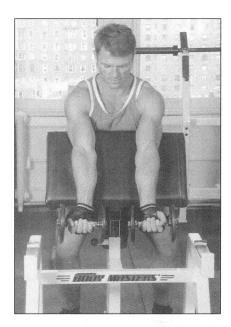

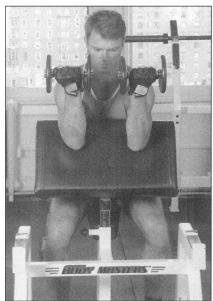

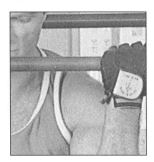

Exercise:
Barbell Preacher Curl

DIFFICULTY: 2
LOWER BACK: LOW RISK
AREA: BICEPS

STARTING POSITION: Lean over a preacher stand with your chest firmly pressed against the edge of the bench and grasp a barbell in a shoulder width, underhand grip. Upper arms should be parallel to each other while lower arms are fully extended. You may stand or sit.

MOVEMENT: Curl the barbell in an upward arc from starting position to a point where the forearms are perpendicular to the ground. Contract your biceps at the top of the movement, then slowly lower the barbell back to starting position.

TRAINER'S TIPS:
• Keep upper arm pressed tight against upper edge of preacher stand throughout the movement.
• Maintain a smooth movement throughout the entire range of motion.
• Avoid cheating movements such as bouncing or "throwing" weight upward.
• Focus your mind on working muscles.
• Do not allow the torso to move up and down.

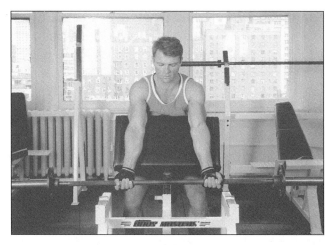

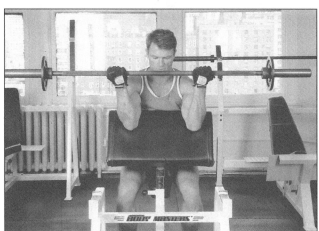

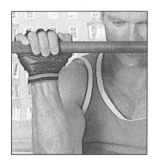

Exercise:
Barbell Preacher Curl, Reverse

DIFFICULTY: 3
LOW BACK: LOW RISK
AREA: BICEPS, FOREARMS

STARTING POSITION: Grasp a barbell in a shoulder width, overhand grip. Lean over preacher bench with your armpits firmly pressed against the edge of the bench. Upper arms should be parallel to each other and the lower arms are fully extended. You may stand or sit.

MOVEMENT: Curl the barbell slowly toward your chin in an upward arc. Contract all arm muscles strongly at the top of the movement, then slowly lower the barbell back to starting position.

TRAINER'S TIPS:
• Keep upper arm pressed tight against upper edge of preacher bench throughout the movement.
• Maintain a smooth movement throughout the range of motion; avoid jerky motions.
• Avoid cheating movements such as bouncing or "throwing" weight upward.
• Focus your mind on working muscles.
• Do not allow torso to move up and down.

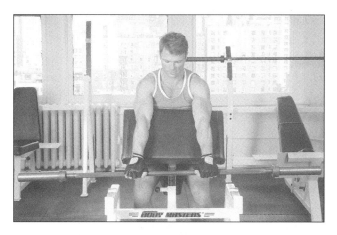

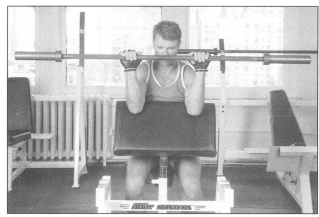

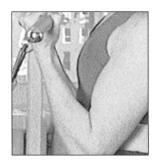

Exercise:
Standing Cable Curl

DIFFICULTY: 1
LOWER BACK: MODERATE RISK
AREA: BICEPS, FOREARM

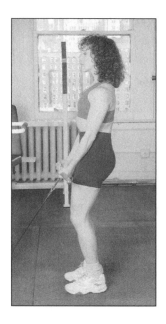
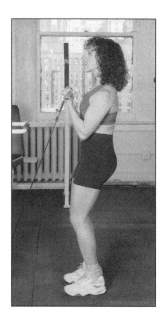

STARTING POSITION: Using the straight bar handle attachment on the floor position pulley, grasp the handle in a shoulder width grip, palms facing up. Stand with feet shoulder width apart, approximately 1½ feet away from floor pulley, body straight and in good lifting posture with knees slightly bent and arms fully extended at your sides. Keep upper arms motionless and pressed against torso throughout movement.

MOVEMENT: Curl the bar handle in an arc to your chest, aiming for the spot just below your chin. Hold the bar at this point. Drop wrists and elevate the elbows slightly while contracting strongly with your concentration on your biceps, then slowly lower the bar handle back to starting position.

    Variations: This exercise can be done with a variety of attachments. You may also stand farther from the floor pulley attachment to vary the exercise. This exercise may be performed in a kneeling position as well as standing.

TRAINER'S TIPS:
- Keep upper arm motionless and pressed close to upper torso throughout the range of movement.
- Upper body should remain motionless throughout the exercise.
- Maintain a smooth movement from bottom to top of range of motion; avoid jerky motions.
- Avoid cheating movements such as bouncing, rocking with hips, or "throwing" weight upward.
- Do not lock out body; keep knees slightly bent.
- Focus your mind on working muscles.

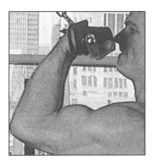

Exercise:
High Cable Curl

DIFFICULTY: 2
LOWER BACK: LOW RISK
AREA: BICEPS

STARTING POSITION: With a straight bar handle attached to the overhead cable, grasp the bar in a close underhand grip, approximately six inches apart. Stand far enough away that arms can be fully extended while allowing weight stack to be elevated.

MOVEMENT: Curl the bar toward your shoulders, keeping your upper arms stationary. Then slowly return the bar handle back to the starting point.

Variations: This exercise can be performed sitting or kneeling on the floor. It is helpful to have a spotter press you into the floor during the movements to avoid rising up with each repetition. It can also be performed one arm at a time.

TRAINER'S TIPS:
• Upper body should remain motionless.
• Body should not lift off floor during exercise.
• Maintain a smooth movement throughout the entire range of motion.
• Avoid cheating by bouncing or "throwing" weight up and down.
• Focus your mind on working muscles.

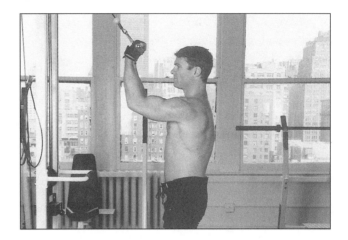

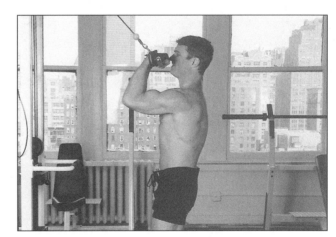

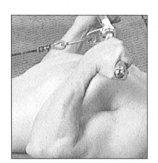

Exercise:
Supine Cable Curl

DIFFICULTY: 2
LOWER BACK: LOW RISK
AREA: BICEPS

STARTING POSITION: Lie on your back on the floor, grasping a straight bar handle attached to a lower cable pulley. With a shoulder width, underhand grip, keep arms fully extended at your sides.

MOVEMENT: Curl the bar up from your thighs to a position just below your chin. Contract your biceps at the top of the motion, then slowly lower the bar handle back to starting position.

    Variations: You may also reverse your grip and perform a Reverse Supine Cable Curl. Exercise can also be done lying on a bench.

TRAINER'S TIPS:
• Keep upper arms motionless and pressed close to upper torso throughout the range of movement.
• Maintain a smooth movement throughout the range of motion.
• Focus your mind on working muscles.

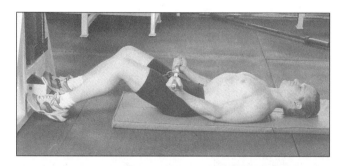

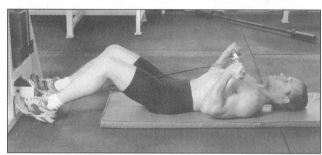

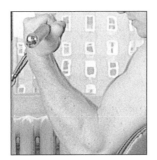

Exercise:
Cable Preacher Curl

DIFFICULTY: 2
LOWER BACK: MODERATE RISK
AREA: BICEPS, FOREARMS

STARTING POSITION: Position a preacher bench about 2½ feet from the floor position pulley, with the angled pad pointing down toward the machine. Using the straight bar handle attachment on the floor position pulley, lean over the bench with your armpits firmly pressed against the edge of the bench and grasp the bar with an underhand grip. Upper arms should be parallel to each other while lower arms are fully extended and leaning down on the angled bench pad in starting position. You may stand or sit.

MOVEMENT: Curl the bar handle slowly toward you in an upward arc from starting position to the spot just below your chin. Contract all arm muscles strongly at the top of the movement, then slowly lower the bar handle back to starting position.

Variations: Grasp the bar with a range of grips to work muscles fully. You may also stand farther back from the floor pulley attachment to vary the exercise.

TRAINER'S TIPS:
- Keep upper arm pressed tight against upper edge of preacher bench throughout the movement.
- Maintain a smooth movement from bottom to top of range of motion; avoid jerky motions.
- Avoid cheating movements such as bouncing or "throwing" weight upward.
- Focus your mind on working muscles.

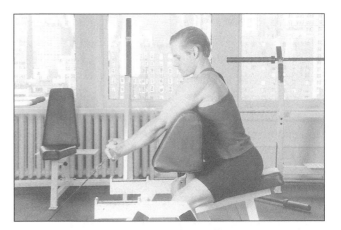

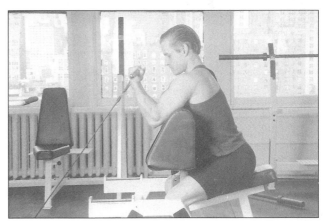

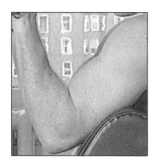

Exercise:
Cable Preacher Curl, Reverse

DIFFICULTY: 3
LOWER BACK: LOW RISK
AREA: FOREARMS

STARTING POSITION: Position a preacher bench about 2½ feet from the lower pulley. Using the straight bar attachment, lean over the bench with your armpits firmly pressed against the edge of the bench and grasp the bar with an overhand grip. Upper arms should be parallel to each other while lower arms are fully extended. You may stand or sit.

MOVEMENT: Curl the bar handle toward your chin. Contract biceps at the top of the movement, then slowly lower the bar handle back to starting position.

TRAINER'S TIPS:
• Keep upper arm pressed tight against upper edge of preacher bench throughout the movement.
• Maintain a smooth movement from bottom to top of range of motion; avoid jerky motions.
• Avoid cheating movements such as bouncing or "throwing" weight upward.
• Focus your mind on working muscles.

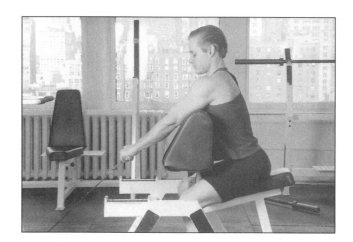

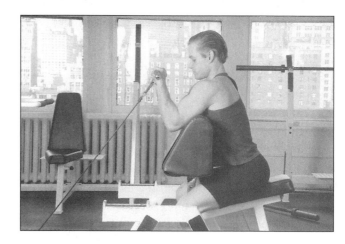

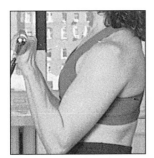

Exercise:
Cable Curl, Reverse

DIFFICULTY: 2
LOWER BACK: MODERATE RISK
AREA: FOREARMS (FLEXOR MUSCLES SECONDARILY), BICEPS, SHOULDERS (BRACHIALIS)

STARTING POSITION: Using a straight bar handle attachment on the floor or other low position pulley, grasp the handle in a shoulder width overhand grip. Stand with feet shoulder width apart approximately six inches away from the pulley in good lifting posture, with knees slightly bent and arms fully extended at your sides. Keep upper arms motionless and pressed against torso throughout movement.

MOVEMENT: Curl the bar handle in an upward arc from the top of your thighs to your chest, aiming for the spot just below your chin. Hold the bar at this point, contracting strongly with your concentration on upper- and forearm muscles, then slowly lower the bar handle back to starting position.

   Variations: Grasp the bar with a range of narrower grips to work muscles fully.

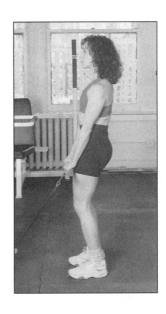 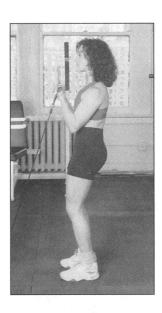

TRAINER'S TIPS:
• Keep upper arm motionless and pressed close to upper torso throughout the range of movement.
• Upper body should remain motionless throughout the exercise.
• Maintain a smooth movement from bottom to top of range of motion; avoid jerky motions.
• Do not lock out body; keep knees slightly bent.
• Avoid cheating movements such as bouncing or "throwing" weight upward.
• Focus your mind on working muscles.

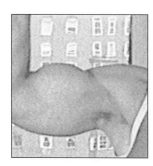

Exercise:
High Cable
Cross Curl

DIFFICULTY: 2
LOWER BACK: LOW RISK
AREA: BICEPS

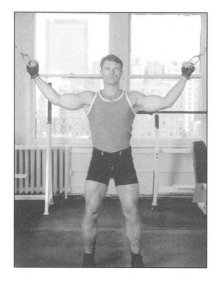

STARTING POSITION: Attach handles to high cable on cable cross machine. Grasping both handles with an underhand grip, position yourself between the two stacks with your shoulders toward the cable weight stacks. Bend knees slightly, with feet shoulder width apart. Arms should be extended at shoulder level.

MOVEMENT: Keeping your elbows static, curl your hands inward until they touch your ears. Return under control to original starting position, keeping your elbows static.

   Variations: Can be performed with one arm, alternating, and with an overhand grip. You can also position yourself on your knees or sit on a bench.

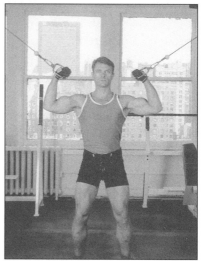

TRAINER'S TIPS:
• Maintain your body position throughout the exercise.
• Keep the elbows static throughout the exercise.
• Focus your mind on the biceps throughout the exercise.
• For added intensity, bring hands behind the head.

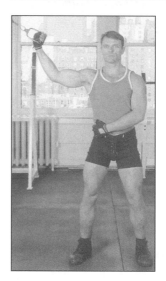
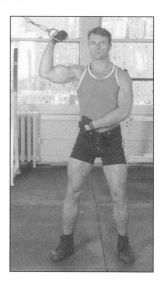

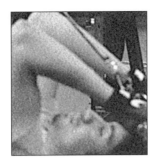

Exercise:
Supine High Cable Curl

DIFFICULTY: 2
LOWER BACK: LOW RISK
AREA: BICEPS

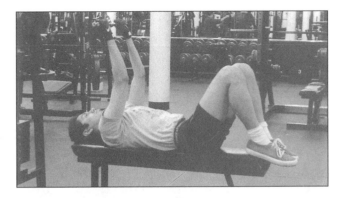

STARTING POSITION: Place a flat work bench about 12 inches away from the weight stack. With your back to the weight stack, grasp attachment (E-Z curl, straight bar, or single handle) with an underhand grip. Assume the supine position (on your back) on the work bench with your arms extended perpendicular to the floor.

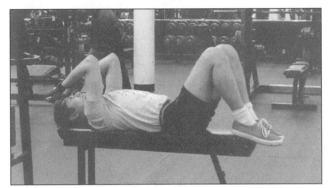

MOVEMENT: Keeping your upper arm static, pull your hands toward you until you touch the top of your head. Return under control to original starting position, keeping your elbows static.

   Variations: Can be performed with one arm, with an overhand grip (reverse grip), or with your head at the other end of the bench.

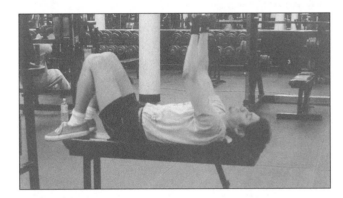

TRAINER'S TIPS:
• Keep body weight distributed on your shoulder blades.
• Keep the upper arm static throughout the exercise.
• Focus your mind on the biceps throughout the exercise.
• Do not allow the torso to raise up.

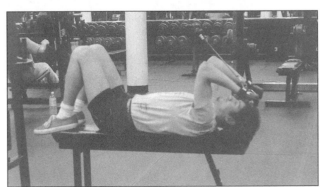

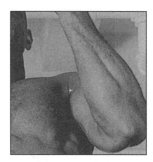

Exercise:
Biceps Chin-Up

DIFFICULTY: 2
LOWER BACK: LOW RISK
AREA: BICEPS

STARTING POSITION: Grasp a chinning bar in a narrow, underhand grip, with hands approximately six inches apart. Hang with arms fully extended. Legs may be straight or bent and crossed.

MOVEMENT: With a smooth motion, pull yourself up so that your chin is above the bar, solely by bending your arms in a curling motion. Contract biceps muscles, then slowly lower your body back to starting position.

  Variations: Biceps chin-ups may also be performed with a reverse or overhand grip.

TRAINER'S TIPS:
• Move hands closer together, even touching, for an increased stress on the biceps.
• Maintain a smooth movement throughout the entire range of motion.
• Focus your mind on the biceps, trying to take the back muscles out of the movement.
• This is a good exercise with which to perform negatives.

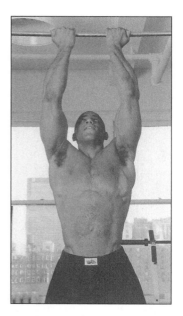

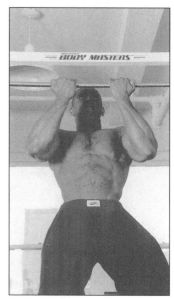

CHAPTER THIRTEEN

The Forearms

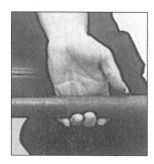

Exercise: Wrist Flexion

DIFFICULTY: 1
LOWER BACK: LOW RISK
AREA: FOREARMS

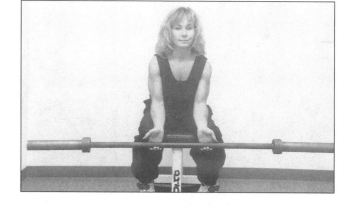

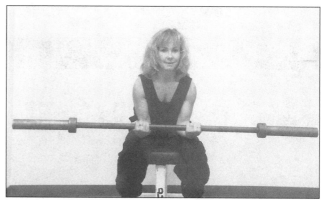

STARTING POSITION: Sit or squat grasping a barbell so that your forearms rest on top of your thighs or on a bench with palms facing up. Hands should hang over the knees.

MOVEMENT: Keeping proper back alignment, lower the bar by allowing your hands to drop until they are perpendicular to your forearm. Once bottom position is reached, move the bar upward by flexing (raising) your hands as far as possible. Repeat for the prescribed number of repetitions.

Variations: Can be performed with dumbbells or machine. This exercise can also be done standing and behind your back.

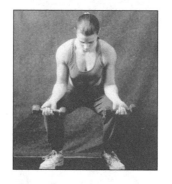
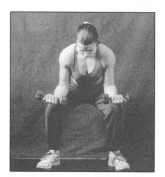

TRAINER'S TIPS:
- Make sure the forearms remain flat on bench or thighs with elbows bent and upper arm perpendicular to the forearms.
- Keep forearms/elbows in contact with thighs or bench through the range of motion.
- If necessary, elevate heels to ensure a full range of motion.
- Concentrate on using the wrist and not the biceps to move the bar.
- Keep good postural alignment.
- Focus your mind on your forearms.

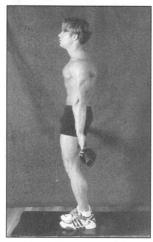
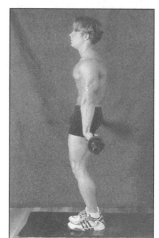

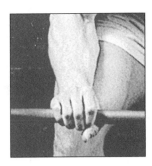

Exercise:
Wrist Extension

DIFFICULTY: 1
LOWER BACK: LOW RISK
AREA: FOREARMS

STARTING POSITION: Sit or kneel grasping a barbell, placing your forearms on top of your thighs or on a bench with palms facing down. Hands should hang over your knees.

MOVEMENT: Keeping proper back alignment, lower the bar by allowing your hands to drop until they are perpendicular to your forearm. Once bottom position is reached, move the bar upward by curling (raising) your hands as far as possible. Repeat for the prescribed number of repetitions.

  Variations: Can be performed with dumbbells or machine.

TRAINER'S TIPS:
- Keep elbows in contact with thighs or bench throughout the range of motion.
- Make sure the forearms remain flat on bench or thighs, with elbows bent and upper arm perpendicular to the forearms.
- If necessary, elevate heels to ensure a full range of motion.
- Keep good postural alignment.
- Focus your mind on your forearms.

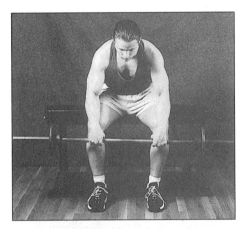

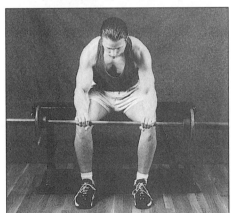

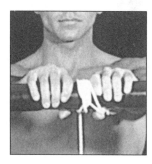

Exercise:
Wrist Roll

DIFFICULTY: 2
LOWER BACK: MODERATE RISK
AREA: FOREARMS

STARTING POSITION: Stand with knees slightly bent, feet shoulder width apart, and arms parallel to the ground. Grasp the ends of the roller with palms facing down.

MOVEMENT: Keeping proper back alignment and with arms straight, roll weights up (away from body or forward), rotating the roller bar one hand at a time, until the resistance is raised to the top of the roller bar. Roll the resistance down in a controlled manner. Repeat for the prescribed number of repetitions.

To work wrist extension, roll weight up by rotating the bar toward your body.

TRAINER'S TIPS:
• Emphasize rolling with the index finger of each hand.
• Use full range of motion.
• Keep good postural alignment.
• Focus your mind on your forearms.

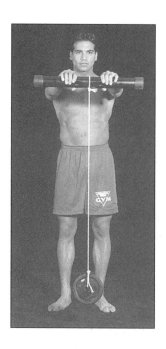
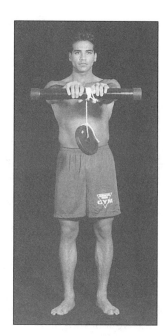

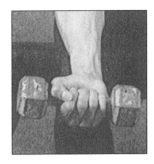

Exercise:
Forearm Rotation Supination/Pronation

DIFFICULTY: 1
LOWER BACK: LOW RISK
AREA: FOREARMS, BICEPS

STARTING POSITION: In a seated position, grasp dumbbell and place forearm on top of your thigh so palm is facing down. Hand should hang over the knee.

MOVEMENT: Keeping proper back alignment, rotate the dumbbell by allowing your palm to face up (thumb moving outside). From this position rotate the dumbbell in the other direction (thumb in) until palm is facing down. Repeat for the prescribed number of repetitions.

   Variations: Can be performed one arm at a time or with two arms.

TRAINER'S TIPS:
• Keep forearm/elbow in contact with thigh or bench throughout the range of motion.
• Control speed of movement.
• If necessary, elevate heels to ensure a full range of motion.
• Keep good postural alignment.
• Focus your mind on your forearms.

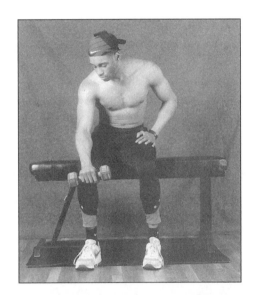

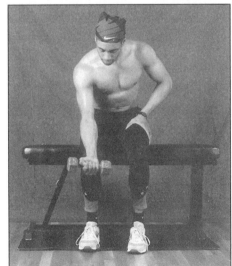

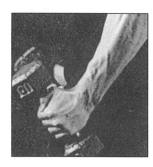

Exercise:
Radial Flexion

DIFFICULTY: 1
LOWER BACK: LOW RISK
AREA: FOREARMS

STARTING POSITION: Stand with knees slightly bent, feet shoulder width apart. Grasp dumbbells with little finger up against the weight plates, palm toward the body. Maintain correct back alignment, while letting arms hang to the side naturally.

MOVEMENT: Relax your hands, allowing the thumb side of the dumbbells to drop. Keeping the arms straight, raise the lowered end as high as possible (so that the far end of the dumbbell moves toward the forearm). Return to starting position in a controlled manner. Repeat for the prescribed number of repetitions.

Variations: Can be performed with one arm at a time.

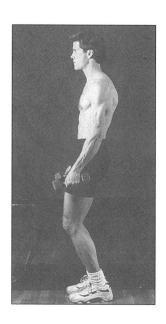
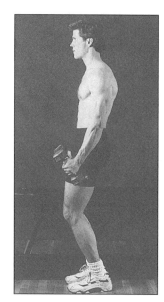

TRAINER'S TIPS:
• Use full range of motion.
• Keep good postural alignment.
• Don't swing arms.

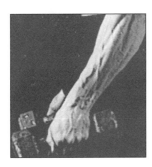

Exercise:
Ulna Flexion

DIFFICULTY: 1
LOWER BACK: LOW RISK
AREA: FOREARMS

STARTING POSITION: Stand with knees slightly bent, feet shoulder width apart. Grasp dumbbells with thumb up against the plates, palm toward the body. Maintain correct back alignment, while letting arms hang to the side naturally.

MOVEMENT: Relax your hand, allowing the little-finger side of the dumbbell to drop. Keeping the arms straight, raise the lowered end as high as possible so that the plates on the lowered end move toward the forearm. Return to starting position in a controlled manner. Repeat for the prescribed number of repetitions.

    Variations: Can be performed with one arm at a time.

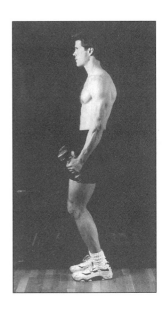 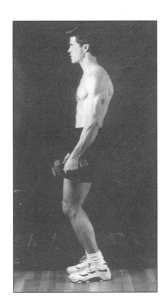

TRAINER'S TIPS:
• Use full range of motion.
• Keep good postural alignment.
• Focus your mind on your forearms.

The Machines

Exercise Machines

This chapter will explain the underlying principles behind proper machine usage, allowing you to feel confident on most of the equipment in health clubs. There are, however, over 20 different manufacturers of exercise equipment. Each brand should display instruction placards for proper use. So make sure you review these instructions for the variations in seat setup, starting positions, and finish positions.

The recent history of exercise machines began with the development of Nautilus equipment. Arthur Jones, the inventor of Nautilus, felt that productive muscular exercise should provide resistance that varies according to the strength of the movement throughout its range of motion. His first attempt at providing this type of changing resistance was done with a bench press. He knew that people were stronger in the last part of this exercise than they were in the first part. This was caused by the increasing biomechanical advantage of the musculoskeletal system toward the end of the lift. In order to increase the resistance at the end of the range of motion, he welded hooks on a barbell and hung heavy chain from it. Thus, as he raised the bar from his chest toward the finish position, he was lifting increasing links of chain from the floor. This led to the idea for variable resistance exercise machines and ultimately the development of Nautilus. As the fitness boom evolved, a variety of machines came on the market with the goal of making weight training safe and productive for the masses.

Exercise Machines Pro and Con

PROS
- Provide variable resistance throughout a full range of motion. This means that as the movement gets easier, the machine automatically increases the resistance.
- Ease of use. The weights are attached (as opposed to free weights) and move in a fixed direction. So you really can't do the movement incorrectly.
- Safety. Since the weights are attached, they can't fall on your head or slide off the bar (it's happened to the best of us). Machines are a safe and effective way for a beginner to build a foundation of strength.
- Isolation of a specific area.
- Ability to limit range of motion for rehabilitation.

CONS
- Size.
- Cost.
- Maintenance.
- Most machines don't work the limbs (shoulders and arms) independently. This means your stronger or dominant arm (your right arm if you're right-handed) is likely to work harder and continue to get bigger and stronger. So it is more difficult to build muscle balance and symmetry on a machine.
- Fixed plane of motion. This is good for safety. But there is not one single fixed plane that is normal or correct for everyone.
- Isolation. Strict isolation doesn't allow the synergistic muscles, which are used to help balance and stabilize the primary working muscle, to get a workout.

Basics Guide for Using Exercise Machines

There are two basic types of machines: those used for isolated movements (one joint) and those used for compound movements (more than one joint).

ISOLATED MOVEMENTS (ONE JOINT)
The key to using these machines is lining up your joint with the axis of rotation of the machine. The axis of rotation is the spot on the machine that the moving part (the exercise arm) rotates around. It is like a joint in a body. You want to line up your axis of rotation for the exercise with the machine's axis of rotation. For a curl, your axis of rotation is your elbow joint. From that joint your arm flexes and extends. You want to line up your elbow with the axis of rotation on the machine for the most effective range of motion. It's as if you become one with the machine.

COMPOUND MACHINES (MORE THAN ONE JOINT)
On this type of machine you want to adjust the height so your starting position allows you to go through a full range of motion. For shoulders, adjust the seat so the starting position of the exercise bar is even with your shoulder joint and creates a slight stretching sensation. Think of yourself as the motor that powers the machine.

Machines for Shoulders and Arms

SHOULDERS
The shoulder, being a ball-and-socket joint, has many degrees of movement. It is therefore impossible to work all the angles on any exercise machine. For that matter, it is impractical to attempt all ranges of motions with a barbell or dumbbell. The two most common exercise machines for the shoulder are the lateral raise and overhead press.

Lateral Raise: When adjusting this machine for individual use, the seat should be set so that the axis of rotation on the machine is aligned with the shoulder socket. The movement is abducting or raising the arms out to the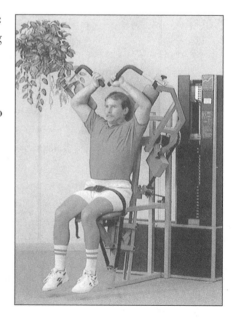

side. Resistance should be applied on the pads that fit the upper arms or forearms. The biggest mistake that people make using this machine is gripping the handles tightly and trying to raise the machine with their hands.

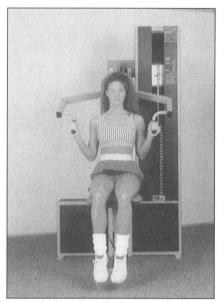

Overhead Press: This is a compound movement that involves the arms being raised through the shoulders and the elbows. Set this machine up by adjusting the height of the seat so the handlebars are even with your shoulder joint. Always, however, let comfort determine how you set up the machine. The exercise is done by pressing the weight overhead and then lowering back to the start position. A drawback to these machines is that you cannot adjust the width of your grip, which can either increase or decrease the range of motion.

BICEPS AND TRICEPS

Control of elbow movement is accomplished by the biceps, which flex or bend the elbow, and the triceps which extend or straighten the arm. This movement is accomplished through one axis of rotation (the elbow).

Arm Curl: Most exercise machines provide a biceps exercise in the preacher curl position. When setting up the machine, align your elbow with the machine's axis of rotation. Adjusting the seat can increase or decrease the movement range of motion. Lowering the seat increases the range of motion, and raising the

seat decreases it. Adjust the seat to a comfortable but full range of motion for you. An advantage to this machine over a dumbbell or barbell is that at the end of the range of motion, the machine is still providing

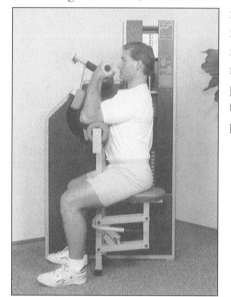

resistance. The rotary resistance mechanism (on most machines) pulls you back to the starting position.

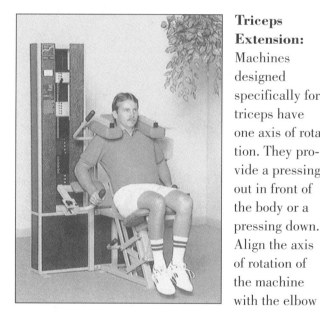

Triceps Extension: Machines designed specifically for triceps have one axis of rotation. They provide a pressing out in front of the body or a pressing down. Align the axis of rotation of the machine with the elbow using the seat height adjustment. Extend the arm under resistance to complete the movement. Keep in mind that the function of this movement is to work the triceps. Do not squeeze the handle grips tightly, as this only increases blood pressure and fatigues the forearms before the triceps reach fatigue.

Exercise machines can provide a quick, effective exercise environment for you. As with any type of resistance, the movement should be slow and smooth, with mental concentration focusing on the muscle groups being worked. Finding which exercises you like to do on machines and which ones you prefer to do with free weights is a matter of trial and error. Enjoy the process.

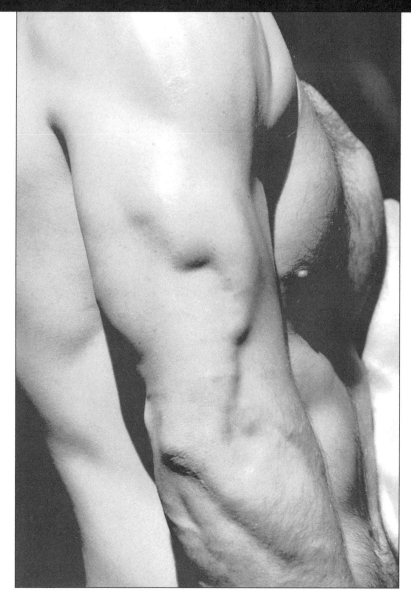

PART FOUR

The Routines

Introduction to the System

To best meet your individual needs, the system has been divided into five programs: shoulders, biceps, triceps, forearms, and trapezius. The programs are the same for both men and women. Muscle is muscle, no matter which sex you are. There will be programs for both home and gym, and a final program for ultimate arm and shoulder development (designed to take you to your highest potential). The gym routines are 24-week programs for developing and strengthening your shoulders and arms. The home routine is designed to allow you to achieve the same development with minimal equipment. The Ultimate Shoulders and Arms program is a highly advanced, nine-week program designed to bring your shoulders and arms to peak potential. You should not begin this program until you have completed all of the previous levels.

These programs do all of the planning for you. They incorporate the training principles discussed in Chapter 3 into each workout. The only thing you have to do is commit to the plan.

Each level of every program is designed to stand on its own while leading progressively to the next level. Depending on your own personal needs and goals, you may complete an entire program, or stop at any level and move to a maintenance routine.

Maintenance Routines

The goal of a maintenance routine is to hang on to the benefits you have worked so hard to achieve. If you finish a level and don't feel the need to move on, it is time to implement a maintenance program. You cannot just stop exercising. Consistency is the key to achieving and keeping the health benefits of exercise. You can maintain your results for each level by following the routine for the last week of the level completed. For example, if you wanted the benefits for any body part at level three, you would follow the workout of the last week for that level. In most cases, maintenance will be a less intense prescription than muscle building. If you want to increase the intensity of our maintenance routine, you can go for two options: increasing the weight or increasing the sets performed. Remember, muscular balance must be maintained between the different muscle groups. If increasing for one group, you should increase for the other groups accordingly.

It is important to note that even though a maintenance program may be effective for a period of time, the body will ultimately grow complacent. The reasons for this are simple: A maintenance program does not adhere to the principles of progression, overload, and variety. There will be regression over a period of time. You cannot sustain the same fitness level if you do not shock the body and force it to adapt.

Advancement

Everyone will progress at different speeds. Each level is designed to move you to the next level. If for some reason you do not feel ready to move on, spend another week, or two weeks if necessary, on your current level. Listen to your body. It will tell you if you're ready to move on. Just don't forget that you must continue to shock the body to achieve growth. Don't stay too long on a level. To be what you have never been, you must do what you have never done. Therefore, you must force yourself to move on.

Remember, there's no slacking off on the lifestyle behaviors that support your weight training program: You need to continuously follow a healthy diet, cut down on your fat content, and do some type of cardiovascular work at least three to four times a week. The combination of all these factors will create the look, feel, and health benefits you want.

Substitutions

If there is an exercise in any of the systems that you can't do for whatever reason—injury, lack of equipment, inability to correctly perform the exercise—then go ahead and substitute. You need to choose an exercise that works the same area(s), has the same difficulty level, and isn't already in the routine. If you have exhausted all options, you can repeat an exercise that is already in the routine that fits these criteria.

Multisets

Multisets are sets comprising two or more exercises in which there is no rest period between the exercises. For example, barbell curls and biceps chins may be grouped in what is called a Super Set. The program may call for three sets of Super Sets, eight repetitions each. This means that you will perform eight repetitions of barbell curls and then without any rest you will perform eight repetitions of biceps chins. You will then rest the required time, and repeat both exercises in the same fashion; then rest again, then repeat the exercise again.

In the different programs, exercises may on occasion be grouped together. These groupings are:

Compound Set: A Compound Set consists of two different exercises in which opposite (agonist/antagonist) sides of a joint are worked. For example, you would do the prescribed number of reps for Triceps Push-Downs (triceps) immediately followed by the prescribed number of reps for Preacher Curls (biceps), followed by rest. These two exercises performed back to back equal one set for each exercise. Then repeat for the prescribed number of sets.

Super Set: A Super Set consists of two different exercises in which the same muscle groups are worked. For example, Supine Triceps Extensions and Close Grip Bench Presses are performed back to back, in the same fashion as the compound set.

Triset: A Triset consists of three different exercises in which the same muscle groups are trained. For example, Standing Dumbbell Curls are performed for the prescribed number of reps, followed by Seated Hammer Curls, then Concentration Curls, each of the latter two performed for the prescribed number of repetitions. After completing all three in a row, you have done one set. Rest and repeat if necessary.

Giant Set: A Giant Set consists of four or more different exercises in which the same muscle groups are trained. For example, Front Raises, Lateral Raises, Rear Delt Raises, and Seated Dumbbell Presses are performed back to back in the same manner as the Super Sets or Tri Sets above.

Recovery Principles

It is important that you allow adequate recovery time for the muscles you have worked out. Current research indicates that you need a minimum of 48 hours recovery in between lifting the same body part. After that time, your guess may be as good as anyone's. Most experts consider 72 to 96 hours to be optimal. Empirically, strength gains have been made with a variety of recovery times. Your guidelines should consist of no less than 48 hours (every other day) and no more than 120 hours (5 days). Experiment, and see where optimal training takes place for you, as your recovery time may be different from someone else's.

Protocols

STRIPPING PROTOCOL

After completing the last set, strip (unload) 10 percent, or the closest equivalent, of the weight off the bar or machine. If exercising with dumbbells, have them already preselected. Once stripped, rest for 15 sec-

onds. Complete the next set to failure. Unload 10 percent, rest for 15 seconds, complete the next set to failure. Repeat the procedure for one final set.

ISOMETRIC CONTRACTION

When prescribed following the last repetition, complete the movement through the full range of motion (finish the positive phase of the movement). From this position hold contraction for prescribed amount of time. Then, using a controlled 10-second eccentric contraction, unload the resistance.

OVERLOAD PROTOCOL

After concentric (positive) failure is reached, perform a strict assisted rep. This is accomplished by having a spotter help you complete the repetition. Once the assisted rep is completed, follow up with a 15-second isometric contraction. This contraction takes place at the end of the positive phase. Rest for 15 seconds. This may be accomplished by racking, handing the spotter the weights, or putting the weights on the floor. After a 15-second rest, perform another concentric movement followed again by a 15-second isometric contraction.

Planning Your Workouts

In some levels you will work out two days a week, in others three. Remember your recovery principles when planning workouts.

The best plan for those levels in which you work out three times a week is to lift on Monday, Wednesday, and Friday. Another option would be to lift Tuesday, Thursday, and Saturday. The best plan for the levels where you work out two times a week is to lift on Monday and Thursday, Tuesday and Friday, Wednesday and Saturday. If intensity levels are high, add another day of recovery. The most important thing is to plan the days and times you know you can work out consistently, and stick with that schedule.

The Home System

This program is designed for your home. You do not need any special equipment such as weight benches, special home gym machines, or gadgets. The only equipment you will need is a set of adjustable dumbbells, which can be purchased for a reasonable price at most sporting good stores and are easily stored.

The system is designed so you can work one body area or all four areas in a workout, depending on your needs. Remember, your goal is always to train for whole-body conditioning: strength, cardio, and stretching.

Phase 1: Building a Foundation

WEEKS 1 AND 2

Train two times a week, taking at least two days off between workouts. In each exercise try to add one rep per workout.

REST:

One minute between exercises.

Shoulders	Sets	Reps
Dumbbell Shoulder Press (page 152)	1	15–20
Traps		
Shrugs (page 168)	1	15–20
Triceps		
Dumbbell Upright Extensions (page 179)	1	15–20
Biceps		
Standing Dumbbell Curls (page 201)	1	15–20

Training tips: As you go into week three, you may be saying to yourself, this workout seems easy, it can't be doing anything. Keep in mind you don't need to do a lot in the beginning to get results. When you're just starting out it doesn't take much to shock the body and cause it to adapt. During the first month concentrate on mastering proper technique and establishing proper workout habits.

WEEKS 3 AND 4

Train three times a week, taking at least ONE day off between workouts. In each exercise try to add one rep per workout. When you work up to 20 reps for each exercise, add a 2½-pound plate to each side of your dumbbells.

REST:

30 to 45 seconds between exercises.

Shoulders	Sets	Reps
Dumbbell Shoulder Press (page 152)	1	15–20
Traps		
Shrugs (page 168)	1	15–20
Triceps		
Dumbbell Upright Extensions (page 179)	1	15–20
Biceps		
Standing Dumbbell Curls (page 201)	1	15–20

Phase 2: Strengthen and Shape

WEEKS 5 AND 6

Train 3 times a week, taking at least ONE day off between workouts. In each exercise try to add one rep per workout. When you work up to 20 reps for each exercise, add a 2½-pound plate to each side of your dumbbells.

REST:

One minute between exercises.

Shoulders	Sets	Reps
Dumbbell Shoulder Press (page 152)	1	15–20
Rear Delt Raises (page 143)	1	15
Traps		
Shrugs (page 168)	1	15–20
Dumbbell Upright Rows (page 158)	1	15
Triceps		
Dumbbell Upright Extensions (page 179)	1	15–20
Bench Dips (page 195)	1 (to failure)	
Biceps		
Standing Dumbbell Curls, Alternating (page 201)	1	15–20
Concentration Curls (page 209)	1	15

WEEKS 7 AND 8

Train 3 times a week, taking at least ONE day off between workouts. During the next two weeks do two sets of each exercise. In each exercise try to add one rep per workout. When you work up to 20 reps for each exercise, add a 2½-pound plate to each side of your dumbbells.

REST:

One minute between exercises.

Shoulders	Sets	Reps
Dumbbell Shoulder Press (page 152)	2	15–20
Rear Delt Raises (page 143)	2	15
Traps		
Shrugs (page 168)	2	15–20
Dumbbell Upright Rows (page 158)	2	15
Triceps		
Dumbbell Upright Extensions (page 179)	2	15–20
Bench Dips (page 195)	2 (to failure)	
Biceps		
Seated Dumbbell Curls, Alternating (page 201)	2	15–20
Concentration Curls (page 209)	2	15

Phase 3: See the Changes

WEEKS 9 AND 10

Train 3 times a week, taking at least ONE day off between workouts. During the next four weeks you'll increase your intensity by using a weight that will only allow you to do 10 reps, before you reach failure. Once you can do 15 reps with that weight, then add 2½ pounds to each side of the dumbbell.

REST:

1 minute between exercises and 30 seconds between sets.

Shoulders	Sets	Reps
Dumbbell Shoulder Press (page 152)	2	10–15
Rear Delt Raises (page 143)	2	10–15
Traps		
Shrugs (page 168)	2	10–15
Dumbbell Upright Rows (page 158)	2	10–15
Triceps		
Dumbbell Upright Extensions (page 179)	2	10–15
Bench Dips (page 195)	2 (to failure)	
Biceps		
Seated Dumbbell Curls, Alternating (page 201)	2	10–15
Concentration Curls (page 209)	2	15

WEEKS 11 AND 12

Train 3 times a week, taking at least ONE day off between workouts. During the next four weeks you'll increase your intensity by using a weight that will only allow you to do 10 reps, before you reach failure. Once you can do 15 reps with that weight, then add 2½ pounds to each side of the dumbbell.

REST:

1 minute between exercises and 15 seconds between sets.

Shoulders	Sets	Reps
Dumbbell Shoulder Press (page 152)	2	10–15
Rear Delt Raises (page 143)	2	10–15
Lateral Raises (page 141)	1	10–15
(Week 12: add another set.)		
Traps	**Sets**	**Reps**
Shrugs (page 168)	2	10–15
Dumbbell Upright Rows (page 158)	2	10–15
Trap Raises (page 175)	1	10–15
(Week 12: add another set.)		

Triceps		
Dumbbell Upright Extensions (page 179)	2	10–15
Bench Dips (page 195)	2 (to failure)	
Dumbbell Kickbacks (page 180)	1	10–15
(Week 12: add another set.)		
Biceps	**Sets**	**Reps**
Seated Dumbbell Curls, Alternating (page 200)	2	10–15
Concentration Curls (page 209)	2	15
Dumbbell 21s (page 216)		

Now that you've established a base of strength, endurance, and solid workout habits, the question is: What's the next step? First you need to evaluate your goals. Do you just want to maintain? Do you want to add strength and size? More definition and endurance? Here are a few tips.

To maintain, all you need to do is stay with the last phase twice a week.

To add strength and size, increase the intensity. This means lower your rep scheme. Stay between 5 and 10 reps. When you reach 10 reps, add weight. But the answer is not quite this simple. You also need to pay close attention to nutrition, caloric intake, and recuperation time. More information on this can be found in Chapters 5 and 18.

For endurance and definition, increase your volume. This means higher reps. Staying within 15 to 20 reps would be a good rule of thumb. But again, you must pay attention to nutrition, caloric intake, and aerobic work.

CHAPTER SEVENTEEN

The System

SHOULDERS GYM

Level 1:
Preparation and Foundation

WEEKS 1-2, TWO TIMES PER WEEK
Concentric phase 2 seconds, eccentric phase 4 seconds.

Exercise	Sets	Reps	Rest
1. Dumbbell Shoulder Press, Bilateral (page 152)	3	15	60 seconds
2. Lateral Raise, Bilateral (page 141)	1	15	
3. Rear Delt Raise, Bilateral (page 143)	1	15	
4. High Cable Internal Rotation (page 160)	1	15	
5. Low Cable External Rotation (page 161)	1	15	

WEEKS 3-4, TWO TIMES PER WEEK
Concentric phase 2 seconds, eccentric phase 4 seconds.

Exercise	Sets	Reps	Rest
1. Lateral Raise, Bilateral (page 141)	3	15	45 seconds
2. Rear Delt Raise, Bilateral (page 143)	3	15	45 seconds
3. Dumbbell Shoulder Press, Bilateral (page 152)	1	15	
4. Low Cable External Rotation (page 161)	1	15	
5. High Cable Internal Rotation (page 160)	1	15	

WEEKS 5-6, TWO TIMES PER WEEK
Concentric phase 2 seconds, eccentric phase 4 seconds.

Exercise	Sets	Reps	Rest
1. Front Raise Dumbbell, Bilateral (page 138)	1	12	
2. Military Press (page 153)	3	12	45 seconds
3. Lateral Raise (page 141)	1	12	
4. Rear Delt Raise (page 143)	2	12	45 seconds
SUPER SET:			
5. Low Cable External Rotation (page 161)	1	12	
6. High Cable Internal Rotation (page 160)	1	12	

Level 2:
Creating Strength and Power

WEEKS 1-3, TWO TIMES PER WEEK
DAY 1

Exercise	Sets	Reps	Rest
1. Behind-the-Neck Press (page 154)	3	8	60 seconds
2. Rear Delt Raise, Unilateral (page 143)	3	8	
3. Front Raise with Plate (page 138)	1	8	
SUPER SET:			
4. Lateral Raise, Unilateral (page 141)	1	8	
5. Internal Cable Rotation (page 164)	1	8	

DAY 2

Exercise	Sets	Reps	Rest
1. Behind-the-Neck Press (page 154)	1	15	
2. Rear Delt Raise, Unilateral (page 143)	2	15	45 seconds
3. Front Raise with Plate (page 138)	2	8	60 seconds
4. Lateral Raise, Unilateral (page 141)	3	8	60 seconds
SUPER SET:			
5. External Cable Rotation (page 165)	1	8	
6. Internal Cable Rotation (page 164)	1	8	

Final set of each exercise is completed with a 10-second isometric contraction for the last repetition.

WEEKS 4-6, TWO TIMES PER WEEK
DAY 1

Exercise	Sets	Reps	Rest
1. Dumbbell Shoulder Press, Bilateral (page 152)	3	5-6	3 minutes
2. Rear Delt Raise, Unilateral (page 143)	3	5-6	3 minutes
3. Lateral Raise, Bilateral (page 141)	1	15	
4. Front Raise with Bar (page 138)	1	15	
5. Overhead Rotation (page 166)	1	5-6	

DAY 2

Exercise	Sets	Reps	Rest
1. Rear Delt Raise, Bilateral (page 143)	1	15	
2. Lateral Raise, Unilateral (page 141)	3	5-6	3 minutes
3. Front Raise with Bar (page 138)	3	5-6	3 minutes
4. Overhead Rotation (page 166)	1	5-6	
5. Dumbbell Shoulder Press, Bilateral (page 152)	1	12	

(continued)

For all exercises, repetitions for the last set are completed with an 8-second eccentric phase. Also incorporate a 15-second isometric contraction for the last repetition of each set.

ONE WEEK ACTIVE REST

Level 3:
Achieving Strength and Power

WEEKS 1–3, TWO TIMES PER WEEK

Exercise	Sets	Reps	Rest
1. Rotation Press, Bilateral (page 155)	3	12	60 seconds
2. Lateral Cable Raise, Bilateral (page 141)	1	12	
3. Rear Delt Cable Raise, Bilateral (page 145)	1	12	
SUPER SET:			
4. High Cable Internal Rotation (page 160)	1	12	
5. Low Cable External Rotation (page 161)	1	12	

WEEKS 4–6, TWO TIMES PER WEEK

Exercise	Sets	Reps	Rest
1. Military Press with Smith Machine (page 153)	3	8	2 minutes
2. Rear Delt Cable Raise, Bilateral (page 145)	2	8	2 minutes
3. Lateral Cable Raise, Bilateral (page 141)	2	8	2 minutes
SUPER SET:			
4. External Cable Rotation (page 165)	1	8	
5. Internal Cable Rotation (page 164)	1	8	

Final set of each exercise is completed with a 10-second isometric contraction for the last repetition.

WEEKS 7–9, TWO TIMES PER WEEK

DAY 1

Exercise	Sets	Reps	Rest
SUPER SET:			
1. Shoulder Press with Cable/ Machine/Dumbbell, Alternating (page 152)	3	5–6	
2. Cable Straight-Arm Pullback (page 146)	3	5–6	3 minutes
3. Upright Row (page 158)	1	15	
4. Lateral Cable Raise, Bilateral (page 141)	1	15	

After completion of last repetition for exercises 2 and 3, proceed with stripping protocol for those exercises (see page 245).

DAY 2

Exercise	Sets	Reps	Rest
1. Cable Straight-Arm Pullback (page 146)	1	15	
2. Upright Row (page 158)	3	5–6	3 minutes
3. Lateral Cable Raise, Unilateral (page 141)	3	5–6	3 minutes
4. Shoulder Press with Cable/ Machine/Dumbbell, Alternating (page 152)	1	15	

For exercises 1 and 2, complete last set with a 10-second isometric contraction for the last repetition.

After completion of last repetition for exercises 3 and 4, proceed with stripping protocol for those exercises (see page 245).

WEEKS 10–11, TWO TIMES PER WEEK

DAY 1

Exercise	Sets	Reps	Rest
SUPER SET:			
1. Behind-the-Neck Press (page 154)	3	5–6	
2. Rear Delt Raise, Bilateral (page 143)	3	5–6	3 minutes
3. Upright Row (page 158)	1	12	
4. Lateral Raise, Unilateral (page 141)	1	12	

After completion of last repetition for exercises 1 and 2, proceed with stripping protocol for those exercises (see page 245).

DAY 2

Exercise	Sets	Reps	Rest
1. Rear Delt Cable Raise, Unilateral (page 145)	1	12	90 seconds
2. Upright Row (page 158)	3	5–6	3 minutes
3. Lateral Cable Raise, Unilateral (page 141)	3	5–6	3 minutes
4. Military Press with Machine (page 153)	1	12	

Final set of each exercise is completed with a 10-second isometric contraction for the last repetition.

Ultimate Shoulders

WEEKS 1–3, TWO TIMES PER WEEK

DAY 1

Exercise	Sets	Reps	Rest
1. Dumbbell Shoulder Press, Bilateral (page 152)	3	12	60 seconds
2. Rear Delt Raise, Unilateral (page 143)	3	12	60 seconds
3. Lateral Raise, Bilateral (page 141)	1	15	
4. Front Raise with Bar (page 138)	1	15	
5. Overhead Rotation (page 166)	1	12	

Complete last set of exercise 1 with purposely slow 8-second concentric contraction repetitions—i.e., movement should take 8 seconds to move through the full concentric range.

DAY 2

Exercise	Sets	Reps	Rest
1. Rear Delt Raise, Bilateral (page 143)	1	15	
2. Lateral Raise, Unilateral (page 141)	3	12	60 seconds
3. Front Raise with Bar (page 138)	3	12	60 seconds
4. Overhead Rotation (page 166)	1	12	
5. Dumbbell Shoulder Press, Bilateral (page 152)	1	15	

Final set of each exercise is completed with a 10-second isometric contraction for the last repetition.

WEEKS 4–5, TWO TIMES PER WEEK

Exercise	Sets	Reps	Rest
1. Compound Press (page 156)	3	8	2 minutes
2. Lateral Cable Raise, Bilateral (page 141)	2	8	2 minutes
3. Rear Delt Cable Raise, Bilateral (page 145)	2	8	2 minutes
SUPER SET:			
4. High Cable Internal Rotation (page 160)	1	8	
5. Low Cable External Rotation (page 161)	1	8	

For all exercises, repetitions for the last set are completed with an 8-second eccentric phase.

A 15-second isometric contraction for the last repetition of each set is prescribed for all exercises.

WEEKS 6–7, TWO TIMES PER WEEK

DAY 1

Exercise	Sets	Reps	Rest
1. Military Press with Smith Machine (page 153)	3	5–6	3 minutes
2. Rear Delt Cable Raise, Bilateral (page 145)	3	5–6	3 minutes
3. Lateral Cable Raise, Bilateral (page 141)	2	12	90 seconds
4. External Cable Rotation (page 165)	1	5–6	
SUPER SET:			
5. Internal Cable Rotation (page 164)	1	5–6	

For exercises 1 and 2, perform overload protocol (page 245).

DAY 2

Exercise	Sets	Reps	Rest
1. Cable Straight-Arm Pullbacks (page 146)	1	15	
2. Upright Row (page 158)	3	5–6	3 minutes
3. Lateral Cable Raise, Unilateral (page 141)	3	5–6	3 minutes
4. Shoulder Press with Cable/ Machine/Dumbbell, Alternating (page 152)	2	15	45

For exercises 2 and 3, perform overload protocol (page 245).

WEEKS 8–9, TWO TIMES PER WEEK

DAY 1

Exercise	Sets	Reps	Rest
SUPER SET:			
1. Behind-the-Neck Press (page 154)	3	5–6	3 minutes
2. Rear Delt Raise, Bilateral (page 143)	3	5–6	3 minutes
3. Upright Row (page 158)	1	12	
4. Lateral Raise, Unilateral (page 141)	1	12	

After completion of last repetition for exercises 1 and 2, proceed with stripping protocol for those exercises (see page 245).

DAY 2

Exercise	Sets	Reps	Rest
1. Rear Delt Cable Raise, Unilateral (page 145)	1	12	
2. Upright Row (page 158)	3	5–6	3 minutes
3. Lateral Cable Raise, Bilateral (page 141)	3	5–6	3 minutes
4. Military Press with Machine (page 153)	1	12	

After completion of last repetition of exercises 2 and 3, proceed with stripping protocol for those exercises (see page 245).

TRAPEZIUS GYM

Level 1: Preparation and Foundation

WEEKS 1–2, TWO TIMES PER WEEK

Concentric phase 2 seconds, eccentric phase 4 seconds.

Exercise	Sets	Reps	Rest
Standing Shrugs with Dumbbell, Bilateral (page 168)	3	15	45 seconds

WEEKS 3–4, TWO TIMES PER WEEK

Concentric phase 2 seconds, eccentric phase 4 seconds.

Exercise	Sets	Reps	Rest
Standing Shrugs with Barbell (page 168)	3	15	45 seconds

WEEKS 5–6, TWO TIMES PER WEEK

Concentric phase 2 seconds, eccentric phase 4 seconds.

Exercise	Sets	Reps	Rest
Standing Angled Shrug with Dumbbell, Bilateral (page 170)	3	12	60 seconds

Level 2:
Creating Strength and Power

WEEKS 1–3, TWO TIMES PER WEEK

Exercise	Sets	Reps	Rest
Standing Angled Shrug with Barbell (page 170)	3	8	60 seconds

The third set is completed with a 15-second isometric contraction for the last repetition.

WEEKS 4–6, TWO TIMES PER WEEK

Exercise	Sets	Reps	Rest
1. Seated Shrug with Barbell (page 171)	2	5–6	75 seconds
2. Front Trap Raise (page 175)	2	5–6	60 seconds

For both exercises, all repetitions for the last set is completed with an 8-second eccentric phase.

Also, incorporate a 15-second isometric contraction for the last rep of each set.

ONE WEEK ACTIVE REST

Level 3:
Achieving Strength and Power

WEEKS 1–3, TWO TIMES PER WEEK

Exercise	Sets	Reps	Rest
Behind-the-Back Shrug (page 172)	3	12	60 seconds

WEEKS 4–6, TWO TIMES PER WEEK

Exercise	Sets	Reps	Rest
SUPER SET:			
1. Wide Shrug (page 169)	3	8	
2. Lateral Trap Raise (page 176)	3	8	90 seconds

Final set of each exercise is completed with a 10-second isometric contraction for the last repetition.

WEEKS 7–9, TWO TIMES PER WEEK

DAYS 1 AND 3

Exercise	Sets	Reps	Rest
SUPER SET:			
1. Seated Shrug with Dumbbell (page 171)	3	5–6	
2. Overhead Shrug with Dumbbell (page 173)	3	5–6	2 minutes

After completion of last repetition of overhead shrugs, proceed with stripping protocol for that exercise (see page 245).

DAY 2

Exercise	Sets	Reps	Rest
SUPER SET:			
1. Seated Shrug with Dumbbell (page 171)	3	12	
2. Overhead Shrug with Dumbbell (page 173)	3	12	90 seconds

WEEKS 10–11, TWO TIMES PER WEEK

DAYS 1 AND 3

Exercise	Sets	Reps	Rest
SUPER SET:			
1. Standing Shrug with Barbell (page 168)	3	5–6	
2. Front Trap Raise (page 175)	3	5–6	2 minutes

After completion of last repetition of shrugs, proceed with stripping protocol for that exercise (see page 245).

DAY 2

Exercise	Sets	Reps	Rest
SUPER SET:			
1. Standing Shrug with Barbell (page 168)	3	15	
2. Front Trap Raise (page 175)	3	15	90 seconds

Final set of each exercise is completed with a 10-second isometric contraction for the last repetition.

Ultimate Trapezius

WEEKS 1–3, TWO TIMES PER WEEK

Exercise	Sets	Reps	Rest
1. Seated Shrug with Barbell (page 171)	2	12	60 seconds
2. Front Trap Raise (page 175)	2	12	60 seconds

Final set of each exercise is completed with a 10-second isometric contraction for the last repetition.

WEEKS 4–5, TWO TIMES PER WEEK

Exercise	Sets	Reps	Rest
SUPER SET:			
1. Wide Shrug (page 169)	3	8	
2. Lateral Trap Raise (page 176)	3	8	90 seconds

For all exercises, repetitions for the last set are completed with an 8-second eccentric contraction.

A 15-second isometric contraction for the last rep of each set is prescribed for all exercises.

WEEKS 6–7, TWO TIMES PER WEEK

DAYS 1 AND 3

Exercise	Sets	Reps	Rest
SUPER SET:			
1. Seated Shrug with Dumbbell (page 171)	3	5–6	
2. Overhead Shrug with Dumbbell (page 173)	3	5–6	2 minutes

For exercises 1 and 2, perform overload protocol (page 245).

DAY 2

Exercise	Sets	Reps	Rest
SUPER SET:			
1. Seated Shrug with Dumbbell (page 171)	3	12	
2. Overhead Shrug with Dumbbell (page 173)	3	12	90 seconds

WEEKS 8–9, TWO TIMES PER WEEK

DAYS 1 AND 3

Exercise	Sets	Reps	Rest
SUPER SET:			
1. Standing Shrug with Barbell (page 168)	3	5–6	
2. Modified Snatch Pull (page 174)	3	5–6	2 minutes

After completion of last repetition of exercise 1, proceed with stripping protocol for that exercise (see page 245).

DAY 2

Exercise	Sets	Reps	Rest
SUPER SET:			
1. Standing Barbell Shrug (page 168)	3	15	
2. Front Trap Raise (page 175)	3	15	90 seconds

Final set of each exercise is completed with a 10-second isometric contraction for the last repetition.

TRICEPS GYM

Level 1: Preparation and Foundation

WEEKS 1–2, TWO TIMES PER WEEK

Concentric phase 2 seconds, eccentric phase 4 seconds.

Exercise	Sets	Reps	Rest
Supine Dumbbell Extension, Bilateral (page 178)	3	15	60 seconds

WEEKS 3–4, TWO TIMES PER WEEK

Concentric phase 2 seconds, eccentric phase 4 seconds.

Exercise	Sets	Reps	Rest
1. Triceps Push-Down (page 186)	3	15	45 seconds
2. Supine Dumbbell Extension, Bilateral (page 178)	1	15	

WEEKS 4–6, TWO TIMES PER WEEK

Concentric phase 2 seconds, eccentric phase 4 seconds.

Exercise	Sets	Reps	Rest
1. Close-Grip Bench Press (page 184)	3	12	60 seconds
2. High Cable Overhead Extension, Reverse Grip, Unilateral (page 191)	2–3	12	45 seconds

Level 2:
Creating Strength and Power

WEEKS 1–3, TWO TIMES PER WEEK

Exercise	Sets	Reps	Rest
1. French Press with Dumbbell, Elbow In (page 182)	3	8	2 minutes
2. Triceps Pull-Down (page 187)	3	8	2 minutes

Final set of each exercise is completed with a 10-second isometric contraction for the last repetition.

WEEKS 4–6, TWO TIMES PER WEEK

Exercise	Sets	Reps	Rest
1. Supine Bar Extension (page 183)	2	5–6	3 minutes
2. Low Cable Upright Extension (page 190)	2	5–6	3 minutes
3. Close-Grip Bench Press (page 184)	2	5–6	3 minutes

For all exercises, repetitions for the last set are completed with an 8-second eccentric contraction.

A 15-second isometric contraction for the last rep of each set is prescribed for all exercises.

ONE WEEK ACTIVE REST

Level 3
Achieving Strength and Power

WEEKS 1–3, TWO TIMES PER WEEK

Exercise	Sets	Reps	Rest
SUPER SET:			
1. French Press with Dumbbell (page 182)	3	12	90 seconds
2. Body Weight Push-Backs (page 197)	3	12–15	90 seconds
SUPER SET:			
3. Dumbbell Kickbacks, Bilateral (page 180)	3	12	
4. Bench Dip (page 195)	3	15–failure	90 seconds

WEEKS 4–6, TWO TIMES PER WEEK

Exercise	Sets	Reps	Rest
SUPER SET:			
1. High Cable Overhead Rope Extension (page 191)	3	8	
2. Dumbbell Kickback, Reverse Bilateral (page 180)	3	8	2 minutes
SUPER SET:			
3. Dumbbell Upright Extension, Elbow In (page 179)	3	8	
4. Supine Dumbbell Extension, Elbow Out (page 178)	3	8	2 minutes

Perform exercises 3 and 4 with one arm, then switch.

Final set of each exercise is completed with a 10-second isometric contraction for the last repetition.

WEEKS 7–9, THREE TIMES PER WEEK
DAYS 1 AND 3

Exercise	Sets	Reps	Rest
SUPER SET:			
1. Supine Bar Extension (page 183)	3	5–6	
2. Close-Grip Bench Press (page 184)	3	5–6	3 minutes

After completion of last repetition of close grip bench, proceed with stripping protocol for that exercise (see page 245).

SUPER SET:			
3. Dumbbell Upright Extension, Out Unilateral (page 179)	3	5–6	
4. Body Weight Push-Back (page 197)	3	15–failure	3 minutes

Perform exercises 3 and 4 with one arm, then switch.

DAY 2

Exercise	Sets	Reps	Rest
1. Cable Cross Pull-Downs (page 193)	2	12	45 seconds
2. Supine Dumbbell Extension, Bilateral (page 178)	2	12	45 seconds

Final set of each exercise is completed with a 10-second isometric contraction for the last repetition.

WEEKS 10–11, THREE TIMES PER WEEK

DAYS 1 AND 3

Exercise	Sets	Reps	Rest
SUPER SET:			
1. Barbell Upright Extension with Cambered Bar (page 185)	3	5–6	
2. Bench Dip, Weighted (page 195)	3	to failure	3 minutes

After completion of last repetition of bench dips, proceed with stripping protocol for that exercise (see page 245).

Exercise	Sets	Reps	Rest
SUPER SET:			
3. High Cable Overhead Extension, Unilateral (page 191)	3	5–6	
4. One-Arm Triceps Pull-Down (page 189)	3	5–6	2 minutes

Perform exercises 3 and 4 with one arm, then switch.

DAY 2

Exercise	Sets	Reps	Rest
1. Close-Grip Bench Press (page 184)	2	12	45 seconds
2. Body Weight Push-Back, Reverse Grip (page 197)	2	12	45 seconds

Final set of each exercise is completed with a 10-second isometric contraction for the last repetition.

Ultimate Triceps

WEEKS 1–3, TWO TIMES PER WEEK

Exercise	Sets	Reps	Rest
1. Supine Bar Extension (page 183)	2	12	60 seconds
2. Low Cable Upright Extension with Cable, Unilateral (page 190)	2	12	60 seconds
3. Close-Grip Bench Press (page 184)	2	12	60 seconds

Perform repetitions for last set of exercise 3 with 8-second purposely slow concentric contractions.

Final set of each exercise is completed with a 10-second isometric contraction for the last repetition.

WEEKS 4–5, TWO TIMES PER WEEK

Exercise	Sets	Reps	Rest
SUPER SET:			
1. Dumbbell French Press (page 182)	3	8	
2. Body Weight Push-Back (page 197)	3	to failure	2 minutes
SUPER SET:			
3. Dumbbell Kickback, Bilateral (page 180)	3	8	
4. Bench Dip, Weighted (page 195)	3	8	2 minutes

For all exercises, repetitions for the last set are completed with an 8-second eccentric contraction.

A 15-second isometric contraction for the last rep of each set is prescribed for all exercises.

WEEKS 6–7, THREE TIMES PER WEEK

DAYS 1 AND 3

Exercise	Sets	Reps	Rest
SUPER SET:			
1. High Cable Overhead Rope Extension (page 191)	3	5–6	
2. Triceps Pull-Down (page 187)	3	5–6	3 minutes

After completion of last repetition of exercise 2, proceed with stripping protocol for that exercise (see page 245).

Exercise	Sets	Reps	Rest
SUPER SET:			
3. Dumbbell Upright Extension, Elbow In (page 179)	3	5–6	
4. Supine Dumbbell Extension, Elbow Out (page 178)	3	5–6	3 minutes

Perform exercises 3 and 4 with one arm, then switch
For exercise 4, perform overload protocol (page 245).

DAY 2

Exercise	Sets	Reps	Rest
1. Close-Grip Bench Press (page 184)	2	12	45 seconds
2. Body Weight Push-Back, Reverse Grip (page 197)	2	12	45 seconds

For exercise 1, perform overload protocol (page 245).

WEEKS 8–9, THREE TIMES PER WEEK

DAYS 1 AND 3

Exercise	Sets	Reps	Rest
SUPER SET:			
1. Supine Bar Extension (page 183)	3	5–6	
2. Close-Grip Bench Press (page 184)	3	5–6	3 minutes

After completion of last repetition of exercise 2, proceed with stripping protocol for that exercise (see page 245).

SUPER SET:			
3. Dumbbell Upright Extension, Bilateral (page 179)	3	8	
4. Triceps Push-Down, Neutral (page 186)	3	8	2 minutes

DAY 2

Exercise	Sets	Reps	Rest
TRISET:			
1. One-Arm Body Weight Push-Back (page 197)	2	12	
2. Supine Dumbbell Extension, Unilateral (page 178)	2	12	
3. Triceps Pull-Down (page 187)	2	12	90 seconds

Perform all exercises with one arm, then switch.

Final set of each exercise is completed with a 10-second isometric contraction for the last repetition.

BICEPS GYM

Level 1:
Preparation and Foundation

WEEKS 1–2, TWO TIMES PER WEEK

Concentric phase 2 seconds, eccentric phase 4 seconds.

Exercise	Sets	Reps	Rest
Standing Dumbbell Curl, Bilateral (page 201)	3	15	60 seconds

WEEKS 3–4, TWO TIMES PER WEEK

Concentric phase 2 seconds, eccentric phase 4 seconds.

Exercise	Sets	Reps	Rest
1. Standing Barbell Curl (page 211)	3	15	45 seconds
2. Standing Dumbbell Curl, Bilateral (page 201)	1	15	

WEEKS 5–6, TWO TIMES PER WEEK

Concentric phase 2 seconds, eccentric phase 4 seconds.

Exercise	Sets	Reps	Rest
1. Hammer Curl, Bilateral (page 203)	3	12	60 seconds
2. Standing Barbell Curl (page 211)	2–3	12	45 seconds

Level 2:
Creating Strength and Power

WEEKS 1-3, TWO TIMES PER WEEK

Exercise	Sets	Reps	Rest
1. Seated Dumbbell Curl, Bilateral (page 200)	3	8	2 minutes
2. Barbell Reverse Curl with E-Z Curl Bar (page 215)	3	8	2 minutes

Final set of each exercise is completed with a 10-second isometric contraction for the last repetition.

WEEKS 4-6, TWO TIMES PER WEEK

Exercise	Sets	Reps	Rest
1. Incline Dumbbell Curl, Bilateral (page 204)	2	5–6	3 minutes
2. Barbell Reverse Curls (page 215)	2	5–6	3 minutes
3. Barbell Preacher Curl with E-Z Curl Bar (page 218)	2	5–6	3 minutes

For all exercises, repetitions for the last set are completed with an 8-second eccentric phase. Also incorporate a 15-second isometric contraction for the last repetition of each set.

ONE WEEK ACTIVE REST

Level 3:
Achieving Strength and Power

WEEKS 1-3, TWO TIMES PER WEEK

Exercise	Sets	Reps	Rest
SUPER SET:			
1. High Cable Cross Curl, Bilateral (page 226)	3	12	
2. Standing Cable Curl, Narrow Grip (page 220)	3	12	60 seconds
SUPER SET:			
3. Hammer Curl, Bilateral (page 203)	2	12	
4. Kung Fu Curl (page 206)	2	12	75 seconds

WEEKS 4-6, TWO TIMES PER WEEK

Exercise	Sets	Reps	Rest
SUPER SET:			
1. Supine High Cable Curl (page 227)	3	8	
2. Supine High Cable Reverse Curl (page 227)	3	8	2 minutes
SUPER SET:			
3. Standing Barbell Curl (page 211)	2	8	
4. Biceps Chin-Up (page 228)	2	8	2 minutes

Final set of each exercise is completed with a 10-second isometric contraction for the last repetition.

WEEKS 7-9, THREE TIMES PER WEEK

DAYS 1 AND 3

Exercise	Sets	Reps	Rest
SUPER SET:			
1. Incline Dumbbell Curl, Alternating (page 204)	3	5–6	
2. Zottman Curl, Alternating (page 207)	3	5–6	3 minutes
SUPER SET:			
3. Barbell Preacher Curl, Reverse (page 219)	2	8	
4. Barbell Concentration Curl (page 212)	2	8	2 minutes

After completion of last repetition of exercise 4, proceed with stripping protocol for that exercise (see page 245).

DAY 2

Exercise	Sets	Reps	Rest
1. Concentration Curl (page 209)	2	12	45 seconds
2. Kung Fu Curl (page 206)	2	12	45 seconds

Final set of each exercise is completed with a 10-second isometric contraction for the last repetition.

WEEKS 10–11, THREE TIMES PER WEEK
DAYS 1 AND 3

Exercise	Sets	Reps	Rest
SUPER SET:			
1. Hammer Curl, Bilateral (page 203)	3	5–6	
2. Barbell Drag Curl (page 214)	3	5–6	3 minutes

After completion of last repetition of exercise 2, proceed with stripping protocol for that exercise (see page 245).

SUPER SET:			
3. Seated Dumbbell Curl (page 200)	2	5–6	
4. Concentration Curl (page 209)	2	5–6	3 minutes

Perform exercises 3 and 4 with one arm, then switch.

DAY 2

Exercise	Sets	Reps	Rest
1. Incline Hammer Curl (page 203)	2	12	45 seconds
2. 21s (page 216)	2	7 each	2 minutes

Final set of each exercise is completed with a 10-second isometric contraction for the last repetition.

Ultimate Biceps

WEEKS 1–3, TWO TIMES PER WEEK

Exercise	Sets	Reps	Rest
1. Incline Dumbbell Curl, Bilateral (page 204)	2	12	60 seconds
2. Barbell Reverse Curl (page 215)	2	12	60 seconds
3. Barbell Preacher Curl with E-Z Curl Bar (page 218)	2	12	60 seconds

Perform repetitions for last set of exercise 3 with 8-second purposely slow concentric contractions.

Final set of each exercise is completed with a 10-second isometric contraction for the last repetition.

WEEKS 4–5, TWO TIMES PER WEEK

Exercise	Sets	Reps	Rest
SUPER SET:			
1. Standing Barbell Curl (page 211)	3	8	
2. Biceps Chin-Up (page 228)	3	8	2 minutes
SUPER SET:			
3. Hammer Curl, Bilateral (page 203)	2	8	
4. Kung Fu Curl (page 206)	2	8	2 minutes

For all exercises, repetitions for the last set are completed with an 8-second eccentric phase.

A 15-second isometric contraction for the last rep of each set is prescribed for all exercises.

WEEKS 6–7, THREE TIMES PER WEEK
DAYS 1 AND 3

Exercise	Sets	Reps	Rest
SUPER SET:			
1. Seated Dumbbell Curl (page 200)	3	5–6	
2. Concentration Curl (page 209)	3	5–6	3 minutes

Perform exercises 1 and 2 with one arm, then switch.

For exercise 2, perform overload protocol (page 245).

SUPER SET:			
3. Barbell Preacher Curl (page 218)	2	5–6	
4. High Cable Reverse Curl with Straight Bar, Facing Stack (page 221)	2	5–6	3 minutes

After completion of last repetition of exercise 4, proceed with stripping protocol for that exercise (see page 245).

DAY 2

Exercise	Sets	Reps	Rest
1. Barbell Drag Curl (page 214)	2	12	45 seconds
2. Zottman Curl (page 207)	2	12	45 seconds

WEEKS 8-9, THREE TIMES PER WEEK
DAYS 1 AND 3

Exercise	Sets	Reps	Rest
SUPER SET:			
1. Standing Barbell Curl (page 211) 3		5-6	
2. Biceps Chin-Up (page 228)	3	5-6	3 minutes

Each rep for exercise 2 should be performed with an 8-second eccentric phase.

Last set of standing barbell curls should follow the protocol for 21s.

Exercise	Sets	Reps	Rest
SUPER SET:			
3. Incline Dumbbell Curl (page 204) 2		5-6	
4. Barbell Preacher Curl, Reverse (page 219)	2	5-6	3 minutes

After completion of last repetition for exercise 4, proceed with stripping protocol for that exercises (see page 245).

DAY 2

Exercise	Sets	Reps	Rest
TRISET:			
1. Standing Cable Curl, Unilateral (page 220)	2	12	
2. High Cable Curl Facing Stack, Unilateral (page 221)	2	12	
3. Concentration Cable Curl (page 209)	2	12	2 minutes

Perform all exercises with one arm, then switch.

Final set of each exercise is completed with a 10-second isometric contraction for the last repetition.

FOREARMS GYM

Level 1:
Preparation and Foundation

WEEKS 1-2, TWO TIMES PER WEEK
Concentric phase 2 seconds, eccentric phase 4 seconds.

Exercise	Sets	Reps	Rest
SUPER SET:			
1. Wrist Flexion Seated with Dumbbell, Bilateral (page 230)	1	20	
2. Wrist Extension Seated with Dumbbell, Bilateral (page 231)	1	20	

WEEKS 3-4, TWO TIMES PER WEEK
Concentric phase 2 seconds, eccentric phase 4 seconds.

Exercise	Sets	Reps	Rest
SUPER SET:			
1. Wrist Flexion Seated with Dumbbell, Bilateral (page 230)	1	12	
2. Wrist Extension Seated with Dumbbell, Bilateral (page 231)	1	12	

WEEKS 5-6, TWO TIMES PER WEEK
Concentric phase 2 seconds, eccentric phase 4 seconds.

Exercise	Sets	Reps	Rest
SUPER SET:			
1. Wrist Flexion Seated with Dumbbell, Bilateral (page 230)	1	8	
2. Wrist Extension Seated with Dumbbell, Bilateral (page 231)	1	8	

Level 2:
Creating Strength and Power

WEEKS 1–3, TWO TIMES PER WEEK

Exercise	Sets	Reps	Rest
SUPER SET:			
1. Wrist Flexion Seated with Barbell (page 230)	1	8	
2. Wrist Extension Seated with Barbell (page 231)	1	8	

Final set of each exercise is completed with a 10-second isometric contraction for the last repetition.

WEEKS 4–6, TWO TIMES PER WEEK

DAY 1

Exercise	Sets	Reps	Rest
SUPER SET:			
1. Wrist Flexion Seated with Barbell (page 230)	1	5–6	
2. Wrist Extension Seated with Barbell (page 231)	1	5–6	

For all exercises, repetitions for the last set are completed with an 8-second eccentric contraction.

A 15-second isometric contraction for the last rep of each set is prescribed for all exercises.

DAY 2

Exercise	Sets	Reps	Rest
SUPER SET:			
1. Wrist Flexion Seated with Barbell (page 230)	1	15	
2. Wrist Extension Seated with Barbell (page 231)	1	15	

ONE WEEK ACTIVE REST

Level 3:
Achieving Strength and Power

WEEKS 1–3, TWO TIMES PER WEEK

Exercise	Sets	Reps	Rest
SUPER SET:			
1. Radial Flexion with Dumbbell (page 234)	1	20	
2. Ulna Flexion with Dumbbell (page 235)	1	20	

WEEKS 4–6, TWO TIMES PER WEEK

Exercise	Sets	Reps	Rest
SUPER SET:			
1. Radial Flexion with Dumbbell (page 234)	1	12	
2. Ulna Flexion with Dumbbell (page 235)	1	12	

Final set of each exercise is completed with a 10-second isometric contraction for the last repetition.

WEEKS 7–9, TWO TIMES PER WEEK

DAY 1

Exercise	Sets	Reps	Rest
SUPER SET:			
1. Wrist Flexion Seated with Barbell (page 230)	1	15	
2. Wrist Extension Seated with Barbell (page 231)	1	15	

DAY 2

Exercise	Sets	Reps	Rest
SUPER SET:			
1. Wrist Roll Extension (page 232)	1	1	
2. Wrist Roll Flexion (page 232)	1	1	

WEEKS 10–11, TWO TIMES PER WEEK

DAY 1

Exercise	Sets	Reps	Rest
SUPER SET:			
1. Wrist Flexion Seated with Barbell (page 230)	1	8	
2. Wrist Extension Seated with Barbell (page 231)	1	8	

DAY 2

Exercise	Sets	Reps	Rest
SUPER SET:			
1. Wrist Roll Extension (page 232)	1	2	
2. Wrist Roll Flexion (page 232)	1	2	

Ultimate Forearms

WEEKS 1–3, TWO TIMES PER WEEK

Exercise	Sets	Reps	Rest
SUPER SET:			
1. Wrist Flexion Seated with Barbell (page 230)	1	12	
2. Wrist Extension Seated with Barbell (page 231)	1	12	

Final set of each exercise is completed with a 10-second isometric contraction for the last repetition.

WEEKS 4–5, TWO TIMES PER WEEK

Exercise	Sets	Reps	Rest
Forearm Rotation Supination/ Pronation (page 233)	1	12	

WEEKS 6–7, TWO TIMES PER WEEK

DAY 1

Exercise	Sets	Reps	Rest
SUPER SET:			
1. Wrist Flexion Standing with Barbell (page 230)	1	8	
2. Wrist Extension Standing with Barbell (page 231)	1	8	

DAY 2

Exercise	Sets	Reps	Rest
SUPER SET:			
1. Wrist Roll Extension (page 232)	1	1	
2. Wrist Roll Flexion (page 232)	1	1	

WEEKS 8–9, TWO TIMES PER WEEK

DAY 1

Exercise	Sets	Reps	Rest
SUPER SET:			
1. Wrist Flexion Seated with Barbell (page 230)	1	5–6	
2. Wrist Extension Seated with Barbell (page 231)	1	5–6	

For exercises 1 and 2, perform overload protocol (page 245).

DAY 2

Exercise	Sets	Reps	Rest
SUPER SET:			
1. Wrist Roll Extension (page 232)	1	2	
2. Wrist Roll Flexion (page 232)	1	2	

TRICEPS AND BICEPS GYM

Level 1:
Preparation and Foundation

WEEKS 1–2, TWO TIMES PER WEEK

Concentric phase 2 seconds, eccentric phase 4 seconds.

Exercise	Sets	Reps	Rest
COMPOUND SET:			
1. Supine Dumbbell Extension, Bilateral (page 178)	3	15	
2. Standing Dumbbell Curl, Bilateral (page 201)	3	15	90 seconds

WEEKS 3–4, TWO TIMES PER WEEK

Concentric phase 2 seconds, eccentric phase 4 seconds.

Exercise	Sets	Reps	Rest
COMPOUND SET:			
1. Triceps Push-Down (page 186)	1	15	
2. Incline Dumbbell Curl, Bilateral (page 204)	1	15	90 seconds
COMPOUND SET:			
3. Supine Dumbbell Extension, Bilateral (page 178)	3	15	
4. Standing Barbell Curl (page 211)	3	15	90 seconds

WEEKS 5–6, TWO TIMES PER WEEK

Concentric phase 2 seconds, eccentric phase 4 seconds.

Exercise	Sets	Reps	Rest
COMPOUND SET:			
1. Close-Grip Bench Press (page 184)	3	12	
2. Hammer Curl, Bilateral (page 203)	3	12	90 seconds
COMPOUND SET:			
3. High Cable Overhead Extension (page 191)	2–3	12	
4. Standing Barbell Curl (page 211)	2–3	12	90 seconds

Level 2:
Creating Strength and Power

WEEKS 1–3, TWO TIMES PER WEEK

Exercise	Sets	Reps	Rest
COMPOUND SET:			
1. Dumbbell Upright Extension, Bilateral, Elbow In (page 179)	3	8	
2. Seated Dumbbell Curl (page 200)	3	8	2 minutes
COMPOUND SET:			
3. Triceps Pull-Down (page 187)	3	8	
4. Barbell Reverse Curl with E-Z Curl Bar (page 215)	3	8	2 minutes

Final set of each exercise is completed with a 10-second isometric contraction for the last repetition.

WEEKS 4–6, TWO TIMES PER WEEK

Exercise	Sets	Reps	Rest
COMPOUND SET:			
1. Supine Bar Extension (page 183)	2	5–6	
2. Incline Dumbbell Curl, Bilateral (page 204)	2	5–6	3 minutes
COMPOUND SET:			
3. Dumbbell French Press (page 182)	2	5–6	
4. Barbell Reverse Curl (page 215)	2	5–6	3 minutes
COMPOUND SET:			
5. Close-Grip Bench Press (page 184)	2	5–6	
6. Barbell Preacher Curl with E-Z Curl Bar (page 218)	2	5–6	3 minutes

For all exercises, repetitions for the last set are completed with an 8-second eccentric contraction.

A 15-second isometric contraction for the last rep of each set is prescribed for all exercises.

ONE WEEK ACTIVE REST

Level 3:
Achieving Strength and Power

WEEKS 1–3, TWO TIMES PER WEEK

Exercise	Sets	Reps	Rest
SUPER SET:			
1. Dumbbell French Press (page 182)	3	12	
2. Body Weight Push-Back (page 197)	3	12–15	60 seconds
SUPER SET:			
3. High Cable Cross Curl (page 226)	3	12	
4. Standing Cable Curl, Narrow Grip (page 220)	3	12	60 seconds
SUPER SET:			
5. Dumbbell Kickback, Bilateral (page 180)	1	12	
6. Bench Dip (page 195)	1	15–failure	
SUPER SET:			
7. Hammer Curl, Bilateral (page 203)	1	12	
8. Kung Fu Curl (page 206)	1	12	

WEEKS 4–6, TWO TIMES PER WEEK

Exercise	Sets	Reps	Rest
SUPER SET:			
1. High Cable Overhead Rope Extension (page 191)	3	8	
2. Barbell Kickback, Reverse Grip (page 180)	3	8	2 minutes
SUPER SET:			
3. Supine Cable Curl (page 222)	3	8	
4. Supine Cable Reverse Curl (page 222)	3	8	2 minutes
SUPER SET:			
5. Dumbbell Upright Extension, Elbow In (page 179)	1	8	
6. Supine Dumbbell Extension, Elbow Out (page 178)	1	8	
SUPER SET:			
7. Standing Barbell Curl (page 211)	1	8	
8. Biceps Chin-Up (page 228)	1	8	

Final set of each exercise is completed with a 10-second isometric contraction for the last repetition.

WEEKS 7–9, THREE TIMES PER WEEK

DAYS 1 AND 3

Exercise	Sets	Reps	Rest
COMPOUND SET:			
1. Supine Bar Extension (page 183)	2	5–6	
2. Incline Dumbbell Curl, Alternating (page 204)	2	5–6	3 minutes
COMPOUND SET:			
3. Close-Grip Bench Press (page 184)	2	5–6	

Upon completion of last repetition of the last set for close grip bench, proceed with stripping protocol for that exercise (see page 245).

4. Zottman Curl, Alternating (page 207)	2	5–6	3 minutes
COMPOUND SET:			
5. Dumbbell Upright Extension, Unilateral (page 179)	2	5–6	
6. Barbell Preacher Curl (page 218)	2	5–6	3 minutes

Upon completion of last repetition of the last set for exercise 6, proceed with stripping protocol for that exercise (see page 245).

DAY 2

Exercise	Sets	Reps	Rest
COMPOUND SET:			
1. Cable Cross Pull-Down (page 193)	2	12	45 seconds
2. Kung Fu Curl (page 206)	2	12	45 seconds

Final set of each exercise is completed with a 10-second isometric contraction for the last repetition.

WEEKS 10–11, THREE TIMES PER WEEK

DAYS 1 AND 3

Exercise	Sets	Reps	Rest
COMPOUND SET:			
1. Barbell Upright Extension with E-Z Curl (page 185)	3	5–6	
2. Hammer Curl, Bilateral (page 203)	3	5–6	3 minutes
COMPOUND SET:			
3. High Cable Overhead Extension (page 191)	3	8–10	
4. High Cable Curl, Facing Stack (page 221)	3	8–10	2 minutes

Upon completion of last repetition of the last set for exercise 4, proceed with stripping protocol for that exercise (see page 245).

COMPOUND SET:			
5. Triceps Pull-Down (page 187)	1	12–15	

Upon completion of last repetition of the last set for exercise 5, proceed with stripping protocol for that exercise (see page 245).

6. Barbell Concentration Curl (page 212)	1	12–15	

DAY 2

Exercise	Sets	Reps	Rest
1. Close-Grip Bench Press (page 184)	2	12	90 seconds
2. 21s (page 216)	2	7	2 minutes

Final set of each exercise is completed with a 10-second isometric contraction for the last repetition.

Ultimate Triceps and Biceps

WEEKS 1–3, TWO TIMES PER WEEK

Exercise	Sets	Reps	Rest
COMPOUND SET:			
1. Supine Bar Extension (page 183)	2	12	
2. Incline Dumbbell Curl, Bilateral (page 204)	2	12	2 minutes
COMPOUND SET:			
3. Dumbbell Upright Extension (page 179)	2	12	
4. Barbell Reverse Curl (page 215)	2	12	2 minutes
COMPOUND SET:			
5. Close-Grip Bench Press (page 184)	2	12	
6. Barbell Preacher Curl with E-Z Curl Bar (page 218)	2	12	2 minutes

Perform repetitions for last set of exercises 1 and 2 with 8-second purposely slow concentric contractions.

Incorporate 10-second isometric contraction for the last rep of the last set for each exercise.

WEEKS 4–5, TWO TIMES PER WEEK

Exercise	Sets	Reps	Rest
SUPER SET:			
1. Dumbbell French Press (page 182)	3	8	
2. Body Weight Push-Back (page 197)	3	12– failure	2 minutes
SUPER SET:			
3. High Cable Cross Curl (page 226)	3	8	
4. Standing Cable Curl, Narrow Grip (page 220)	3	8	2 minutes
SUPER SET:			
5. Triceps Push-Down (page 186)	1	8	
6. Bench Dip, Weighted (page 195)	1	8–failure	
SUPER SET:			
7. Hammer Curl, Bilateral (page 203)	1	8	
8. Kung Fu Curl (page 206)	1	8	

For all exercises, repetitions for the last set are completed with an 8-second eccentric phase.

A 15-second isometric contraction for the last rep of each set is prescribed for all exercises.

WEEKS 6–7, THREE TIMES PER WEEK

DAYS 1 AND 3

Exercise	Sets	Reps	Rest
COMPOUND SET:			
1. Supine Bar Extension (page 183)	2	5–6	
2. Incline Dumbbell Curl, Alternating (page 204)	2	5–6	3 minutes

For exercises 1 and 2, perform overload protocol (page 245).

COMPOUND SET:			
3. Close-Grip Bench Press (page 184)	2	5–6	

Upon completion of last repetition for exercise 3, proceed with stripping protocol for that exercise (see page 245).

4. Zottman Curl, Alternating (page 207)	2	5–6	3 minutes
COMPOUND SET:			
5. Dumbbell Upright Extension, Bilateral (page 179)	2	5–6	
6. Barbell Preacher Curl (page 218)	2	5–6	3 minutes

Upon completion of last repetition of the last set for exercise 6, proceed with stripping protocol for that exercise (see page 245).

DAY 2

Exercise	Sets	Reps	Rest
COMPOUND SET:			
1. Cable Cross Pull-Downs (page 193)	2	12	45 seconds
2. Kung Fu Curl (page 206)	2	12	45 seconds

WEEKS 8–9, THREE TIMES PER WEEK

DAYS 1 AND 3

Exercise	Sets	Reps	Rest
COMPOUND SET:			
1. Barbell Upright Extension with E-Z Curl (page 185)	3	5–6	
2. Hammer Curl, Bilateral (page 203)	3	5–6	3 minutes
COMPOUND SET:			
3. High Cable Overhead Extension, Reverse Grip (page 191)	3	8–10	
4. High Cable Curl (page 221)	3	8–10	2 minutes

Upon completion of last repetition of the last set for exercise 4, proceed with stripping protocol for that exercise (see page 245).

COMPOUND SET:			
5. Triceps Pull-Down (page 187)	1	12–15	

Upon completion of last repetition of the last set for exercise 5, proceed with stripping protocol for that exercise (see page 245).

6. 21s (page 216)	1	7	

DAY 2

Exercise	Sets	Reps	Rest
1. Close-Grip Bench Press (page 184)	2	12	90 seconds
2. Concentration Curl (page 209)	2	12	90 seconds

Final set of each exercise is completed with a 10-second isometric contraction for the last repetition.

Routines from the Pros

Strength and Power Development in the Shoulders for Basketball by Al Vermiel

Al Vermiel is head strength and conditioning coach for the Chicago Bulls.

Strength and power in the shoulders and arms is essential for rebounding and finishing shots in basketball. The following programs are used by the Bulls. Some exercises involve jumping as part of the activity. Younger players who cannot dunk the ball should set up a vertical target that challenges their jump instead of a basket (unless they have access to a lower basket). They should also use a lighter medicine ball or basketball.

PRESS AND DUNK SUPER SET

Exercise	Sets	Reps	Comments
Push Press (page 157)	3	4	
Medicine Ball Dunk	3	3–5	4–6 lb. medicine ball

Additional comments: Perform the two exercises as a super set going from a set of the Push Press to a set of the Medicine Ball Dunks. The Medicine Ball Dunks are the same motion as a two-arm power dunk.

COMPLEX

Exercise	Sets	Reps	Comments
Upright Row (page 158)	2–3	6	
Snatch (page 174)	2–3	6	
Push Press (page 157)	2–3	6	

Additional comments: This complex is performed as a giant set. In other words, you would perform one set of each exercise in the sequence in order, rest, and then perform another set.

Training Shoulders & Arms for Tennis
by Jim Landis

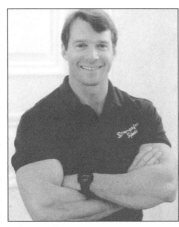

Jim Landis has been a personal trainer and fitness consultant for the last sixteen years. He has worked with business executives, television and film personalities, and professional athletes. In the tennis world he has trained Martina Navratilova, Chris Evert, Gigi Fernandez, and Natalia Zvereva, to name a few.

He is a member of the National Strength and Conditioning Association and has been featured in *Sports Illustrated, The New York Times, Lears, Ski Magazine,* and *Longevity.*

(This program assumes an individual has completed an introductory strength program of at least 8 to 12 weeks.)

Training the shoulders and arms to improve one's tennis requires specific considerations of the highly dynamic and ballistic nature of the sport. Proper preparation will require some loading that is ballistic so the tissues will not only perform more effectively but also be much more injury resistant. This explains the need for a well-developed strength base and some proficiency with these exercises before attempting the more vigorous movements ultimately recommended on some exercises.

This program takes into consideration not only those large movers of the joints such as the deltoids, biceps, and triceps but also the critically important smaller muscles—those muscles that make up the rotator cuff of the shoulder joint, as well as the small muscles of the forearm.

Also, notice that most exercises employ dumbbells, while standing, using single-arm (unilateral) movements. This offers a more specific recruitment of the nervous system in relation to tennis than does the use of barbell or machines.

Done consistently, this program will improve strength, power, and a highly increased resistance to injury so common in tennis. Practically put, this will translate into hitting the ball harder, quicker racket preparation for shots (i.e., getting the racket in position faster for an overhead smash), and more overall racket control.

NOTES

Rotary Lateral: Standing, start with dumbbells at sides with palms facing body (neutral grip). Raise dumbbells vigorously but under control directly out to sides, externally rotating as you raise the weights. Stand in front of a mirror and make sure palms are facing mirror by the time the dumbbells are shoulder height. Continue raising dumbbells until they are directly overhead, at which time the palms should be facing the mirror or each other. This external rotation is critical when abducting the shoulder completely overhead so no impingement will occur inside the shoulder joint. This is excellent for getting the racket up for serves and all overhead shots. Target: medial and anterior deltoids and supraspinatus.

Exercise	Sets	Reps
Upright Rows (page 158)	3	8–10
Lateral Raises, One-Arm (page 141)	3	8–10
Rotary Laterals (page 270)	3	8–10
Front Raises (Alternating) (page 138)	2–3	8–10
Rear Delt Raises (page 143)	3	8–10
Hammer Curls (page 203)	3	8–12
Dumbbell Upright Extensions (page 179)	3	8–12
Lying Internal/External Rotations (page 163)	2–3	10–15
Standing External Rotations (page 163)	2–3	10–15
Wrist Curls (Flexion) (page 230)	2	10–15
Reverse Wrist Curls (Extension) (page 231)	2	10–15
Pronation/Supination (page 233)	2	10–15
Ulnar (page 235) and Radial Flexion (page 234)	2	10–15

Injury Prevention for the Rotator Cuff Strain
by Bill Fabrocini, PT, CSCS

Bill Fabrocini is a physical therapist at the Aspen Club Fitness & Sports Medicine Institute in Aspen, Colorado.

The rotator cuff consists of four small muscles that run from the upper portion of the shoulder blade to the top of the arm. Together they act to stabilize your shoulder by pressing the ball portion of the arm bone (humeral head) into the shoulder socket whenever you raise your arm. Two of the rotator cuff muscles, the teres minor and the infraspinatus, work together to produce external rotation motion—arm rotation away from the body (page 212).

One of the most common shoulder injuries in sports is the rotator cuff strain. This muscle injury occurs quite frequently with high-speed sports motions, such as pitching in baseball or serving in tennis. These types of forceful, high-speed motions can result in a sudden elongation of the rotator cuff muscles, particularly the infraspinatus, teres minor, and supraspinatus. These muscles, which originate behind the shoulder on the top of the shoulder blade, can easily tear when they are weak in relation to the muscles that insert to the front of the shoulder, such as the pectoralis major and latissimus dorsi. These muscles in the front part of the shoulder produce the forceful, high-speed internal rotation motions (arm rotation toward the body) that is observed with overhead shoulder actions such as throwing and serving. Repetition of these forceful motions can easily strain a weak rotator cuff. It is a quite similar situation to a hamstring pull sustained with sprinting or jumping, in which the powerful quadriceps on the front of the thigh overpowers the weaker hamstrings behind the thigh.

Strategy to prevent a rotator cuff strain is similar to the prevention of all types of muscle strains. The basic program includes proper warm-up, stretching before and especially after sporting events and exercise bouts, and a specific strengthening program to isolate the rotator cuff muscles.

WARMING UP

The physiological benefits of warming up for injury prevention have been known for years. Warm-up exercises will help to increase circulation to cold, stiff muscles and begin to raise their temperature so that they can stretch more easily. For the shoulders, warming up may simply involve a few minutes of raising your arms up and down or side to side. Gentle sport-specific motions, such as swinging your tennis racket with the cover on or lightly swinging a couple of baseball bats, is another effective warm-up tool. It is always wise to perform a few specific-sport motions at half speed, such as serving or throwing, before exerting full effort.

STRETCHING

One of the most effective ways to stretch the rotator cuff and the back of the shoulder joint is to pull your involved arm across your chest. Pulling your involved arm behind your back with a towel is also a good stretch. Remember to hold the stretch for approximately one minute and not to bounce at the end of the stretch.

STRENGTHENING

Isolation of the rotator cuff external rotators can easily be performed by keeping a bent elbow at your side while externally rotating your arm so that your forearm moves away from your body. This motion can be performed by standing with resistance coming from a rubber coil, or by lying on your side with the resistance coming from a weight. Lifting a straight arm up and rotating it so that your thumb points upward while lying on your stomach is also a good exercise.

As with any strengthening program, three sets of 10 to 12 repetitions, with enough resistance to produce close to muscle failure, is an effective method for strengthening. Adding variety to the number of repetitions, sets, and rest periods, as described with periodization concepts in this book (Chapter 19), will lead to optimal results.

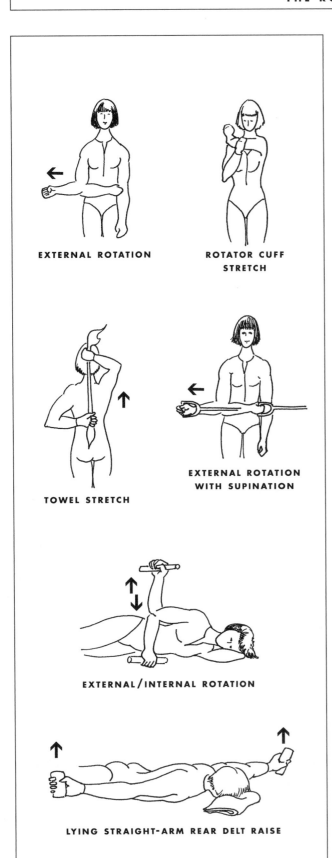

EXTERNAL ROTATION

ROTATOR CUFF STRETCH

TOWEL STRETCH

EXTERNAL ROTATION WITH SUPINATION

EXTERNAL/INTERNAL ROTATION

LYING STRAIGHT-ARM REAR DELT RAISE

Exercise	Sets	Reps	Comments
Warm-up			
Stretch			
External Rotation			
(page 163)	3	10–12	
Lying Straight-Arm Rear Delt Raise			
(page 143)	3	10–12	

Additional comments: Remember to add variety after 4–6 weeks on this program by changing your sets, or reps, or rest periods.

Concerns for the Older Population by Deborah M. Holmes, M.S.

As the body ages there are a few prevention concerns that become important when performing any exercise program. Exercises that should be avoided are those that place undue stress on any part of the body; knees, hips, back, and shoulders are the most susceptible areas.

It is extremely important to pay special attention to the shoulder and back. These areas are extremely susceptible to injury with increased aging. You will find it valuable to use a variety of exercises, allowing the joint to strengthen and move throughout its entire range of motion. Concentrate on exercises that help daily life functions, such as getting up out of a chair, carrying, bending over, placing objects on a high shelf. These are basic movements that become more difficult as our joints and muscles age.

In order to assure safety, it is important to concentrate on the duration of exercise instead of intensity. Encourage them to work toward increased numbers of repetitions instead of increasing the difficulty levels of the exercises. With strong seniors who have no joint or muscle difficulties, there are no increased dangers with any routine that is designed for them.

SUGGESTED EXERCISES FOR THE OLDER POPULATION

Shoulders

LATERAL RAISES: Machines are the safest for the senior population; however, the use of dumbbells would be recommended for those who are uncomfortable in a machine.

DUMBBELL SHOULDER PRESS (SEATED): It is safest to perform overhead presses while seated with back support, as the increased weight load on the aging spine could be of concern. Begin with an extremely light weight; often the motion itself is enough workload for beginners.

UPRIGHT ROWS: Make sure that there is no swaying while performing the lift. Always watch form.

SUGGESTED TRAINING ROUTINE: Choose 2 of the above exercises.

Beginners:	1 set of each	12–15 repetitions
Intermediate:	2 sets of each	15–20 repetitions
Advanced:	2 sets of each	12–15 repetitions to failure

Arms

SEATED DUMBBELL CURLS: Usually it is best to start the seniors with dumbbells. There are really no concerns with most of the standard biceps curls. Avoid exercises that take the elbow out of alignment with the anterior deltoid.

DUMBBELL UPRIGHT EXTENSION: Most of the exercises for the triceps are acceptable for this population. Avoid exercises that would put you in any kind of compromising positions, e.g., close grip push-ups, close grip triceps curl to forehead (while lying on back). Avoid exercises that take the elbow out of alignment with the shoulder.

FOREARMS: No real concerns with the basic movements as long as the wrist is kept in alignment with the elbow, and that there are no preexisting concerns with the client being trained.

SUGGESTED TRAINING ROUTINE: Choose 1 or 2 exercises for each muscle

Beginners:	1 set of each	12–15 repetitions
Intermediate:	2 sets of each	15–20 repetitions
Advanced:	2 sets of each	12–15 repetitions to failure

Following these general guidelines, you can choose exercises from the book that suit your needs.

Hand-Held Weights and Rubber Bands: Rubber bands tend to be more difficult for this population to use. The way rubber bands increase the workload through the range of motion is often hard on the joints associated with the exercise. Hand-held weights are usually a better choice.

Definition Program by Mike Brungardt

To bring out the cuts in your body, you have to eliminate body fat. Although a certain amount of body fat is necessary for good health, many people carry too much body fat. As you reduce body fat, more muscle definition reveals itself. The best way to eliminate body fat is through a proper diet (Chapter 5) and a combination of consistent resistance and aerobic training (four times a week for aerobic training).

A good way to incorporate this into your weight workout is circuit training. In this type of routine you lift for designated amounts of time and also rest for a designated time. Upper body and lower body exercises are alternated (lower body work helps keep your heart rate up). The following is an example of a shoulder and arm routine that incorporates the circuit principle. All steps (1 to 5) are to be completed in one training session.

1. Five-minute stationary bike or Stairmaster (or as long as it takes to get you to your target heart rate).
2. Dumbbell Shoulder Press (30 seconds)—rest 20 seconds—Triceps Push-Downs (30 seconds)—rest 20 seconds—Dumbbell Curls (30 seconds)—one-minute bike or Stairmaster. Perform routine three times.

3. Lateral Raise (30 seconds)—rest 20 seconds—Bench Dips (30 seconds)—rest 20 seconds—Dumbbell Hammers (30 seconds)—rest 20 seconds—one-minute bike or Stairmaster. Perform routine three times.
4. Rear Delt Raise (30 seconds)—rest 20 seconds—Dumbbell Kickbacks (30 seconds)—rest 20 seconds—Concentration Curls (30 seconds)—one-minute bike or Stairmaster. Perform routine three times.
5. Front Raise (30 seconds)—one-minute bike or Stairmaster. Perform routine three times.

Body Tech Routine
by Donna Cyrus

In this day and age, when women are no longer content to just jump up and down in aerobics classes, there are a greater number of women lifting weights. At Club Body Tech we have an international clientele of women, and they all want to know how to tone their upper body without looking like Ms. Arnold Schwarzenegger. The easiest way to achieve this look is by using less weight and more repetitions in your upper-body workout. What follows is a basic upper-body toning segment to tone the triceps, shoulders, back, and biceps area of the body.

I would suggest using a five-pound weight set to start off. As you increase to 15 reps, you can move into 8 or 10 pounds. This set should be repeated three times.

1. Dumbbell Shoulder Press (page 152)
2. Dumbbell Curl (page 201)
3. One-Arm Rear Deltoid Raise (page 143)

Remember to always exhale on the effort and have a good time!

The Rugby Routine
by Kirk Miller

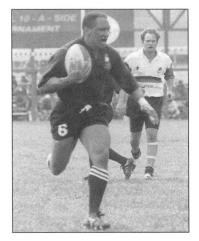

Kirk Miller is a world-class rugby player, a champion power lifter, and a personal trainer.

Strong shoulders are essential for full-contact sports like rugby and football. This is especially true for rugby, since players are not allowed to use any type of protective gear—muscle is your only pad. Weight training will not only improve performance, it will also decrease chances of injury. The following is a basic shoulder routine that will work all three heads of the deltoid (front, side, and rear).

Dumbbell Shoulder Press (page 152): This is the core exercise for shoulders, and it works both the front and sides of your deltoids. For power and strength I recommend doing between 5 and 10 reps. This means once you can do 10 reps, increase to a weight that will allow you to do 5 reps; then work up to 10 reps and add weight again.

Rear Delt Raise (page 143): This exercise works the rear portion of your deltoids. I recommend a repetition scheme between 10 and 15 reps. Follow the same procedure for adding weight as described above.

Medicine Ball Routine
by Dave Johnson

Dave Johnson is a personal trainer and a poet.

Using the medicine ball is one of the most efficient ways to train for specific sports that require your hands held above your head and/or away from your body. This routine will help develop both endurance and explosiveness. It should be performed three times a week.

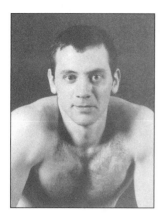

Step 1: Place feet shoulder width apart with hands palming the ball on the sides (east–west direction). Hold the ball in front of the body, resting it on the chest, elbows bent. Straighten arms, keeping them at shoulder level. Return to the starting position. Repeat for 15 reps.

Step 2: Extend arms down in front of your waist, hands on the side of the ball; raise arms until they are perpendicular to your torso (shoulder level). Return the ball to the starting position. Repeat for 15 reps.

Step 3: From the same starting position as step 2, raise the ball diagonally to the left until it is perpendicular to your body. Return to the starting position. Then swing the ball diagonally up and out to the right. Repeat for 10 reps on each side.

Step 4: From the same starting position as step 2, raise the ball above your head, making a straight line with ball, arms, and torso. Return to starting position. Repeat for 15 reps.

Step 5: With the ball above your head, bend your elbows, allowing the ball to drop to your upper chest. Then extend the arms and move the ball back to its starting position. Repeat for 15 reps.

Step 6: With the ball above your head, arms extended, bend your elbows, letting the ball drop behind your head, until your lower arms are perpendicular to your upper arms. Keep your upper arms static and vertical. Then extend your arms and move the ball back to the starting position. Repeat for 15 reps.

Step 7: Repeat steps 1 through 6.

Variations: Repeat steps 1 through 6 three times. Experiment with repetitions and pace of routine.

Barbell, Dumbbell, Cable Routine by Steven Wilde

Steven Wilde is a personal trainer and screenwriter. He lives in Los Angeles.

This routine works the biceps from a variety of angles and uses three different pieces of equipment to guarantee the best development.

STANDING BARBELL CURLS (PAGE 211)

Do three sets of this exercise. For the first two sets, use a grip that is slightly wider than shoulder width. For the first set use a moderate weight to warm up the muscle. On the second set, use a weight that will allow you to do 5 reps. On the last set, lower the weight (use a weight that will allow you to do 12 reps) and use an extra-wide grip.

INCLINE DUMBBELL CURLS (PAGE 204)

Do three sets of this exercise on an incline bench.

HIGH CABLE CURLS (PAGE 221)

Do two sets of this exercise, one arm at a time.

Martial Arts Push-Up Routine by Steven Rittersporn

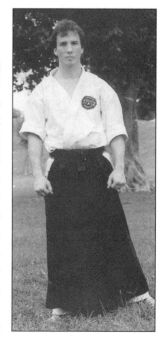

Steven Rittersporn has been involved in martial arts for over 17 years. He is a fourth-degree black belt in Okinawan Shobayashi Shorin-ryu Karate and first-degree black belt in Eizan-ryu Jujitsu. He studies and teaches at the Shobayashi Shorin-ryu Karate in New York City. He maintains the Okinawan Shobayashi Shorin-ryu Karate Homepage on the World Wide Web. The

URL is http://www.inch.com./~sritter. He is also a computer graphics specialist.

The following push-ups are the same as a traditional push-up except for the hand variations. The emphasis on these movements is to strengthen the hands and forearms.

1. *Knuckle Push-ups*—Make a fist and support yourself on your top two knuckles and the balls of your feet. Then straighten your arms just short of locking out, and lower your body till your chest is about a quarter of an inch from the floor. Return to starting position and repeat.
2. *Fingertip Push-ups*—Follow the same procedure as above, but this time support your body with your fingertips.
3. *Wrist Push-ups*—Follow the same procedure as above, but this time support yourself on the tops of your wrists by pointing your fingers in toward each other (palms up). It's as if you are handless and you are doing push-ups on the tops of your wrists.
4. *Handstand Push-ups*—Using a wall for support, stand on your head. From this position elevate your body straight up by extending your arms. Then lower yourself until your head almost touches the floor and repeat. You can also do this exercise using the knuckle or fingertip position.

For the first three exercises, work up to three sets of 25. For the fourth exercise, try to work up to three sets of 10 reps. For all exercises, hands should be slightly wider than shoulder width apart.

BASEBALL

The physical skills of baseball require refined neuromuscular skills, combined with explosive strength and power. Additional components of conditioning for baseball would include injury prevention and metabolic efficiency. Although this fifteen-week program is limited to the shoulders and arms, it satisfies these requirements with a specific methodology. Because of the refined neuromuscular components involved in baseball (i.e., swinging, throwing), mimicking these movements in the weight room would be an ineffective way to train and would be detrimental to performance. Instead, the principle of specificity will be adhered to by looking at the muscles involved in the sport-specific movements and training these muscles at appropriate angles and speeds to improve strength and power and reduce the potential for injury. Skill acquisition, or practice, is used to enhance proficiency of components like bat and arm speed. These abilities will also be enhanced by improved strength and power. Remember, skill acquisition is the highest priority, practice skills prior to a strength training session.

The joints of the upper body (shoulder, elbow, and wrist) are common areas of injury. Many exercises included in this routine are specifically designed to reduce the potential for injury in these areas (rotator cuff exercises; elbow and wrist joint stabilizers).

To achieve your highest level of performance you must integrate these aspects of skill and conditioning, along with flexibility, proper nutrition, and mental preparation.

Guidelines

OFF-SEASON
Follow frequency guidelines for the prescribed routine. Allow at least 48 hours recovery time between training sessions, with optimal recovery time being 72 to 96 hours.

This routine trains opposing muscle groups. In accordance with the principle of whole-body training, other body parts should be trained in the same way to ensure optimal recovery. The following would be an appropriate format to follow:

Day 1: Chest/Back/Abs
Day 2: Legs/Forearms
Day 3: Shoulders/Triceps/Biceps/Abs
Day 4: Rest
Repeat

Every two weeks take a day off between day 2 and day 3.

Each exercise should be preceded by a warm-up set followed by the prescribed number of sets and reps at very high intensity.

IN-SEASON

Attempt to follow the frequency guidelines. Optimal recovery would be 48 hours before competition, with a minimum of 36 hours. If the competition schedule is too busy, training once a week is acceptable.

Strength training following competition is an optimal time to train.

If training plateaus occur, refer to Off-Season, Weeks 1–3 for a three-week period.

During the in-season, follow a 4-weeks on 1-week-off whole-body strength training schedule.

Rest between sets is dictated by intensity or repetition scheme.

15 repetitions and above	60 seconds
12 repetitions	90 seconds
8 repetitions	2 minutes
5–6 repetitions	3 minutes

Off-Season

WEEKS 1–3, TWO TIMES PER WEEK

Concentric phase 2 seconds, eccentric phase 4 seconds.

Exercise	Sets	Reps
COMPOUND SET:		
1. Dumbbell Shoulder Press, Bilateral (page 152)	2	15
2. Dumbbell Shrug (page 168)	2	15
3. Lateral Raise, Bilateral (page 141)	2	15
4. Rear Delt Raise, Bilateral (page 143)	2	15
SUPER SET:		
5. External Cable Rotation (page 165)	1	15
6. Internal Cable Rotation (page 164)	1	15
COMPOUND SET:		
7. Supine Dumbbell Extension, Bilateral (page 178)	2	15
8. Standing Dumbbell Curl, Bilateral (page 201)	2	15
SUPER SET:		
9. Wrist Flexion with Dumbbell, Bilateral (page 230)	1	20
10. Wrist Extension Dumbbell, Bilateral (page 231)	1	20

WEEKS 4–6, TWO TIMES PER WEEK

Concentric phase 2 seconds, eccentric phase 4 seconds.

Exercise	Sets	Reps
1. Front Raise with Dumbbell, Bilateral (page 138)	1	12
COMPOUND SET:		
2. Military Press (page 153)	2	12
3. Barbell Shrug (page 168)	2	12
4. Lateral Raise (page 141)	2	12
5. Rear Delt Raise (page 143)	2	12
SUPER SET:		
6. External Cable Rotation (page 165)	1	12
7. Internal Cable Rotation (page 164)	1	12
COMPOUND SET:		
8. Triceps Push-Down (page 186)	3	12
9. Hammer Curl, Bilateral (page 203)	3	12
SUPER SET:		
10. Wrist Flexion with Dumbbell, Bilateral (page 230)	1	12
11. Wrist Extension with Dumbbell, Bilateral (page 231)	1	12

WEEKS 7–9, TWO TIMES PER WEEK

Exercise	Sets	Reps
COMPOUND SET:		
1. Behind-the-Neck Press (page 154)	2	8
2. Standing Barbell Shrug (page 168)	2	8
3. Rear Delt Raise, Unilateral (page 143)	3	8
4. Front Raise with Plate (page 138)	1	8
5. Lateral Raise, Unilateral (page 141)	2	8

SUPER SET:

Exercise	Sets	Reps
6. External Cable Rotation (page 165)	1	8
7. Internal Cable Rotation (page 164)	1	8

COMPOUND SET:

Exercise	Sets	Reps
8. Dumbbell Upright Extension, Bilateral, Elbow In (page 179)	3	8
9. Reverse Curl with E-Z Curl Bar (page 215)	3	8

COMPOUND SET:

Exercise	Sets	Reps
10. Triceps Pull-Down (page 187)	1	8
11. Incline Dumbbell Curl (page 204)	1	8
12. Supination/Pronation (page 233)	1	8

SUPER SET:

Exercise	Sets	Reps
13. Wrist Flexion with Barbell (page 203)	1	8
14. Wrist Extension with Barbell (page 231)	1	8

Third set completed with a 10-second isometric contraction for the last repetition for all exercises.

WEEKS 10–12, TWO TIMES PER WEEK

DAY 1

Exercise	Sets	Reps
1. Dumbbell Shoulder Press, Bilateral (page 152)	3	5–6
2. Rear Delt Raise, Unilateral (page 143)	3	5–6
3. Lateral Raise, Bilateral (page 141)	1	15
4. Front Raise with Bar (page 138)	1	15

SUPER SET:

Exercise	Sets	Reps
5. Internal Rotation (page 162)	1	5–6
6. External Rotation (page 163)	1	5–6

DAY 2

Exercise	Sets	Reps
1. Rear Delt Raise, Bilateral (page 143)	1	15
2. Lateral Raise, Unilateral (page 141)	3	5–6
3. Front Raise Bar (page 138)	3	5–6
4. Dumbbell Shoulder Press, Bilateral (page 152)	1	12

DAYS 1 AND 2

Exercise	Sets	Reps

COMPOUND SET:

Exercise	Sets	Reps
1. Supine Bar Extension (page 183)	3	5–6
2. Barbell Reverse Curl (page 215)	3	5–6

COMPOUND SET:

Exercise	Sets	Reps
3. Cable Cross Pull-Down (page 193)	1	12
4. Concentration Curl (page 209)	1	12
5. Supination/Pronation (page 233)	1	10

SUPER SET:

Exercise	Sets	Reps
6. Radial Flexion (page 234)	1	5
7. Ulna Flexion (page 235)	1	5

Peaking (Off-Season)

WEEKS 13–15, TWO TIMES PER WEEK

DAY 1 (SHOULDERS)

Exercise	Sets	Reps

SUPER SET:

Exercise	Sets	Reps
1. Behind-the-Neck Press (page 154)	3	5–6
2. Rear Delt Raise, Bilateral (page 143)	3	5–6
3. Upright Row (page 158)	2	12
4. Lateral Raise, Unilateral (page 141)	2	12

DAY 2 (SHOULDERS)

Exercise	Sets	Reps
1. Rear Delt Cable Raise, Unilateral (page 145)	1	12
2. Upright Row (page 158)	3	5–6
3. Lateral Cable Raise, Unilateral (page 141)	3	5–6
4. Military Press with Machine (page 153)	1	12

SUPER SET:

Exercise	Sets	Reps
5. Internal Rotation, Unilateral (page 162)	1	5–6
6. External Rotation, Unilateral (page 163)	1	5–6

DAY 1 (ARMS)

Exercise	Sets	Reps

COMPOUND SET:

Exercise	Sets	Reps
1. Triceps Push-Down (page 186)	3	5–6
2. Kung Fu Curl (page 206)	3	5–6

COMPOUND SET:

Exercise	Sets	Reps
3. Triceps Pull-Down (page 187)	1	15
4. Hammer Curl, Alternating (page 203)	1	15

DAY 2 (ARMS)

Exercise	Sets	Reps

COMPOUND SET:

Exercise	Sets	Reps
1. Triceps Pull-Down (page 187)	3	8
2. Hammer Curl, Alternating (page 203)	3	8

COMPOUND SET:

Exercise	Sets	Reps
3. Body Weight Push-Back (page 197)	1	failure
4. Biceps Chin-Up (page 228)	1	failure

DAY 1 (FOREARMS)

Exercise	Sets	Reps

SUPER SET:

Exercise	Sets	Reps
1. Wrist Roll Extension (page 232)	1	1
2. Wrist Roll Flexion (page 232)	1	1

DAY 2 (FOREARMS)

Exercise	Sets	Reps

SUPER SET:

Exercise	Sets	Reps
1. Radial Flexion (page 234)	1	5
2. Ulna Flexion (page 235)	1	5

In-Season

DAY 1 (SHOULDERS)

Exercise	Sets	Reps
SUPER SET:		
1. Behind-the-Neck Press (page 154)	2	5–6
2. Rear Delt Raise, Bilateral (page 143)	2	5–6
3. Upright Row (page 158)	1	12
4. Lateral Raise, Unilateral (page 141)	1	12

DAY 2 (SHOULDERS)

Exercise	Sets	Reps
1. Rear Delt Cable Raise, Unilateral (page 145)	1	12
2. Upright Row (page 158)	2	5–6
3. Lateral Cable Raise, Unilateral (page 141)	2	5–6
4. Military Press with Machine (page 153)	1	12

DAY 1 (ARMS)

Exercise	Sets	Reps
COMPOUND SET:		
1. Triceps Push-Down (page 188)	2	5–6
2. Kung Fu Curl (page 206)	2	5–6

DAY 2 (ARMS)

Exercise	Sets	Reps
COMPOUND SET:		
1. Triceps Pull-Down (page 189)	1	12
2. Hammer Curl, Alternating (page 203)	1	12
COMPOUND SET:		
3. Body Weight Push-Back (page 197)	1	failure
4. Biceps Chin-Up (page 228)	1	failure

DAY 1 (FOREARMS)

Exercise	Sets	Reps
SUPER SET:		
1. Wrist Roll Extension (page 231)	1	1
2. Wrist Roll Flexion (page 230)	1	1

DAY 2 (FOREARMS)

Exercise	Sets	Reps
SUPER SET:		
1. Wrist Flexion (page 234)	1	8
2. Wrist Extension (page 235)	1	8

Skill Enhancement

Skills are trained before a strength training session. Skill training, if specific to the body parts being worked on during the strength-training session, may be considered warm-up. Start skill training after the first four weeks of strength training.

Bat Speed

WEEKS 1–2, TWO TIMES PER WEEK

Train with arms and shoulders
Warm-up: general to specific

Form swing	1 set	50 reps

Refine general techniques of the swing
Last 10 reps should be full speed

WEEKS 3–15

Warm-up
Overspeed swing training: use a bat

2–3 ounces lighter than competition bat	1 set	25 reps

Resistance swing training: use a bat

2–3 ounces heavier than competition bat	1 set	25 reps

The last 10 swings of both sets should be target swings, i.e., low-outside, high-inside, etc.

All swings for both sets should be full speed combined with mental imagery

GOLF

Improved performance and no injury or pain while playing the game—what golfer wouldn't want this? This workout is designed to increase muscular power and endurance. This in turn will enhance club-head speed and enjoyment of the game, while eliminating the nagging joint problems that are associated with golf.

Implementation

For many individuals there may be no off-season for golf, but there are times when an individual wants to peak. The thirteen-week (off-season) training program may be implemented in a time frame that allows the individual to achieve his or her personal goals.

Please remember that strength training is only one aspect of improving performance. To achieve your highest level of performance you must incorporate all aspects of training—flexibility, conditioning, concentration, nutrition, and skill—with skill acquisition (practice) being the highest priority. On days when weight training, always practice prior to the training session.

Golf is a sport that requires the use of a variety of muscles in complex neuromuscular sequences. As with other sports that involve fine motor skills, this routine will train the specific muscles that are involved while not attempting to copy the sport movement patterns with added resistance.

Guidelines

OFF-SEASON

Follow frequency guidelines for the prescribed routine. Allow at least 48 hours of recovery time between training sessions, with optimal recovery time being 72 to 96 hours.

This routine trains opposing muscle groups. In accordance with the principle of whole-body training, other body parts should be trained in the same way to ensure optimal recovery. The following would be an appropriate format to follow:

Day 1: Chest/Back/Abs
Day 2: Legs/Forearms
Day 3: Shoulders/Triceps/Biceps/Abs
Day 4: Rest
Repeat

Every two weeks take a day off between day 2 and day 3. Each exercise should be preceded by a warm-up set followed by the prescribed number of sets and reps at very high intensity.

IN-SEASON

Attempt to follow the frequency guidelines.

Strength training following practice or competition is an optimal time to train.

If training plateaus occur refer to Off-Season, Weeks 1–3 for a three-week period.

During the in-season, follow a 4-weeks-on 1-week-off whole-body strength training schedule.

Rest between sets is dictated by intensity or repetition scheme.

15 repetitions and above	60 seconds
12 repetitions	90 seconds
8 repetitions	2 minutes
5–6 repetitions	3 minutes

Off-Season

WEEKS 1–2, TWO TIMES PER WEEK

Concentric phase 2 seconds, eccentric phase 4 seconds.

Exercise	Sets	Reps
1. Dumbbell Shoulder Press, Bilateral (page 152)	1	15
2. Lateral Raise, Bilateral (page 141)	1	15
3. Rear Delt Raise, Bilateral (page 143)	1	15
SUPER SET:		
4. High Cable Internal Rotation (page 160)	1	15
5. Low Cable External Rotation, Bilateral (page 161)	1	15
COMPOUND SET:		
6. Supine Bar Extension, Bilateral (page 183)	1	15
7. Standing Dumbbell Curl, Bilateral (page 201)	1	15
SUPER SET:		
8. Wrist Flexion Dumbbell (page 230)	1	20
9. Wrist Extension Dumbbell (page 231)	1	20

WEEKS 3–4, TWO TIMES PER WEEK

Concentric phase 2 seconds, eccentric phase 4 seconds.

Exercise	Sets	Reps
1. Front Raise Dumbbell, Bilateral (page 138)	1	12
2. Military Press (page 153)	2	12
3. Lateral Raise, Bilateral (page 141)	1	12
4. Rear Delt Raise, Bilateral (page 143)	2	12
SUPER SET:		
5. External Cable Rotation (page 165)	1	12
6. Internal Cable Rotation (page 164)	1	12
COMPOUND SET:		
7. Triceps Push-Down (page 186)	2	12
8. Hammer Curl, Bilateral (page 203)	2	12
SUPER SET:		
9. Wrist Flexion Dumbbell, Bilateral (page 230)	1	12
10. Wrist Extension Dumbbell, Bilateral (page 231)	1	12

WEEKS 5–7, TWO TIMES PER WEEK

Exercise	Sets	Reps
1. Behind-the-Neck Press (page 154)	2	8
2. Rear Delt Raise, Unilateral (page 143)	2	8
3. Front Raise with Plate (page 138)	1	8
4. Lateral Raise, Unilateral (page 141)	2	8
SUPER SET:		
5. External Cable Rotation (page 165)	1	8
6. Internal Cable Rotation (page 164)	1	8

COMPOUND SET:		
7. Dumbbell Upright Extension, Bilateral, Elbow In (page 179)	3	8
8. Barbell Reverse Curl with E-Z Curl Bar (page 215)	3	8
SUPER SET:		
9. Radial Flexion (page 234)	1	20
10. Ulna Flexion (page 235)	1	20

Last set completed with a 10-second isometric contraction for the last repetition for all exercises.

WEEKS 8–10, TWO TIMES PER WEEK

Concentric phase 2 seconds, eccentric phase 4 seconds.

DAY 1

Exercise	Sets	Reps
1. Dumbbell Shoulder Press, Bilateral (page 152)	3	5–6
2. Rear Delt Raise, Unilateral (page 143)	3	5–6
3. Lateral Raise, Bilateral (page 141)	1	15
4. Front Raise with Bar (page 138)	1	15
5. Internal Rotation (page 162)	1	5–6

DAY 2

Exercise	Sets	Reps
1. Rear Delt Raise, Bilateral (page 143)	1	15
2. Lateral Raise, Unilateral (page 141)	3	5–6
3. Front Raise Bar (page 138)	3	5–6
4. External Rotation (page 163)	1	5–6
5. Dumbbell Shoulder Press, Bilateral (page 152)	1	12

DAYS 1 AND 2

Exercise	Sets	Reps
COMPOUND SET:		
1. Supine Bar Extension (page 183)	2	5–6
2. Straight Bar Reverse Curl (page 215)	2	5–6
SUPER SET:		
3. Radial Flexion Dumbbell (page 234)	1	12
4. Ulna Flexion Dumbbell (page 235)	1	12
5. Supination/Pronation (page 233)	1	12

Peaking (Off-Season)

WEEKS 11–13, TWO TIMES PER WEEK
Concentric phase 2 seconds, eccentric phase 4 seconds.

DAY 1

Exercise	Sets	Reps
SUPER SET:		
1. Behind-the-Neck Press (page 154)	3	5–6
2. Rear Delt Raise, Bilateral (page 143)	3	5–6
3. Upright Row (page 158)	1	12
4. Dumbbell Lateral Raise, Unilateral (page 141)	1	12

DAY 2

Exercise	Sets	Reps
1. Rear Delt Cable Raise, Unilateral (page 143)	1	12
2. Upright Row (page 158)	3	5–6
3. Lateral Cable Raise, Unilateral (page 141)	3	5–6
4. Military Press with Machine (page 153)	1	12

DAY 1

Exercise	Sets	Reps
COMPOUND SET:		
1. Triceps Push-Down (page 186)	3	5–6
2. Kung Fu Curl (page 206)	3	5–6

DAY 2

Exercise	Sets	Reps
COMPOUND SET:		
1. Triceps Pull-Down (page 187)	1	15
2. Hammer Curl, Alternating (page 203)	1	15

DAYS 1 AND 2

Exercise	Sets	Reps
SUPER SET:		
1. Forearm Wrist Roll Extension (page 232)	1	1
2. Forearm Wrist Roll Flexion (page 232)	1	1

Last set completed with a 10-second isometric contraction for the last repetition for all exercises.

In-Season

TWO TIMES PER WEEK
Concentric phase 2 seconds, eccentric phase 4 seconds.

DAY 1

Exercise	Sets	Reps
SUPER SET:		
1. Behind-the-Neck Press (page 154)	3	5–6
2. Rear Delt Raise, Bilateral (page 143)	3	5–6
3. Upright Row (page 158)	1	12
4. Dumbbell Lateral Raise, Unilateral (page 141)	1	12
COMPOUND SET:		
5. Triceps Push-Down (page 186)	3	5–6
6. Kung Fu Curl (page 206)	3	5–6
SUPER SET:		
7. Forearm Wrist Roll Extension (page 232)	1	1
8. Forearm Wrist Roll Flexion (page 232)	1	1

DAY 2

Exercise	Sets	Reps
1. Dumbbell Front Raise, Bilateral (page 138)	1	12
2. Military Press with Bar (page 153)	2	12
3. Lateral Raise (page 141)	1	12
4. Rear Delt Raise (page 143)	2	12
5. Overhead Rotation (page 166)	1	12
COMPOUND SET:		
6. Triceps Push-Down (page 186)	2	12
7. Hammer Curl, Bilateral (page 203)	2	12
SUPER SET:		
8. Radial Flexion (page 234)	1	12
9. Ulna Flexion (page 235)	1	12

Getting Bigger/Bulking Up

Before we decide how to get bigger, let's define what getting bigger means. By getting bigger do we mean just adding weight, or do we mean adding lean body mass (increased cross-sectional size of the muscle fiber, increased bone density, etc.) and positively enhancing body composition? To be honest, any time getting bigger is the goal, you will probably do a little of both, you will add weight by both increasing lean tissue and body fat. The key here is to add a higher percentage of lean tissue.

To be successful you must utilize a systematic approach. This approach includes two components: nutrition and resistance training.

NUTRITIONAL GUIDELINES

To add weight we must generally consume more calories than we expend. This combined with a high-intensity training program will bring about increases in muscle growth. To gain a pound of muscle we must increase our caloric intake by 2500 kcals (2500 kcals equals what a pound of muscle has in potential energy) per week. How we increase these calories is the key to adding muscle mass.

- Add weight gradually
- Caloric intake should not exceed caloric expenditure by more than 1000 kcals a day
- Caloric increases should only take place on days you train
- Eat small frequent meals
- Avoid large meals
- Plot weight gain
- Follow macronutrients guidelines listed in this series of books

RESISTANCE TRAINING

One goal of any resistance program is to positively enhance body composition. If our goal is to really bulk up, let's say put on twenty pounds of quality lean tissue for a specific competition in six months, then your approach needs to be very calculated and precise.

Training Guidelines: The most commonly asked question is what set-repetition scheme will bring about the most muscle growth? Let's first look at what specific set-rep schemes are designed to do.

Sets	Repetitions	Adaptations
3	8–15	Best for developing hypertrophy
3–5	4–7	Strength and power
4–7	1–3	Peaking and maximum strength

Looking at the above chart and following the training principle of specificity, one would assume that performing sets of 8–15 repetitions would be best for promoting muscle growth. That assumption would be true for a period of time. A repetition scheme of 8 to 15 reps, give or take a rep or two, is specifically designed to bring about muscle hypertrophy. But if we persisted in this protocol you would plateau or move into an overtraining syndrome. The best way to promote long-term gains in muscle mass, which will naturally be the greatest, is to incorporate a properly periodized program that involves a variety of specific set-rep schemes (such as the ones described previously) over specific periods of time (see "Creating Your Own Routine," page 285).

You might ask yourself, If a variety of schemes works best, why not incorporate these into one workout? This concept, called pyramiding, is very effective for the short term, but this approach is nonspecific and doesn't allow for complete adaptations. You would soon plateau and have no variance to turn to. Your only alternative would be to take time off or work at a very low intensity. Both scenarios are unacceptable for your goal. Quality gains in lean muscle tissue take time. The best way to achieve this is to be able to train long and hard without having to take time off for overtraining. A program that follows the concepts of periodization will allow you to achieve your ultimate goal.

Another key training component is that of intensity. You must train with intensity to add lean tissue. The component that most positively or negatively affects the ultimate outcome of the exercise is the intensity of the exercise. You must reach momentary muscular exhaustion (MME) for the prescribed number of repetitions.

Let's face another fact, at one time or another all of us have stopped short of MME, consciously or not. MME is uncomfortable if not downright painful and reaching it is an acquired skill. Push yourself and learn this skill with the help of the following guidelines:

For every 4 reps you can perform at a specific weight, add 2 reps to help you reach true MME. For example, the exercise prescription calls for 1 set of Triceps Push-Downs to be performed for 12 reps. In this instance you would want to use a weight that previously would have brought you to MME in 8 reps (two groups of 4 would mean 4 additional reps). Or make your new goal 16 reps. Push yourself, get fired up, enjoy the good pain. The results you see will be worth it. Train with and acquire the skill of intensity—this is the key. Also remember to be progressive; add weight or resistance when needed. Don't be satisfied with your accomplishments.

The final guideline is just as important: Make sure your recovery time is optimal. Allow at least 48 hours but no more than 120 hours recovery time before training the same body part.

Creating Your Own Routine

Yes, there will come a time when you need to leave the nest and create your own training routine. This may cause anxiety, and that's expected. Don't worry, this chapter will give you the tools you need to design your own routine, turning you into your own personal trainer.

Part One: The Design Model

When creating a shoulders and arms routine you need a basic design model or blueprint to work from. You will need to divide the shoulders and arms into five separate areas—shoulders, triceps, biceps, traps, and forearms. These areas can be worked separately or in conjunction with other body parts.

To build a routine, you need to think about how you want to shape and strengthen each area. This will depend on your individual needs and goals: weak areas, aesthetics, sport-specific training, etc. It is always important to remember that you must create balance and symmetry between these areas—not only in appearance but also in strength.

Since the exercises in this book are categorized according to these five areas, you'll find it easy to plug in exercises and personalize your routine.

Part Two: Basic Concepts

Setting up a shoulders and arms training program requires preparation and attention to detail. An understanding of the basic concepts of training is necessary for your design to be successful.

The following are key concepts (along with the principles in Chapter 3) you will need to consider when building your routine.

VOLUME

Volume is the number of repetitions performed. Fifteen repetitions is a higher volume than 10 reps. Total volume for a workout can be defined by total *sets × repetitions*. If you did 9 sets of shoulder exercises and 10 reps in each set, your total volume would be 90 reps. When creating a progressive series of routines, you want to keep an eye on total volume, making sure you're doing enough but not too much. Total volume should usually never exceed 100 repetitions per muscle group. Volume is also important as it relates to intensity. These two components are inversely related: If volume goes up, intensity goes down, and vice versa.

INTENSITY

Intensity can most easily be measured by the amount of weight lifted. Intensity is dependent upon goals, specificity, training stage, and experience or maturity of the individual. The intensity that different people can handle will vary greatly. The beginner or novice should not attempt to handle high-intensity training until he or she has established a training base. Intensity can also be affected by total volume of work. High-volume training, numerous exercises, sets, etc., may increase intensity.

Intensity is the key to successful training. *An individual should use an intensity that will produce momentary muscular fatigue in the prescribed number of repetitions.*

VARIATION

Variation is often the most neglected training principle. Training needs to be varied for the following reasons: to prevent overtraining, to avoid training plateaus, to alleviate the boredom of monotony, and to bring about the best possible training results.

The most important aspect of variation is related to intensity and volume. When you first started working out, it was easier to shock your muscles and cause adaptations. As you become more advanced you will need to change your workouts more frequently. One way to do this is to increase your intensity (weight) and decrease your repetitions (volume). Another way to create variety is to do the opposite: increase volume (repetitions) and decrease your intensity (weight). When you're considering variations in volume and intensity, you may want to vary similar training days within a training week. You will have a day of high-intensity training (heavy) and one of low-intensity training (light). The terms *heavy* and *light* can be misnomers. On both "light" and "heavy" days you should push yourself to momentary muscular failure.

EXERCISE ORDER

In general, the best order for exercises is from largest muscles to the smallest (see anatomy). Staying with the same exercise order for extended periods of time may cause plateaus (no adaptations), which means less than optimal or no gains.

The order can also be affected by individual goals and the need for variety. For the muscle groups in this book, that would mean training your shoulders, trapezius, triceps, biceps, and forearms, in that order.

Alternative Exercise Order

Prioritizing: If your primary goal is to shape your shoulder muscles, one way to achieve this would be to target or exercise them first. This can be applied to any muscle group.

Pre-exhaustion: Pre-exhaustion is a technique used to fatigue assisting muscles in order to better isolate a specific muscle. To preexhaust your deltoids, you would train your trapezius and triceps first.

ENERGY SYSTEMS

Exercises and exercise prescriptions are not all created equal. To ensure the best development, you need to include three different energy systems: a routine of high intensity and short duration; a routine of medium intensity and medium duration; and a routine of low intensity and longer duration. All three of these should be included at one time or another. In other words, you need to include exercises that are arduous and exhaust you quickly, and exercises that are less strenuous and allow you to train for longer intervals.

Including these three basic energy systems will ensure the best overall shoulder and arm development. This type of training involves a variety of muscle fiber types, while introducing specificity into the training regimen. Being aware of energy metabolism ensures that you train for muscular endurance and/or strength.

REPETITION GUIDELINES

Short duration—Training in a range of 1 to 4 repetitions maximum, using a weight that brings about failure in this repetition range.

Medium duration—Repetition maximums that range from 5 to 15 repetitions. Supersetting or Compound setting of exercises would be included in this time frame.

Long duration—Forced slow contraction (lowering and raising the weight in a exaggerated, slow motion), mega-rep schemes (over 20), trisets, quadsets, etc. would all be ways to train at this level.

INJURY PREVENTION AND REHABILITATION

The greatest benefit of strength training is that of injury prevention. Strengthening the muscles and connective tissue (through proper strength training) around a specific area helps the skeletal structure. Bone density is also improved through increased retention of calcium. This decreases the potential of injury in that area.

If an individual is unlucky enough to be injured and has been involved in a proper strength training program, that person will recover from the injury more quickly than a person who was not involved in a strength training program.

With the obvious benefits of injury prevention, quicker recovery, and more complete rehabilitation, exercises that address these areas should be included in your training routine. On the other hand, exercises that aggravate specific areas should be avoided.

PERFORMANCE

When formulating a shoulders and arms training program you need to analyze performance needs. Is there a specific sport or activity in which you wish to improve performance? Examine the movements of the sport or activity. Is there throwing, pushing, or pulling? I'll bet there is! Based on this analysis you can choose exercises and create a shoulder and arm routine that will enhance these specific movements.

MUSCLE BALANCE

Muscle balance must be considered when choosing exercises. Shoulder and arm muscles (see anatomy) work together in a variety of movements, as well as in maintaining proper posture. The movements used in training need to include all the muscle groups, while working these muscle groups at a variety of angles.

All muscles should be trained in an effort to maintain muscular balance. When a muscle or muscle group becomes considerably stronger than others, the potential for injury is greatly increased.

In the same respect, never neglect one muscle area to work on weaker areas. Simply shift stronger areas onto more of a maintenance regimen while continuing to follow a growth-oriented resistance program with weaker body parts.

Movements should also include combination (or compound) exercises (exercises that work two or more muscle groups at the same time).

The training routines included in this book are designed with these principles of movement in mind, in order to give you optimal gains. Pick and choose or create your own.

SAID

Specificity or the SAID principle (Specific Adaptations to Imposed Demands) is a very important training concept. Exercises should be chosen to fit your specific needs. The following elements will guide you.

Training Stage: Exercise choice will be affected by your training stage: a preconditioning stage, a maintenance stage, a peak performance stage, etc.

Sport or Activity: The specific needs of your sport are a major consideration in exercise selection. You need to train for specific kinds of movements as well as the type of energy output used in the sport.

Personal Goals: When choosing exercises, you have to be aware of your specific goals: what you want and how much time you are willing to spend. If you are a bodybuilder, your goals are going to be much different from those of someone who wants to firm up a little and not get winded from a stroll down the beach.

Part Three: Periodization

Periodization is a systematic and progressive training method designed to aid in planning and organization. This cyclical training method encompasses all of the basic training principles. It is utilized by the greatest athletes and strength coaches in the world (many of whom are included in this book) and is designed to bring training to a peak. The scope of this book does not allow for a detailed discussion of the many intricacies of periodization, but the following summary will help you in creating your own shoulder and arm routines.

The basis for periodization is derived from the General Adaptation Syndrome (GAS), which was developed during the 1930s. It was intended to describe a person's ability to adapt to stress. There are three distinct phases to the GAS:

1. *Alarm Stage*—This relates to the individual's initial response to training. This could represent itself as a temporary drop in performance due to stiffness/soreness.
2. *Resistance Stage*—This stage represents itself as the period when the athlete or individual adapts to the training stimulus by making certain adjustments. These adjustments may include physiological, mechanical, structural, and psychological adaptations.
3. *Exhaustion or Overwork Stage*—If total stress placed upon the athlete is too great, then the third stage, overtraining, manifests itself.

Overtraining can represent itself in the following ways:

• a loss of strength or plateauing of performance
• chronic fatigue
• loss of appetite
• loss of body weight, or lean body mass
• increased illness potential
• increased injury potential
• decreased motivation and low self-esteem

During the exhaustion stage, desired training adaptations are not likely to occur. Outside stresses—social life, improper nutrition, lack of sleep, long work hours—also need to be considered to avoid overtraining.

The goal then is to remain in the resistance stage of training, with periodic moves into the alarm stage. This allows your body to make the compensations to the stresses while continually improving. This is done through careful manipulation of certain training principles and detailed planning.

OBJECTIVES

Defining your objectives is the first step in creating your own routine.

1. Identify areas of importance. Obviously the muscles of the shoulders and arms (see Chapter 2, "Body Basics") are of primary importance. Individual muscles within this group may take priority (see Exercise Order and Variation), but remember not to neglect any muscle group. If an area is being rehabilitated, this area should take precedence.
2. Distinguish between training that is effective and that which is ineffective. In many cases this comes down to a mental attitude. You must perform the exercises that are most effective, not those that are fun and comfortable to perform.
3. Work toward a definite time when you should peak. This may be for a competition or just for looking good at the beach. During this designated time all facets of your endeavor should be peaking: training, diet, etc.

Remember, very few things are set in stone, especially when it comes to fitness training. Periodic evaluation and changing of objectives along with procedures and prescriptions is essential to make any long-term program successful.

THE CYCLES

Once your goals and objectives have been defined, the next step is planning, which can be divided into four training phases.

Macrocycle: The macrocycle is the longest of the training phases. Its length varies depending on the goals. In general, the macrocycle lasts from the end of one peaking period to another. The macrocycle defines long-term goals, and a specific time frame in which you want to peak: six weeks, six months, or one year. The macrocycle contains three components: preparation, peaking, and transition.

Mesocycle: The next largest phase is the mesocycle. Mesocycles make up a macrocycle. A mesocycle is a phase that has very specific goals (see system). For example, the goal of the first mesocycle may be that of preparation. This would include training of high volume and fairly low intensity to build a base of strength and muscular endurance.

The next mesocycle's goals would include an increase in intensity (increased weight, more difficult exercises, shorter rest periods, etc.). This action would necessitate a lowering of volume prescriptions.

The next mesocycle's goal may be oriented for strength (increase in intensity—decrease in volume).

The final mesocycle in which you reach peak condition might include more intensive evaluation: what areas are weak and need *more intense* work, what areas are strong, what has worked best in the past, diet, mental state, etc.

Depending upon specific goals, peaking for the shoulders and arms will differ for each individual. Someone whose goal is strength may continue to increase intensity and lower volume, while concentrating on optimal recovery for competition. Bodybuilders may increase volume and lower relative intensity while peaking for competition. Athletes may spend more time on sport-specific movements, metabolic specificity, and skill acquisition when peaking for a compet-

itive season (there may be several peaking phases within a competitive season). The better the preparation—i.e., the better the condition you are in—the longer you will be able to maintain your peak.

Microcycle: Within each mesocycle are smaller units called microcycles. Microcycles further refine the objectives by manipulating training variables on a daily basis. One day may include training of high intensity and low volume, while the next day may include training of low intensity and high volume. Or it may become even more complex as in our ultimate shoulder and arms section, varying day to day from specific muscle groups and also in the training stimulus (volume, intensity, and specificity). In most cases a microcycle will last from one to four weeks.

The Peaking Period: This is the period when all your training culminates, bringing out the best possible results. This will, of course, be different for everybody, depending on individual goals. For the elite athlete, this can be very complicated, because several variables have to come together at once: strength, endurance, sport-specific skills, diet, mental state, etc. The same is true for a bodybuilder. Things become somewhat more simplified if it's just the shoulders and arms you're concerned about. If you want your shoulders and arms to reach a peak for a vacation on the beach, you should be focusing on three variables, your weight training routine, diet, and cardiovascular training. Again, the peaking period is when you bring all these elements together at their highest level.

Transition: Unfortunately, maintaining peak anything for a long period of time can be very difficult. The cycle or period of time following a peaking period is the transition phase.

Transition is designed to introduce variety into the program while bringing about recovery and recuperation, both mentally and physically. And as the term *transition* applies, this phase allows you to start at a higher training level for the next macrocycle, or whatever your goals may entail.

Ultimately the rigors of continuing to peak will lead

us into stage 3 of the GAS, which is that of overtraining and exhaustion. The body needs some time off from the peaking phase and training in general. Diet restriction and high intensity will eventually lead to overtraining.

When most people think of recuperation they think of sitting on their butt and doing nothing. In the transition phase you will continue to engage in activities but at low volumes and intensities. These activities can be physical activities that you enjoy. In conjunction with these activities, light weight training once a week may be undertaken (following correct training guidelines). Depending upon your goals and the next peaking period, the transition phase will usually last from one to two weeks.

Correct application of the concepts of periodization takes the guesswork out of training. Periodization allows you to identify and isolate the variables necessary to obtain the ultimate shoulders and arms. Using the design model in part one of this chapter and following the basic concepts outlined here and in Chapter 3, you can choose exercises from the book and create your own customized routine. Then, following the natural cycles of periodization, you can create a series of progressive routines, staying as long as possible in the growth and peaking phases, achieving the shoulders and arms you envision.

A Case Study

You want to peak for a tennis tournament over the Labor Day weekend, and it is now June 1. Ideally, you would plan a three-month macrocycle.

The next step is to break this down into one-month mesocycles. These in turn would be divided into two-week microcycles for the first two months and one-week microcycles the last month as you prepare to peak. If you plan to play other tournaments during the summer, that is okay, but let's say that this tournament is the most important one of the summer and this is when we want your shoulders and arms to peak.

Your breakdown may go something like this:

First month: This would be your preparation period. You would build a safe foundation doing low-intensity training with high volume. Your first microcycle would include basic strength training exercises to create muscular balance, and would promote joint integrity. During your second microcycle, intensity would increase (causing volume to decrease), and the introduction of multijoint exercises would be important. At this point in time, skill acquisition is very important and should be undertaken when fresh (preferably before weight training).

Second month: During this period the primary goal is to increase the intensity of your training; consequently your volume is going to have to drop. You may add some more specific exercises during the first two-week microcycle. During the second microcycle, the plan for your shoulders and arms would be the same, higher intensity and lower volume (repetition scheme 5 to 8). Again skill acquisition is paramount.

Third month: You now move into one-week microcycles. The first week, volume is increased and intensity is lowered (volume is the same as the first week of the second microcycle; if all is going well the intensity should be greater). During the second week, intensity is increased, volume decreased, and the repetition scheme should be lowered to eight for each exercise.

The third week the progression continues: increased intensity/lower volume for the first day of training the shoulders and arms. The rep scheme would be at 5 reps. The second day of shoulder and arm training would be considered a light day, with high volume—12 reps and lower intensity. If during this time you are scheduled to play other tournaments, consider the last tournament played as a training day; any previous tournaments are considered off days.

The last week should consist of one high-intensity day. This should take you up to the week of the tournament. At least 72 hours before the tournament, go through a workout that includes one set per body part. Use a repetition prescription of 8. As always, to be a better tennis player you must play tennis; skill acquisition is top priority.

Good luck with your advanced principles. The applications of these principles will lead to your ultimate success and longevity in training.

Major Contributors

Kurt Brungardt is a writer, personal trainer, and a member of Strength Advantage Inc. He is the author of the best-selling fitness book, *The Complete Book of Abs* and coauthored *The Complete Book of Butt and Legs.* His video *Abs of Steel for Men* was a *Billboard* Top-10 selection, selling more than 150,000 units. He has been featured in numerous national magazines and programs, including: *Men's Fitness, Details, Vogue, Newsweek, The Wall Street Journal, USA Today, Total Fitness, Fitness Plus, Hard Copy, CBS This Morning, The Today Show,* and QVC. The last four years he has toured the country appearing on local radio, television shows, and giving seminars on fitness-related issues.

   Mike Brungardt is the strength and conditioning

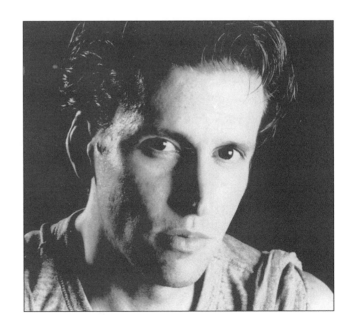

coach for the San Antonio Spurs. He is a coauthor of *The Complete Book of Butt and Legs* and *The Strength Kit*. He is a cofounder of Strength Advantage Inc. He has given clinics for fitness educators and coaches in schools and health clubs throughout the country. Mike has been involved in sports and coaching for over twenty-five years. He writes a weekly column for the *Austin American Stateman*.

Brett Brungardt is a cofounder of Strength Advantage Inc. He is a coauthor of *The Complete Book of Butt and Legs* and *The Strength Kit*. He is a former strength and conditioning coach at the University of Houston and the University of Wyoming. As a fitness consultant, he has designed programs for professional and college athletes, corporations, and the elderly. He is a certified strength and conditioning specialist with the National Strength and Conditioning Association. He has his master's degree in exercise science from the University of Houston.

Bryon Holmes is a fitness expert and strength coach specializing in preventive care and rehabilitation for the lower back. He has given seminars and clinics on the lower back for health professionals and corporations throughout the world. He has authored over 40 articles and abstracts on lower-back care and rehabilitation. He is a member of the American College of Sports Medicine. He has a B.S. and M.S. in exercise physiology from the University of Florida.

Debbie Holmes is a fitness educator, teacher, and personal trainer. She is the former coordinator for the adult fitness program at San Diego State University and the founder of one of the largest in-home training operations in southern California. She is currently developing a newsletter and a fitness website. She is on the advisory board of the American Council on Exercise for fitness certification. She is a member of the American College of Sports Medicine and the American Council on Exercise. She has a B.S. and M.S. in health science and education from the University of Florida.

Becky Chase is a registered dietician. She currently maintains a private practice through her company, Alpine Nutritional Services. Becky specializes in sports nutrition and eating disorders. Becky has written many articles for newspapers, magazines, and hospital publications. She is currently working on a book based on her Market Smarts program. Becky has B.S. and M.S. degrees in clinical diatetics from Texas Women's College.

Models

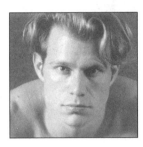

Elizabeth Jonas is a personal trainer and fitness instructor at Crunch Fitness in New York City.

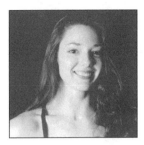

Noah Brody is a model, computer whiz, and actor. He lives in New York City.

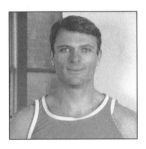

Michael Mahana is a fitness enthusiast and writer. He lives in New York City.

Geoffry Goodridge is a photographer and weight lifter—in that order.

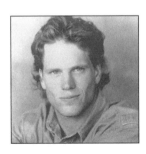

Jonathan Schaefer is a personal trainer and actor.

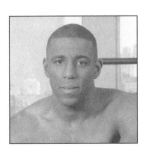

Adolphus is a personal trainer and owner of Adolphus Fitness Inc. in New York City.

Lisa Mackechnie is a personal trainer and body-builder. She lives in New York City.

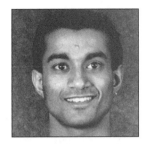

Kenny Mahadeo is a model and personal trainer at Crunch Fitness.

Dave Johnson is a personal trainer and poet. He lives in New York City.

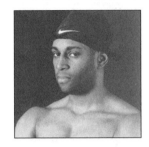

Doug Dickerson is a personal trainer and member of the U.S. Olympic track team for the 200 meters.

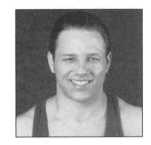

Raymond Jarrell is an actor. He lives in New York City.

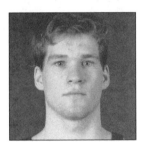

Greg Pike is a personal trainer, massage therapist, and author of *Sports Massage for Peak Performance*.

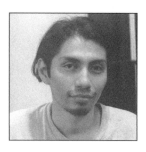

Abel Castro is a model and filmmaker. He lives in New York City.

Ralph Sosa is an actor, model, and fitness enthusiast.

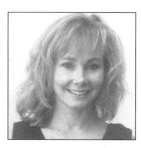

Becky Henni is an aerobics instructor, nurse, and mother of two. She lives in Grand Junction, Colorado.

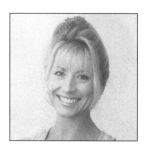

Rebecca Cork is a personal trainer and mother. She lives in Grand Junction, Colorado.

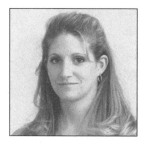

Jennifer Licke is a model and studies exercise science at Mesa State College.

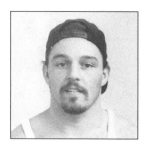

Corey Coleman is a bodybuilder and personal trainer. He is the father of two.

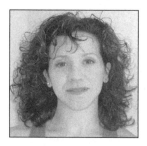

Sharon Jackson is a personal trainer and writer.

Andrew Brucker is a New York photographer. He specializes in portraits and nudes. His work has appeared in numerous journals, magazines, and books, including: *Interview, Details, Rolling Stone, New York Woman,* and *Manner Vogue.* He also did the photography for *The Complete Book of Abs* and *The Complete Book of Butt and Legs.*

Lisa MacKechnie is a personal trainer.

INDEX